Guide to Medical Billing

Insurance Career Development Center

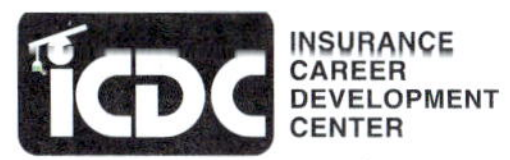

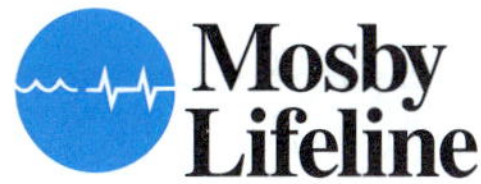

St. Louis Baltimore Boston Carlsbad Chicago Naples New York Philadelphia Portland
London Madrid Mexico City Singapore Sydney Tokyo Toronto Wiesbaden

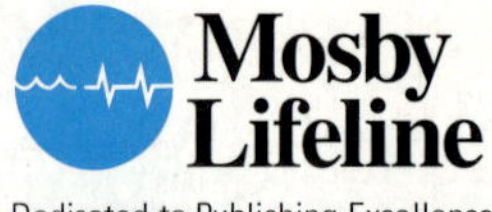

Publisher: David T. Culverwell
Editor-in-Chief: Richard A. Weimer
Editor: Eric Duchinsky
Senior Developmental Editor: Cecilia F. Reilly
Developmental Editor: Nancy Peterson
Assistant Editors: Christine Ambrose; Carla Goldberg
Book Design and Production: Reuter & Associates
Manufacturing Supervisor: Betty Richmond
Cover Design: Avenue K, St. Louis

Fourth edition

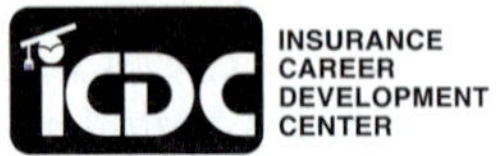

Printed in the United States of America

Composition by:
Reuter & Associates

Printing/Binding by:
William C. Brown

Mosby–Year Book, Inc.
11830 Westline Industrial Drive
St. Louis, Missouri 63146

International Standard Book Number 0-8151-4810-0

95 96 97 98 99/ 9 8 7 6 5 4 3 2 1

Disclaimer

This text is a guide for learning the medical billing and health claims examining fields. Decisions should not be based solely on information within this guide. Decisions impacting the practice of medical billing and health claims examining must be based on individual circumstances including legal/ethical considerations, local conditions and payor policies.

The information contained in this text is based on experience and research. However, in the complex, rapidly changing medical environment, this information may not always prove correct. Data used are widely variable and can change at any time. Readers should follow current coding regulations outlined by official coding organizations.

CPT is a listing of descriptive terms and five-digit numeric identifying codes and modifiers for reporting medical services performed by physicians. This presentation includes only CPT descriptive terms, numeric identifying codes and modifiers for reporting medical services and procedures that were selected by Mosby Lifeline for inclusion in this Publication

The most current CPT is available from the American Medical Association.

No fee schedules, basic unit values, relative value guides, conversion factors or scales or components thereof are included in CPT.

Mosby Lifeline has selected certain CPT codes and service/procedure descriptions and assigned them to various specialty groups. The listing of a CPT service or procedure description and its code number in this Publication does not restrict its use to a particular specialty group. Any procedure or service in this Publication may be used to designate the services rendered by any qualified physician.

The American Medical Association assumes no responsibility for the consequences attributable to or related to any use or interpretation of any information or views contained in or not contained in this Publication.

The publisher and author do not accept responsibility for any adverse outcome from undetected errors, opinion and analysis contained in this text that may prove inaccurate or incorrect, or the reader's misunderstanding of an extremely complex topic. All names used in this book are completely fictitious. Any resemblance to persons or companies, current or no longer existing, is purely coincidental.

Acknowledgements

Many people have contributed to the development and success of *Guide to Medical Billing.* We extend our thanks and deep appreciation to the many students and classroom instructors who have provided us with helpful suggestions for this edition of the text.

We would like to express our thanks to the following individuals who believed in the program in its initial stages and helped us work through the glitches associated with any new product:

Jolene Buck, Ameritech College, Van Nuys, CA
Anna B. Little, Ladera Career Paths, Los Angeles, CA
Hollis Anglin and Colleen Wheatley, Dawn Training Institute, New Castle, DE
Tami Freedman, College America, San Francisco, CA
Bob Malone and Gloria Stender, Grand Rapids Educational Centers, Grand Rapids, MI
Ruby Herold, Heritage College of Health Careers, Denver, CO
Donna Montfoort, BSN, Carolyn Dykes, C.P.C. and Patti Overman, C.P.C., John Alden Life Insurance Company, Phoenix, AZ
Jennifer L. Spalding, R.N., MPA, Annis Collins, R.N., MS and Femi Daramola, United Health Plan, Inglewood, CA
Lowell P. Theard, PH.D, MD, and Katherine Rogers, MHA, Culver Healthcare Associates, Culver City, CA

We would like to thank those Insurance Career Development Center consultants who helped with this text, Mayra I. Caraballo and especially Caitlind L. Alexander for her loyalty and commitment, which was instrumental in bringing this edition to successful completion.

Thanks to the CPA firm of Miller, Kaplan, Arase and Company. To Mannon Kaplan, C.P.A., thank you for believing in and supporting ICDC, for all of your knowledge and wisdom. A special thank you to George Nadel Rivin, C.P.A,. and Joseph C. Cahn, C.P.A., for their valued consultation. For having the faith and commitment to see it through, we truly appreciate you and your partners, Jeffrey S. Slomiak, C.P.A., Edwin Kanemaru, C.P.A., Kenneth R. Holmer, C.P.A., Douglas S. Waite, C.P.A., James E. Veale, C.P.A., Charles Schnaid, C.P.A., and Donald G. Garrett, C.P.A..

We also wish to express our thanks to the expert staff at Mosby Lifeline who gave freely of their support. An extra special thank you to Editor Eric Duchinsky for realizing the need to publish such a text and for having the courage to undertake this project. Thanks to Editor-in-Chief Richard A. Weimer, Senior Developmental Editor Cecilia F. Reilly, Developmental Editor Nancy Peterson, and Assistant Editors Christine Ambrose and Carla Goldberg.

And finally, to Thomas, Sean and Sydney Adams, thank you for allowing me to spend the time and energy required to concentrate on this project. To Floree Brown, thank you for all of your love and support. I would like to dedicate this book to the memory of my father, Nathaniel Brown Sr.

Sharon E. Brown, President
Insurance Career Development Center, Inc.

Preface

Health claims examining and medical billing are two of the fastest-growing employment opportunities in the United States today. Insurance companies, medical offices, hospitals and other health care providers are in great need of trained personnel to create and process medical billing claims.

With the aid of this textbook, you can learn the skills necessary to become a successful health claims biller or examiner. The material has been designed to be comprehensive, yet user-friendly. The text follows a logical learning format by beginning with a broad base of information and then, step by step, following the course of a health claim from billing to examining.

This text is intended to be used with Insurance Career Development Center's Health Claims Examiner/Medical Biller Curriculum Program, which is divided into eight modules consisting of 100 hours each.

Special Features

Some special features of the text enhance understanding and retention of the material covered:

Each chapter begins with **learning objectives** to focus the student on the most pertinent topics covered in that chapter. The straightforward, **easy-to-understand writing style** presents information clearly and concisely. **Questions for Review** at the end of each chapter reinforce key concepts. Answering questions without looking back into the chapter will help students determine if they have grasped the principles within the chapter or if there is a need for further study. They also serve to prepare students for exams. Answers are contained in the instructor materials for this course. **Exercises** provided with most chapters give students the opportunity to put their knowledge into practice. These hands-on, real-life exercises will ensure competence in medical billing.

The most important ingredient to success in this course is the desire to learn, without which the learning process is ineffective. The desire to learn can lead you to a rewarding career in the medical billing or health claims examining fields.

Contents

1

Introduction to Medical Claims

In this chapter you will learn:

- The basic forms used in a medical office.
- How to keep patient charts and records in the billing office.
- Proper collections procedures.
- What constitutes special services and how they are billed.

Eventually everyone visits a doctor's office or clinic or uses the services of a hospital. This means that the services received will generate a claim or bill for processing or payment. Whether the patient has insurance coverage or will be responsible for payment of the services themselves, a claim or bill for the services will be prepared.

In this chapter we will walk you through the initiation of a claim from a provider of services, the submission of that claim to the payor or billing to the patient, and the receipt of payment for the claim or bill by the provider of services.

When a patient walks into a provider's office for the first time, a patient file must be established and several forms must be filled out. These forms provide all the information the provider will need to treat and bill the patient. The most commonly used forms include the following:

- The Patient Information Sheet
- The Release of Information Form
- The Assignment of Benefits Form
- The Patient History Form

Each form has a distinct purpose and, in one style or another, will be present in nearly every provider's office. However, sometimes two or more items are combined on a single form. This is most often true of the Release of Information Form, the Assignment of Benefits Form, and the Patient Information Sheet.

Filling out these forms is relatively simple because the information called for is basic and self-explanatory.

Let's look at each of the forms in greater detail.

Patient Information Sheet

The Patient Information Sheet is used to collect general information regarding the patient (see Figure 1-1). The medical biller should always ensure that the information obtained on the Patient Information Sheet is complete and accurate, since this information will be used for billing and collection and for notifying family members in case of emergency. The Patient Information Sheet should be updated periodically to ensure its accuracy. There are various versions of this form, but they all usually request the following basic information:

- Name: first, middle initial, and last
- Address and telephone number
- Business address, telephone number, and occupation
- Date of birth
- Social Security number
- Person responsible for account, or insured's name
- Spouse's name and occupation
- Information about patient referral
- Driver's license number
- Close relative or friend to contact in case of emergency
- Insurance billing information

Obtain the names, addresses, and policy and group numbers of all carriers insuring the patient. This is important because of the coordination of benefits clauses written into most health insurance policies. If the patient has an insurance card, make a copy of the card to keep in the patient's file. Insurance coverage should be verified prior to rendering services. The insurance information should be rechecked every 6 months, since this information may change.

Release of Information Form

The Release of Information Form is used to request additional information from other providers of service (see Figure 1-2). If the doctor is submitting an insurance claim for the patient, the patient must sign a Release of Information Form before information may be given to an insurance company, attorney, or other third party. According to the Privacy Act, it is illegal to release any information regarding a patient without the patient's knowledge and written consent. The patient's signature is usually good for 1 year from the date the release is signed. If the patient is a child, the parent or guardian must sign the release. Often a release of information statement is included on the actual claim form describing treatment. This brief statement does not

Patient Information Sheet

Date: ______________ Acct #: ______________ ID #: ______________

Name: (Last, First, Middle) ______________

Address: (Number, Street, Apt. #) ______________

City: ______________ State: ______________ Zip: ______________

Home Phone: ______________ Work Phone: ______________ Birth Date: ______________

Sex: ______________ Marital Status: ______________ Social Security #: ______________

Employer Name/Address: ______________

Referred by: ______________

FINANCIALLY RESPONSIBLE PERSON

Name: (Last, First, Middle) ______________

Address: (Number, Street, Apt. #) ______________

City: ______________ State: ______________ Zip: ______________

Home Phone: ______________ Work Phone: ______________

Employer Name/Address: ______________

Other Person to Notify in Emergency: ______________ Phone: ______________

MEDICAL INSURANCE COVERAGE

Name of Primary Ins. Co.: ______________ Ins. Address: ______________

ID/Policy #: ______________ Grp #/Name: ______________ Policy Holder Name: ______________

Name of Secondary Ins. Co.: ______________ Ins. Address: ______________

ID/Policy #: ______________ Grp #/Name: ______________ Policy Holder Name: ______________

Name of Other Ins.: ______________ Ins. Address: ______________

ID/Policy #: ______________ Grp #/Name: ______________ Policy Holder Name: ______________

ACKNOWLEDGEMENT AND AUTHORITY FOR TREATMENT AND PAYMENT

I consent to treatment as necessary or desirable to the care of the patient named above, including but not restricted to whatever drugs, medicine, performance of operations and conduct of laboratory, x-ray, or other studies that may be used by the attending doctor, his/her nurse or qualified designate.

I further understand that the qualified designate in some cases will be the Assistant to the Primary Care Physician, also called a PA. An Assistant to the Primary Care Physician means a person who is a graduate of an approved program of instruction in Primary health care and approved by the Board to perform direct patient care services under the supervision of a Primary Care Physician.

I also acknowledge full responsibility for the payment of such services and agree to pay for them, in full, AT THE TIME OF SERVICE. If the physician must use a collection agency/attorney or court to collect its charges, then I will pay reasonable attorney fees and costs incurred in collecting same, regardless of insurance coverage.

I hereby authorize payment directly to ______________ of the Medical Expense benefits otherwise payable to me but not to exceed my indebtedness to said physician on account of the enclosed charge.

Insured's Signature ______________ Date ______________

Signed (Patient) ______________

Signed ______________

Figure 1-1: Patient Information Sheet

Any Doctor's Office
1234 Drive Way • Any City, Any State 56789 • (555) 555-0009

AUTHORIZATION TO OBTAIN INFORMATION

I AUTHORIZE any physician, medical practitioner, hospital, clinic, other medical or medically related facility, insurance or reinsuring company, the Medical Information Bureau, Inc., consumer reporting agency, or employer having information available as to diagnosis, treatment and prognosis with respect to any physical or mental condition and/or treatment of me or my minor children and any other nonmedical information of me and my minor children to give to the group policy holder, my employer, or its legal representative, any and all such information.

I UNDERSTAND the information obtained by the use of the Authorization will be used by to determine eligibility for insurance, and eligibility for benefits under any existing policy. Any information obtained will not be released by/to any person or organization EXCEPT to the group policyholder, my employer, reinsuring companies, the Medical Information Bureau, Inc., or other persons or organizations performing business or legal services in connection with my application, claim, or as may be otherwise lawfully required or as I may further authorize.

I KNOW that I may request to receive a copy of this Authorization.

I AGREE that a photographic copy of this Authorization shall be as valid as the original.

I AGREE this Authorization shall be valid for one year from the date shown below.

Signed this ____________ day of ____ 19 ____________.

Name of Minor Child ________________________ Signature of Insured ___________________________

Name of Minor Child ________________________ Signature of Spouse ___________________________

Figure 1-2: Release of Information Form

take the place of having a completed and signed release of information statement in the patient's file.

Assignment of Benefits Form

The Assignment of Benefits Form is a request for all payments from payors to be directed to the provider holding the assignment (see Figure 1-3). Most providers consider this a necessity for those patients who have insurance, because the assignment ensures that monies paid for services provided are issued directly to the provider and not to the patient or subscriber. Assignment of Benefits indicates that the payor is authorized to send payment directly to the provider of services. The Assignment of Benefits Form should be signed, dated, and attached to the insurance form and preferably stamped and printed on the insurance form.

Patient History Form

The Patient History Form is important to the physician (see Figure 1-4). It helps in identifying previous incidents of illness that are important in treating the patient's present condition. This form is usually a detailed form with basic health questions requiring only "yes" or "no" answers. The provider generally gives the patient a complete history and physical upon entering the exam room.

The Patient Chart

After the required forms are completed, they are assembled together into a patient chart. If the patient has an insurance card or other proof of coverage, a photocopy of the card or other proof is included with the above forms.

During the course of treatment, the physician may add additional forms to the patient chart, such as a history and physical form, progress notes, or a medication flow sheet for tracking prescribed medicine. If the patient is a child, a pediatric chart should be assembled. This requires additional forms such as an immunization record to track immunizations given and forms for hearing and vision exams.

After the patient has become established and has had several visits, lab and x-ray results and consultation reports may be submitted from other providers. These results should be reviewed by the physician or, in some offices, by a nurse. If reviewed by a nurse, abnormal lab or x-ray or urgent results or requests will be forwarded directly to the physician for an immediate response. After review, these results should be stamped with the date and signed off by the physician prior to being filed in the patient chart.

Billing for Services

After the patient has seen the doctor, the doctor will complete a charge slip or fee ticket. The *charge slip* is a form used by the provider to indicate which services were rendered, the diagnosis for the visit, and whether a return visit is needed (see Figure 1-5). This form usually has a list of service descriptions along with the corresponding numeric billing codes and a list of diagnoses and diagnosis codes. The charge slip is given to the patient after the visit is complete. The patient will in turn give the charge slip to the receptionist for payment to be made and a return visit to be scheduled. At that time, the receptionist collects any amounts that the patient owes. For cash patients (those without insurance or responsibility by a third party payor), the entire amount is often collected or a payment plan is set up. For many patients covered by insurance, a small payment will be required. The receptionist issues a receipt for any monies collected and lists the amount received and the form of payment (cash or check) on the charge slip.

The *ledger card* is used to indicate a chronologic record of all services rendered to a patient (see Figure 1-6).

Mike Moriarty, M.D.
0123 Any Way • Anytown, USA 12345 • (123) 456-7890

ASSIGNMENT OF BENEFITS

I authorize payment directly to the above named provider of medical expense benefits otherwise payable to me but not to exceed my indebtedness to said provider for any services furnished to me by that provider.

The signature on this form or a photocopy is valid one year from the date indicated.

Signature____ Date ________

Figure 1-3: **Assignment of Benefits Form**

This card is used by the biller for billing services and recording payments and adjustments. In the pegboard system, once the payment is received by the receptionist at the time services are rendered, the receptionist records the payment on the charge slip, which is automatically posted to the ledger card when inserted under the charge slip by the carbon in the forms provided. When the medical biller receives the ledger card, the information on the services rendered and the charge is added with information from the patient chart. These items combined should provide all the required information for a biller to complete a billing form.

If the services rendered are complicated, the medical biller may need to refer to the medical record for a report to substantiate the amount charged for the services. The physician is required to dictate a report if this information is necessary for billing.

When billing the carrier, double check to make sure the CPT, ICD-9, and DRG codes are accurate (coding will be discussed in detail in Chapters 15 and 17). Improper coding is the most common error made on billing forms, and it can result in improperly paid as well as delayed claim payments. Since the coding can change on a regular basis, it is important that the most up-to-date information and reference books are available and kept within easy reach of the medical biller.

Also, make sure that all the necessary information has been filled in on a claim form prior to mailing it to the carrier. Medical billers and front office personnel are flooded with tasks and responsibilities, which leaves the situation ripe for minor errors like forgetting valuable information on a form or forgetting to call for pre-authorization of services. Organize your office in such a way that the opportunity for these mistakes is at a minimum. Take the time to do things correctly. It saves having to correct it later.

When the above information has been used and the claim form is complete, the claim form is then mailed to the insurance carrier. The patient is also sent a copy of the billing information. If the charge slip or superbill has carbon copies, one of these may be used as a bill for the patient.

Patient History

Date______________________________

Patient Name __________________________ Age__________

Any allergies to food or medicine? No Yes
If yes: Allergic to: __________________________

Have you ever been hospitalized? No Yes
If yes: Indicate date and reason:__________________________

Have you ever been diagnosed or experienced:

Bladder Infections	_______	Underweight	_______	Anemia	_______
Ear Infections	_______	Epilepsy	_______	Overweight	_______
Sinus Infections	_______	Seizures	_______	Hay Fever	_______
Vision Problems	_______	Mumps	_______	Chickenpox	_______
Frequent Headaches	_______	Sickle Cell	_______	Heart Murmur	_______

Other______________________________

Are you currently taking any medication?
If yes: Name of medication:__________________________

Date of last TB and/or Tetanus shot: __________________________

Check any of the following that any blood relative has or has had:

Anemia	_______	Heart Disease	_______	Thyroid Problems	_______
Sickle Cell	_______	Heart Attack	_______	Diabetes	_______
Stroke	_______	Birth Defects	_______	Asthma	_______
Cancer	_______	Mental Retardation	_______	Kidney Disease	_______
Tuberculosis	_______	Alcoholism	_______	High Blood Pressure	_______

Figure 1-4: Patient History Form

Charge Slip

Date of Service: ____________ Account Number: ____________

Name (Last, First): ____________

X	Code	Description	Fee	X	Code	Description	Fee	X	Code	Description	Fee
Initial				**Established**				**Special Procedures**			
	99204	Extended Exam	100.00		99211	Minimal Exam	35.00				
	99205	Comprehensive Exam	110.00		99212	Brief Exam	40.00				
					99213	Limited Exam	45.00				
					99214	Intermediate Exam	60.00				
					99215	Comprehensive Exam	90.00				
Consultations				**Laboratory**				**Prescriptions**			
	99244	Comprehensive	150.00		36415	Venipuncture	15.00				
					81000	Urinalysis	10.00				
					82948	Glucose Fingerstick	18.00				

X	Code	Diagnosis	X	Code	Diagnosis	X	Code	Diagnosis
	466	Bronchitis, Acute		401	Hypertension		460	Upper Resp Tract Infection
	428	Congestive Heart Failure		414	Ischemic Heart Disease		599.0	Urinary Tract Infection
	431	CVA		724.2	Low Back Syndrome		616	Vaginitis
	250.0	Diabetes Mellitus		278.0	Obesity		**ICD-9**	**Other Diagnosis**
	625.3	Dysmenorrhea		715	Osteoarthritis			
	345	Epilepsy		462	Pharyngitis, Acute			
	0009.0	Gastroenteritis		714	Rheumatoid Arthritis			
	784.0	Headache		477	Rhinitis, Allergic			
	573.3	Hepatitis		471	Sinusitis, Acute			

Remarks/Special Instructions	New Appointment	Statement of Account
		Old Balance
		Today's Fee
Referring Physician	**Recall**	Payment
		New Balance

Figure 1-5: Charge Slip

Ledger Card

RESPONSIBLE PARTY: ______________________________

ADDRESS: ______________________________

TELEPHONE #: ______________________________

PATIENT NAME: ______________________________ PATIENT #: ______________________________

SPECIAL NOTES: ______________________________

Date	Description of Service	Charge	Payments	Adjustments	Remaining Balance

Figure 1-6: Ledger Card

Billing Forms

Billing forms are usually one of three types: the superbill, the HCFA-1500, and the UB-92. These forms are covered briefly in the next sections. The HCFA-1500 and the UB-92 will be covered in depth in Chapters 18 and 19.

The medical biller will be required to use several types of billing forms, depending on the type of services rendered and to whom the bill is being submitted for payment.

Superbill

Superbills are billing forms used by many providers of service and suppliers. The superbill serves as a charging slip to speed the process of medical insurance reimbursement. The standard superbill has three carbonless copies: one copy for the office, one for insurance filing, and a third for the patient's record. As long as a superbill contains the required information, many insurers will accept it for payment; however, Medicare will not.

A superbill is an invoice and, as such, is subject to the same accountability requirements as other standard billing forms.

The superbill is different, depending on the provider of service and the form it chooses to use, therefore we will not discuss the completion of these forms. However, the types of information required by payors are generally the same as those found on the previous medical billing forms.

HCFA-1500

The Health Care Financing Administration (HCFA) 1500 is the basic form prescribed by HCFA for billing services from physicians and suppliers. The medical biller uses the HCFA-1500 form when billing for payment from insurance carriers and Medicare programs. The medical biller can extract the necessary information to properly complete the form for submission from the patient's record or operative report. When billing Medicare, the most current version of the HCFA-1500 is required to be used.

UB-92

The Uniform Billing-92 (UB-92) is used for billing hospital services. Information for completing the UB-92 can be taken from the hospital medical records or from triage reports. Triage reports are generated in the emergency rooms of hospitals or at the scene of an accident (see Chapter 20 for a discussion on triage reports).

Patient Claim Form

In addition to the billing forms, a medical biller or provider may occasionally receive a Patient Claim Form (see Figure 1-7). This form is provided by insurance companies for the purpose of updating the patient's/insured's records.

The information contained on this form is self-explanatory. The fields entitled Patient Information, Subscriber Information, and Other Insurance Information should be filled out by the patient or insured. The Medical Information field may be completed by the patient or by a medical biller. The Prescription Drugs field may be completed by the patient or by a pharmacist.

Electronic Claims Submission

Electronic claims submission is a process whereby insurance claims are submitted via computerized data (either by data diskette or modem) directly from the provider to the insurance company. Since some providers (especially hospitals and large medical offices) generate numerous claims per day, this means of submission is much easier than creating numerous pieces of paper, signing, and mailing them.

Claims submitted electronically contain fewer errors since they eliminate the need for data entry personnel to reenter the information. Payment is also generated more quickly since the claims don't sit around waiting for someone to enter them. In addition, insurance car-

PATIENT CLAIM FORM

Initial claim form to be completed and returned to above address. Information must be **printed** or **typewritten**.

MEDICARE PEOPLE 1. File your claim with Medicare FIRST! We cannot process your claim until you send us their payment information.
2. **Are you actively employed in any profession?** ☐ **Yes** ☐ **No**

TO BE COMPLETED BY MEMBER

1. Information Pertaining to Member

Name ___ Last ___ First ___ M.I. | Sex ☐ M ☐ F | Date of Birth _ – _ – _ | Social Security No. _ – _ – _

Home Address ___ Street ___ City ___ State ___ Zip | Telephone No.

2. Marital Status ☐ Divorced ☐ Legally Separated ☐ Single ☐ Married ☐ Widowed | Name of Spouse | Date of Birth _ – _ – _ | Spouse's Social Security No. _ – _ – _

Is Spouse Employed? ☐ Yes ☐ No | If Yes, Name, Address & Phone Number of Employer

3. Information Pertaining to Patient

If Claim is for ☐ Spouse or ☐ Dependent, Name of Spouse or Dependent | Sex ☐ M ☐ F | Date of Birth _ – _ – _ | Social Security No. _ – _ – _

Home Address ___ Street ___ City ___ State ___ Zip | Telephone No.

Dependent Employed? ☐ Yes ☐ No ☐ Part Time ☐ Full Time | Relationship to Employee

4. If Child is Over 19 Years Old, is Child a Full Time Student? ☐ Yes ☐ No | Name of School Attended

5. Information Pertaining to Nature of Current Disability
Were the expenses incurred due to: Illness ☐ Pregnancy ☐

Brief description of illness ___

6. WAS PATIENT'S INJURY INCURRED ON THE JOB OR THE ILLNESS CAUSED BY THE PATIENT'S WORK? ☐ Yes ☐ No

7. TO BE COMPLETED IF YOU OR YOUR DEPENDENT INJURED

Date of Accident | Where? | Was Patient at Work When Accident Happened? ☐ Yes ☐ No — If So, For Whom

How Did Accident Happen?

8. Information Pertaining to Other Group Insurance Benefits
Are you, your spouse or your dependent children covered by any other group insurance or medical service plan: ☐ **YES** ☐ **NO**
If yes, furnish the following information for each additional group policy: Insured's Name ___

___ Name of Insured's Employer ___ Employer's Address

___ Name of Insurance Company ___ Policy No. ___ Contract Code No.

___ Address Where Claims Are Sent

9. Patient's or Authorized Person's Signature
I Certify that the Above Information is True and Correct and I Authorize the Release of any Medical Information Necessary to Process this Claim to the Directors Guild of America Pension, Health and Welfare Trust/CNA Insurance Trust.

Date ___ Date ___

Member's Signature ___ Spouse's Signature ___

10. Assignment of Benefits
I Assign Payment of Medical Benefits to the following Physician or Supplier of Services ___

___ Signed (Insured or Authorized Person) ___ Date

DG-3

Figure 1-7: Front of Patient Claim Form

TO BE COMPLETED BY PHYSICIAN

11. Patient's Name: ____________________

12. Is condition due to: ☐ injury, ☐ sickness
Was injury or sickness work incurred? ☐ Yes ☐ No
Pregnancy? ☐ Yes ☐ No
If yes, approximate date pregnancy commenced. Date:

13. Diagnosis or nature of illness or injuries: (If diagnosis code other than ICDA* used, give name):

Date of Service	†Place of Service	Description of Medical Services or Supplies Furnished (If Hospital Confined, Name of Hospital)	CPT Procedure Code	ICDA Diagnosis Code	Amount of Charges
				Total Charges	
				Amount Paid	
				Balance Due	

†O — Doctor's Office   IH — Inpatient Hospital   NH — Nursing Home
H — Patient's Home   OH — Outpatient Hospital   OL — Other Location
*ICDA — International Classification of Diseases

14. Date symptoms first appeared or accident happened: ____________________

15. Date patient first consulted you for this condition: ____________________

16. Patient was continuously disabled (unable to work): ☐ Yes ☐ No From __________ Thru __________
If still disabled, date patient should be able to return to work: ____________________

17. Patient still under your care for this condition? ☐ Yes ☐ No

18. Patient ever had same or similar condition? ☐ Yes ☐ No If "Yes", when and describe:

19. Does patient have other health coverage? ☐ Yes ☐ No If "Yes", please identify;

20. UNDER SECTION 6109 OF THE INTERNAL REVENUE CODE, RECIPIENTS OF MEDICAL AND HEALTH CARE PAYMENTS ARE REQUIRED TO FURNISH IDENTIFYING NUMBERS TO PAYERS WHO MUST REPORT SUCH PAYMENTS TO THE INTERNAL REVENUE SERVICE.

INDIVIDUAL HEALTH CARE PRACTITIONERS ENTER YOUR SOCIAL SECURITY NUMBER → ☐☐☐
ALL OTHERS ENTER YOUR EMPLOYER IDENTIFICATION NUMBER → ☐☐

Date   Physician's Name (Print or Type)   Signature   Degree   Telephone

Street Address   City   State   Zip

GENERAL INFORMATION REGARDING THIS CLAIM FORM

A. **Employee**—The Employee is to refer to Sections 1 through 10 and complete those sections which are applicable.

B. **Physician**—The physician is to complete Sections 11 through 20 on each claim form or he may furnish the same information on his own form.

C. **Assignment**—If you would like to have payment made directly to the provider of the service, you must sign and date Section 10.

D. **Additional Charges**—You are required to fill out only one claim form for each illness or injury. An additional bill may be submitted without filling out a claim form. If possible, the bill should be an original and must reflect the patient's name, social security number, diagnosis, type of service, date of service and amount of charge.

E. **Coordination with Medicare Benefits**—If you are eligible for Medicare, then the benefits payable under the DGA policy are coordinated with Medicare benefits. Therefore, if you are eligible for Medicare, it is necessary to **file the Medicare claim form first.** Send us the DGA claim form, the itemized bill and the Medicare "Explanation of Benefits Paid" form **after** you or your doctor have received reimbursement from Medicare. There is an **exception** to this filing routine. If you are **over 65 and are working full time,** then DGA becomes your primary carrier and Medicare becomes your secondary carrier. You should **first** file your claim with DGA and **then** with Medicare. **Remember** this is **only** for members who are over 65 and working full time.

F. **When to File**—The insurance policy provides that a claim must be filed within the ninety (90) day period following the date that the expense was incurred or as soon as it is reasonably possible. **In no event shall claims be filed later than one year from the date that the expense was incurred.**

Figure 1-7: Back of Patient Claim Form

riers reduce their management and overhead costs by allowing electronic claims submission.

Generally, electronic claims submission is done on a weekly basis. Once a week the medical biller calls the insurance carrier on the computer and downloads the information. Electronic claims submission can also be done by the computer service for the medical office.

If any claims are rejected or there is a request for further information, the insurance carrier can contact the medical office by telephone, fax, or via computer modem directly back into the medical office's computer. This allows a medical biller to know immediately if a claim has been rejected or if more information is needed. They can then correct the information and resubmit the claim.

It is important to have the groundwork laid before attempting to submit claims electronically. The format of the claim form must be approved by the carrier, and also an agreement must be in place between the medical office and the insurance carrier. This agreement contains the basic understanding on the means of submitting data and the correct procedure coding system. Since electronic claims submission does not allow the opportunity for the physician to sign the claims, a physician's signature on the agreement will be accepted in lieu of a signature on the claim form. It is also imperative to have a patient signature on file for Authorization to Release Information and Assignment of Benefits.

Occasionally, some data transmission problems will arise, due to systems being incompatible, static or other problems on the telephone lines, or other software or hardware problems. For this reason, always keep a back-up copy of the information transmitted until the claim has been processed.

Also try to submit claims to the insurance carrier early in the morning or late at night. In this way you miss the peak times, during which your call may be jammed by too many other providers trying to submit at the same time.

If electronic submission is not used, the medical office must generate a claim, have it signed by the physician, and mail it to the insurance carrier. The insurance carrier must then receive and log the claim, categorize it according to plan and type, screen claims for incomplete information, make a microfilm copy of the claim for future reference, review the claim and make any necessary adjustments, and keypunch the claim into the computer.

As you can see, electronic submission not only cuts down on errors, it dramatically decreases the time needed for payment of the claim and also prevents loss of claims through the mail or other courier service (see Chapter 10 for a discussion of computer basics).

Accounting and Bookkeeping

The main function and purpose of any bookkeeping system is to provide a way to keep an accurate account of money being received and paid out. Money being received is considered Accounts Receivable and money paid out is referred to as Accounts Payable. Since the medical office provides a service and also functions as a business, one of the responsibilities of the medical biller includes the continued updating of books, or financial records.

Several bookkeeping systems may be used in the medical office to keep track of incoming and outgoing finances. Some systems are computerized and some are manual.

The pegboard system is one of the most frequently used manual systems because it is the simplest to use. Ledger cards, charge slips, and daily journal sheets all are used in the pegboard system. This system uses NCR (no carbon required) material on its forms for recording of information written on one form to be recorded on all the rest.

The charge slip and ledger card are used by the receptionist for recording the needed information regarding payment and services rendered. These forms are not used for accounting purposes. The daily journal is the only form from the pegboard system that is used for accounting. The charge slip and ledger card are used for audit trails in case the daily journal does not balance.

The daily journal is used as a balance sheet. This form indicates the patient's name, the individual fee charged for the day, any payments made, and the cur-

Daily Journal

Mike Moriarty, M.D.
0123 Any Way
Anytown, USA 12345
(123) 456-7890

Date	Name	Description of Service	Charge	Payments	Adjustments	Remaining Balance

Figure 1-8: Daily Journal

rent balance (see Figure 1-8). All receipts for the day and any insurance or other payments should equal the cash/check total collected on the daily journal.

Most offices have a petty cash fund to start the business day. This fund is used for giving change to customers who are making payment and for buying miscellaneous small supplies. This fund should be kept track of on a daily basis. Paid-out receipts are used when money is taken from the petty cash fund for anything other than for making change (see Figure 1-9). Any paid-out receipts should be entered in the daily journal on a separate entry line.

Payment from the insurance carrier should be received within 4 to 6 weeks. When the payment is received, the amount of payment should be compared with the actual claim originally sent to determine whether any balance needs to be billed to the patient. The payment is posted to the patient's ledger card.

Balancing the Daily Journal

At the end of the day, the daily journal will need to be balanced. The beginning line on the daily journal should be the petty cash total for the day. All entries should be made on the journal for insurance payments, cash payments, or any other miscellaneous payments or adjustments. To balance, make a total of the cash receipts for the day, any petty cash paid-out amounts, and the petty cash on hand. A receipt should be made for all payments in the office or by mail. Total all insurance payments received. Combine the receipts total and the insurance payments total. Total the payments column on the daily journal. This total is equal to the combined insurance payments, cash receipts, and petty cash totals.

All checks should be stamped on the back with a bank deposit stamp and entered on a deposit slip for deposit to the bank (see Figure 1-10).

Be sure to fill out the correct deposit slip. Several companies have more than one bank account. The deposit slip has space for coin, cash, and check deposits. Add up the amount of money you have in coins and enter it in the first box. Next, add up the amount of cash you have and list it in the second box.

Checks are listed individually. Fill in the bank number of the check. This is a four- to six-digit number with a hyphen in the middle (ie, 66-123). This number refers to the bank and the branch of the bank that the check is drawn on. Next to this number and below the previous amounts, list the amount of the check. If you run out of room for all of your checks, there is usually additional space on the back of the deposit slip.

When all amounts have been entered, total them and put the amount at the bottom. Then, list any amounts you wish to receive in cash. Finally, subtract any amounts received in cash from the total. This will give you the total amount of your deposit.

Following are some additional forms and reports that may be used in a computerized medical office for billing and accounting purposes.

Accounting Control Summary

The accounting control summary is a weekly or monthly report form that shows each day's charges, payments, and adjustments for the period indicated. The medical biller uses this form to double check the figures with his or her records. This ensures that all information that is to be input reaches the computer properly and has been entered correctly. It also lists items that were not entered.

Items may not be entered or "held in suspense" for a variety of reasons, including wrong account numbers, incorrect spellings, missing code numbers, and no master record for the family.

Cumulative Trial Balance

The cumulative trial balance lists each patient alphabetically and shows any charges, payments, or adjustments to the patient's account. This allows the medical office to keep track of all accounts and the amounts that are owed and have been paid.

Insurance Request Form

Often, computer information on charges is entered into the computer on the same day the patient is seen. However, insurance forms may not always be printed on the day they are entered. There may not be enough claims to print, or you may want to hold off printing a report until additional charges have been added.

RECEIPT Date ______________ 19____ No.

Received From ______________________________

Address ______________________________

______________________________ Dollars $ ________

For ______________________________

ACCOUNT			HOW PAID		
AMT. OF ACCOUNT			CASH		
AMT. PAID			CHECK		
BALANCE DUE			MONEY ORDER		

By ______________________________

Figure 1-9: Receipt

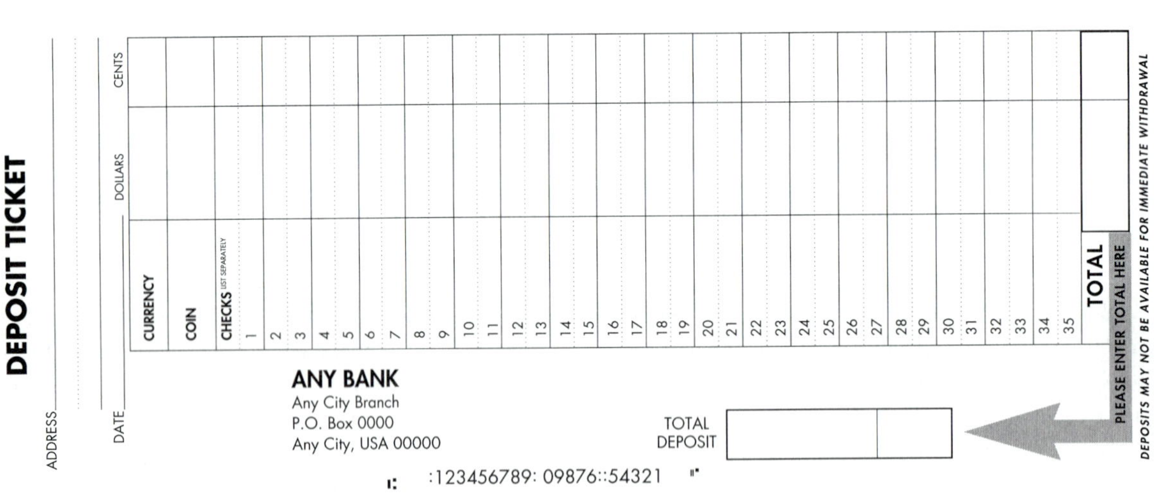

DEPOSIT TICKET

ADDRESS ______

DATE ______

	DOLLARS	CENTS
CURRENCY		
COIN		
CHECKS LIST SEPARATELY 1		
2		
3		
4		
5		
6		
7		
8		
9		
10		
11		
12		
13		
14		
15		
16		
17		
18		
19		
20		
21		
22		
23		
24		
25		
26		
27		
28		
29		
30		
31		
32		
33		
34		
35		
TOTAL		

PLEASE ENTER TOTAL HERE

DEPOSITS MAY NOT BE AVAILABLE FOR IMMEDIATE WITHDRAWAL

ANY BANK
Any City Branch
P.O. Box 0000
Any City, USA 00000

TOTAL DEPOSIT

:123456789: 09876::54321

Figure 1-10: Deposit Ticket

When requested, the Insurance Request Form lists all of the claims that have been entered into the computer, but have not yet been printed onto claim forms. In addition, this form will list them by type by cross-referencing the claim form with the type of form listed on the master file. Since many insurance carriers require different forms for HMO, PPO, Medicare, and other patients, the insurance requests separate the different types and prints the total number included in each group.

To clear a report from the insurance request form, simply get a list of the claim information that was entered into the system on a given day. This information is listed by date, then by patient and social security number. Access the patient's file and print the claim form. This will clear the information from the Insurance Request Form.

Patient Statements

A patient statement is an individual summary (either by patient or by family) that lists all the services, charges, payments, adjustments, and balance due that occurred during the month. This statement is sent to the patient every month. It acts as both a statement of his or her account and as a bill.

Often these statements contain a "dun" notice, which is a statement reminding the patient or insured to make a payment on their account. There are certain days that are more appropriate for sending out patient statements. These dates are usually between the 8th and the 12th of the month and between the 20th and the 27th of the month. Sending out patient statements on these dates receives a higher response, since most people receive their paychecks on the 15th and the 30th or 31st of the month.

Follow-Ups

A claim may be denied or pended (held for further information) if there are omissions or errors on the form. The most common reasons why claims are denied include missing or incomplete diagnosis, diagnosis not corresponding with services rendered, incorrect dates, charges not itemized, incorrect patient insurance information, incorrect procedure codes, and documentation not submitted to substantiate services rendered.

If the claim was denied or pended for these or any other reasons, complete or correct the information and resubmit the claim.

If the payment was denied on all or part of a bill and you feel the denial is incorrect, write to the insurance carrier and ask for a review or appeal of the claim. Every insurance carrier has an appeals process and will give you the required directions and information or forms to use.

Make sure that you have a good system set up to remind you when to follow up on a claim. If you have not heard from the carrier 8 weeks after you have filed a claim, it is definitely time to follow up.

Collections

The patient is always financially responsible for payment of services rendered, regardless of whether or not he or she is covered by insurance. The following are two exceptions: (1) if the patient is a minor, in which case the financial responsibility lies with the parent(s) or legal guardian; or (2) if the patient was injured on the job and the services rendered are related to this injury. In this case (2), the company's workers' compensation carrier would be responsible for payment.

After the claim is paid by the insurance carrier and the payment is posted to the patient account, any remaining balance is billed to the patient. If no payment has been received within 30 days, a follow-up reminder should be sent.

If payment is not received within 15 days of the second notice, send a courteous collection notice reminding the patient that payment is now seriously delinquent, followed by a courtesy call 10 days later. Keep accurate records of when each contact was made and the outcome of that contact. Also list the date you should follow-up if you have not received payment.

Delay in following up (with both the provider and the patient) can result in disputed claims, denied claims, delayed payments, and lost revenue.

The longer an account ages, the less likely you will be to recover the money. This can be as much as 40% or less 6 months after the bill is overdue.

Often providers are wary of becoming "bill collectors" because the image is not consistent with that of a healer. However, if revenues are not collected in a timely manner, it can be difficult for the provider to meet the cost of overhead and other obligations.

Therefore, a balance must be achieved that allows for the collection of revenues without the tarnishing of the provider's image. The best way to achieve this is to set reasonable credit limits and to stress to patients that they are responsible for payment of the bill. Create a credit agreement, then ask each patient to sign and date it. Also make sure that the patient understands that by signing the credit agreement, he or she agrees to abide by its terms.

Don't make your credit policy too stringent. You don't want to lose patients because they can't afford your terms.

If you need to put a little pressure on clients without alienating them, try blaming a third party (eg, your CPA).

Get a commitment from the client. Clients will often try to put off the payment until the arrival of a check or until their cash flow increases. If there is no choice but to wait for the check's arrival, try getting a postdated check from the customer. In this way they are committed to the payment. However, you must remember that the law holds you responsible for ensuring that the check is good before you deposit it.

If the patient cannot pay the entire bill when contacted and your company allows it, payment arrangements should be made. If the payment requires more than four installments, the federal Truth in Lending Act will apply. Regulation Z of the Truth in Lending Act requires that a written disclosure be made. When the installment plan is being discussed, the following important points should be covered:

- The amount of the debt
- The amount of the down payment
- The estimated date of final payment
- The amount of each installment
- The date each payment is due

When collections are being made by telephone, there are also laws to be followed under the Communication Act. Harassing, frightening, or abusive calls are a violation of this act, along with calling during odd hours, or calling friends or neighbors.

A Statute of Limitation is the maximum time that a debt can be collected from the time it has been incurred. For example, if the Statute of Limitations within your state is 4 years, the entire debt must be paid off within 4 years or the debtor will forfeit any amounts remaining unpaid. The Statute of Limitations varies from state to state, so check with your state legislation.

When all other methods of collection are exhausted, a collection agency may be retained to collect delinquent accounts. Most collection agencies charge a percentage of the account once the debt is collected.

FIRST NOTICE

Dear Sir/Madam:

We are currently showing a past due amount on your account. According to our records your payment of $______ was due on/by _________. As of this date payment has not been received.

Please remit payment as soon as possible. If you have recently sent payment, please disregard this notice.

Sincerely,

Account Executive

Figure 1-11: First Notice

Therefore, usually only large amounts are sent to a collection agency.

Many companies use a standard collection letter. A sample of a standard collection letter is shown in Figure 1-11. If this does not gain a response, a delinquent notice should be sent (see Figure 1-12).

Tracing a Skip

A skip is defined as a person who has received services without payment and has moved and left no forwarding address. Skips can usually be determined by mail being returned to the office and postmarks by the post office of "return to sender" or "address unknown." In attempting to trace a skip, use the information on the patient information sheet. The person's name completed in the "person to contact in case of emergency" space should be contacted. Another source is the local Department of Motor Vehicles. If the patient owns a car, it must be registered. The motor vehicle department may be able to provide information regarding the patient's whereabouts. Under no circumstances should information regarding the patient's medical condition be given to the third party.

Tracing a skip is a very tedious and challenging task, which requires tact as well as patience. If the methods just mentioned prove to be futile, the account may be written off or turned over to a collection agency.

Bankruptcy

In bankruptcy, the debtor becomes a ward of the court and, in doing so, has the court's protection. Therefore, if the patient declares the outstanding physician's fees as part of the bankruptcy, the fees owed are canceled and do not have to be paid. If the provider's office decides to continue to see the patient, he or she may choose to see the patient on a "cash only" basis. The patient must be informed of the physician's policy at the time the account has been filed in bankruptcy. In some cases a physician may decide not to treat the patient again. In this case a certified letter, with a return receipt requested, should be sent to the patient. The letter must specify a certain date from which time the patient should seek another physician.

Special Services

Physicians may bill charges other than medical services. Some medical offices charge for completing insurance or claim forms, late charges on past due amounts, charges for missed appointments, and charges for phone calls by or from patients. These services are usually not covered by insurance carriers and are the sole responsibility of the patient.

A Professional Courtesy is when a doctor renders

DELINQUENT NOTICE

Dear Sir/Madam:

Your account is seriously delinquent. According to our records we have not yet received your payment of $_______. This payment was due by _______ and reflects services that were rendered on ________.

If payment is not received by _______ we may be forced to send your bill to collections. Doing so may damage your credit rating.

If you are unable to pay the full amount, please contact our office immediately to set up a payment plan.

Sincerely,

Collections Representative

Figure 1-12: Delinquent Notice

medical services to another professional, such as a doctor, pharmacist, or nurse, or to a relative. Billing procedures vary from no charge to these persons to a percentage of the physician's usual charges. You should familiarize yourself with the provider's billing procedures prior to billing for these services.

Additional Suggestions

The following are four additional suggestions for the medical biller.

1. Give the patient a copy of the bill when he or she leaves the medical office. This can be a superbill, a copy (not the original) of the HCFA-1500, or a listing of the charges incurred during this visit.
2. If an Assignment of Benefits Form is not on file or if the patient's insurance carrier requires it, have the patient sign the Assignment of Benefits box on the claim form before leaving the office.
3. Batch Medicare, Medicaid, HMO, and PPO forms in separate groups before sending them to the computer center. This way each of these types of forms will be done at one time and you will have a separate batch total for each type.
4. Make sure that the forms that the medical office or the computer service generates are compatible with the required submission format for the insurance carrier. If your office is considering a new form, send a copy of it to all the insurance carriers you deal with and ask them to send you a written approval of the form. Requesting the approval in writing can solve problems later. It may take 6 weeks or more to get approval, so check before switching to a new form or system.

There are a number of things to keep in mind when dealing with customers. Of course, customer service should always be your first and foremost concern, but at the same time you need to have regard for the medical office. It is important to obtain all necessary information from the patient. Remember that the primary objective of the medical biller is to minimize the amount of time between the physician's service and the complete payment of the bill. The information that can facilitate this process may include the following:

- Ask the patient to fill out all necessary forms for setting up the patient file. Give the patient sufficient time to fill out the reports and check that they are complete before accepting them. Many offices mail the form to the patient prior to the visit to ensure their completeness.
- Be sure you understand the policies of the office you work for regarding the completion of forms and payment for bills. This way you can explain it accurately to the patient.
- Use the office forms consistently and accurately so that the tracking of information runs smoothly, regardless of who entered the information.
- Secure all the details of the insurance information. If the patient or insured has a card, make a copy of it for your files. Make sure the information contains the subscriber's name, the policy number, the effective date, the company that holds the policy or the name of the policy, and the insurance carrier's address.
- Make sure the patient understands the policy regarding any amounts that the insurance carrier does not pay or does not cover.
- Complete all insurance forms accurately and completely. This is the most important paper to ensure the prompt payment of claims by the insurance carrier. Also, use the forms preferred by the insurance carrier. Use of other forms can result in information being left out and a delay in the processing of the claim.
- Make sure the claims and all necessary papers have been signed by the physician, nurse, and any other necessary people.
- Maintain a copy of all paperwork and claims submitted to the insurance carrier and the date of submission.

Summary

The medical biller has numerous responsibilities. These may include creating the patient chart with all the appropriate forms, billing for services rendered, submitting claims, either manually or electronically, accounting and bookkeeping, collections, following up on delinquent payments, and billing special services.

Assignments

Complete the Questions for Review.
Complete Introduction to Medical Claims Exercises 1-1 and 1-2.

Questions for Review

Directions: Answer the following questions without looking back into the material just covered. Write your answers in the space provided.

1. List five items that should be included on the patient information sheet.
   a. ______
   b. ______
   c. ______
   d. ______
   e. ______
2. List the six most common reasons claims are denied.
   a. ______
   b. ______
   c. ______
   d. ______
   e. ______
   f. ______
3. Name two instances in which financial responsibility for a bill does not lie with the patient.
   a. ______
   b. ______
4. What is a professional courtesy? ______
5. List five items that should be discussed with the debtor when setting up a payment plan.
   a. ______
   b. ______
   c. ______
   d. ______
   e. ______

If you were unable to answer any of the questions, refer back to the section and then fill in the answers.

Exercise 1-1

Directions: Complete a Patient Information Sheet and a ledger card to set up charts for the following five patients. These forms can be found in the student exercise manual. These patients will be used throughout the remainder of this course. Please keep track of all information collected. We suggest that individual folders (preferably with pockets or clasps) be used to keep information for each patient.

Patient #1—Name: Abby Addison
5678 Any Avenue
Alverville, AK 99087
Home: (765) 890-4321; Work: (765) 123-4567
DOB: 12/12/68
Marital Status: Single
Social Security Number: 001-00-0001
Referred by: Friend
Responsible Party: Self
Person to Contact in Emergency: Alice Avery (Friend)
(765) 123-7689
Employer: Artistic Aardvarks, 1234 Any Blvd, Alverville, AK 99087
Insurance Carrier: Atlantic Assurance, 4444 Alice Avenue, Alverville, AK 99087

Patient #2—Name: Bobby Bumble
93485 Bumpkiss Court
Barkingville, DC 23456
(210) 938-4756
DOB: 1/1/44
Marital Status: Married
Social Security Number: 002-02-0020
Referred by: Spouse
Responsible Party: Self
Person to Contact in Emergency: Barbara Bumble (Spouse)
Employer: Bumbling Bureaucrats, 2345 Bumbreed Blvd, Barkingville, DC 23456
Insurance Carrier: Barkerville Assurance Company, PO Box 2345 Beaver Lane, Beaverville, DC 23457

Patient #3—Name: Cathy Crenshaw
9876 Cranbury Lane
Crabapple, CT 06192
(086) 421-3579
DOB: 2/4/43
Marital Status: Single
Social Security Number: 003-03-0030
Referred by: Friend
Responsible Party: Self
Person to Contact in Emergency: Carmen Castro (Sister)

Employer: (Part-time) Creative Creations Corporation, 1234 Creature Lane, Crevise, CT 06192

Insurance Carrier: No insurance (Cash patient)

Patient #4—Name: Daisy Doolittle
1234 Daffy Lane
Danbury, DE 19876
(098) 765-4311
DOB: 8/1/59
Marital Status: Married
Social Security Number: 004-04-0040
Referred by: Dr. Daniel Dobby
Responsible Party: Self
Person to Contact in Emergency: Danny Doolittle (Spouse)

Employer: None

Insurance Carrier: Medicaid, PO Box 0098, Danbury, DE 19876

Patient #5—Name: Edward Edmunds
8888 Every Lane
Evansville, CA 90012
(123) 456-7890
DOB: 1/10/27
Marital Status: Widow
Referred by: Dr. Edith Evan
Responsible Party: Self
Person to Contact in Emergency: Edgar Edmunds (Brother)

Employer: Retired

Insurance Carrier: (Medicare) Blues of America, PO Box 1234, Evansville, CA 90012

Exercise 1-2

Directions: Complete all the steps necessary up to the submission of the claim. Complete a charge slip, receipts, post to ledger and daily journal, and balance the daily journal. Finally, complete the slip for the bank deposit.

1. The following services were billed for: Abby Addison

   Date of Service 9/19/9x

   99204–Extended Exam

   82948–Glucose Fingerstick

   81000–Urinalysis

   Patient made a cash payment of $60.00 on this visit.

2. The following services were billed for: Bobby Bumble

   Date of Service 9/19/9x

   99205–Comprehensive Exam

   81000–Urinalysis

   36415–Venipuncture

   Patient made a payment by check of $75.00 on this visit.

3. The following services were billed for: Cathy Crenshaw

   Date of Service 9/19/9x

   99204–Extended Exam

   81000–Urinalysis

   Patient made a payment by check of $110.00 on this visit.

2
Legal Issues

In this chapter you will learn:

- To define and explain the two types of damages that can be awarded in a bad faith action.
- To define malice, fraud and oppression.

There are several legal issues that affect the medical biller and health claims examiner on a daily basis. These include privacy regulations, rules and regulations regarding allowable collections procedures, and fraud.

Privacy Guidelines

The very nature of health benefits administration requires a great deal of personal information to be gathered and maintained about many individuals. Therefore, the needs of the company must be carefully weighed against the person's right to privacy so as to avoid unwarranted invasions of that right.

In particular, medical information is considered to be privileged and confidential in the context of the physician-patient relationship, and unauthorized disclosure of information may represent a violation of that confidentiality.

The confidentiality of medical records has assumed a new importance for several reasons:

- People are becoming more litigation-minded.
- Health plans are reimbursing for more "sensitive" services that were excluded in the past, for example, alcohol detoxification, mental health treatment, and AIDS-related problems.
- More employers are self-administering or self-funding their health plans, which means that highly personal medical information is, in some instances, routinely handled by fellow employees.

General Rules

Following are 10 general guidelines for ensuring that privacy guidelines are met:

1. Gather only the information that is necessary and relevant to the billing or processing of the claim.
2. Use only legal and ethical means to collect the information required. Whenever permission is necessary, obtain written authorization from the insured or claimant (guardian or parent if the claimant is a minor).
3. When requested, and subject to any applicable legal or ethical prohibition or privilege, the insured or claimant concerned should be advised of the nature and general uses to be made of the information.
4. Make every reasonable effort to ensure that the information upon which an action is based is accurate, relevant, timely, and complete.
5. Upon request, the claimant or insured should be given the opportunity to correct or clarify the information given by him or her, and the file should be amended to the extent that it is fair to both the insurer and the insured or claimant. Requests for review or clarification of medical information will be accepted only from the health care provider from whom the information was obtained.
6. In general, disclosures of information to a third party (other than those described to the insured or claimant) should be made only with the written authorization of the member or claimant. This includes disclosure to the employer and any family members or former spouses.
7. All practical precautions should be taken to ensure that claim files are physically secure and that access to the use of such files is limited to authorized personnel.
8. All personnel involved in the processing of claims should be advised of the need to protect the Right of Privacy in obtaining required information and the need to treat all individually identifiable information as confidential. Willful abuse of the privacy of any insured or claimant by an employee may be cause for dismissal.
9. The disclosure of a diagnosis should never be made to a member or his or her family. If the member requests this information, refer the member to the physician. There may be a reason the patient does not know his or her diagnosis.
10. Never, never release any information to an ex-spouse. This includes the member's address, phone number, when a claim was paid, to whom, and other information. The ex-spouse should be instructed to contact the member directly.

If in doubt as to whether specific information should be released, check with your supervisor before, not after, releasing it.

The guidelines just listed are just that. The final decisions are up to you. Use common sense and put yourself in the place of the claimant or member.

Fraud

Fraud is defined as intentional misrepresentation of a fact with the intent to deprive a person of property or legal rights. The most common instance of fraud that occurs in the health claims industry is doctors or other providers of service billing for goods or services that were not actually provided.

Because of the high incidence of abuse, all services billed for **must** be documented in the medical record to prove that they were actually given. The "law of documentation" states that "if it wasn't documented, it didn't happen." Billing for services not given is a serious offense and constitutes fraud. If a person is convicted, the penalties are extremely stiff. In addition, both the physician and the medical biller can be held liable for the filing of fraudulent claims.

Collections Procedures

The medical biller often needs to work as a bill collector in order to obtain reimbursement for amounts not covered by insurance or other sources. Usually, these amounts need to be collected from the patient. Occasionally, due to an error on a previous claim payment, it may become necessary for a claims examiner to recover monies that were paid in error. For these reasons, we will cover the basic laws and regulations regarding collections.

Although the specific laws and regulations vary from state to state, you should become familiar with several general guidelines. These include the following four guidelines:

1. You are never allowed to make frightening or abusive calls. This includes making any threats to the person, calling names, or making derogatory statements. Racial or ethnic statements should never be made.
2. It is illegal to call people at odd times of the day. In most states, this means any time between 8:00 PM and 8:00 AM. In some states, it is also illegal to contact people at their place of employment.
3. It is illegal to request collection through another party, including friends or neighbors. This means that you are not allowed to leave a message with anyone other than the debtor concerning details of the collection attempt. This includes, but is not limited to, the amount you are trying to collect, any payment amounts or details that may have been worked out, and the nature of the bill. If you call the debtor and reach a family member or roommate, you are allowed to leave a message giving your name, company and phone number, and a request that the person you are trying to contact return your call.
4. You are not allowed to harass the person from whom you are trying to collect. The legal definition of harassment varies from state to state; however, it is always illegal to do things such as call and speak to the person several times a day or even several times a week. For this reason, it is important that you remind them of the debt and then ask when you can expect to receive payment. If they are unable to pay in full and if your company allows payment plans, try to work out a payment plan with the customer, and then make detailed notes of the conversation. You should not contact the person again until after the date on which you expected payment.

Payment Plans

If a payment plan was worked out—whether over the phone or in person—it is advisable to write down the terms of the agreement and have it signed by both parties (the debtor and a representative of the company to which the money is owed). If the payment requires more than four installments, Regulation Z of the Truth in Lending Act requires that a written disclosure be made.

When the installment plan is being discussed, the following important points should be covered:

- The amount of the debt
- The amount of the down payment
- The estimated date of final payment
- The amount of each installment
- The date each payment is due

A Statute of Limitations is the maximum time a debt can be collected from the time it is incurred. Remember that the Statute of Limitations varies from state to state, so please check with your state legislature. You should always be aware of the Statute of Limitations within your state since the entire debt must be paid off prior to this time or the physician will forfeit any amounts remaining unpaid.

Legal Damages

Legal damages are monetary awards that a plan member may attempt to recover, which are above and beyond the benefits provided by the group plan.

In the legal climate today, it is not uncommon for plan members to seek legal channels to obtain benefits or to obtain greater benefits than provided by a plan of benefits. Usually, such cases are based on what is known as "bad faith."

An insurance policy or a health and welfare plan of benefits is considered a legal contract. Under contract law, the claimant can only recover benefits up to the policy or plan limits.

However, with the development of consumerism, the courts have become more liberal. In some states there has developed a body of law that says that there is an implied obligation of good faith and fair dealings in every contract. If this obligation is breached, it is termed as "bad faith." Generally, the law of bad faith allows an insured to attempt to recover various types of damages above and beyond the benefits provided by the plan.

Usually the courts will look at two concepts to determine whether a plan has met the obligation of good faith and fair dealing:

1. Did the plan give the claimant's interest equal consideration with that given the company's interest?
2. Was the claim handled or denied in accordance with the plan provisions and in a timely manner?

The following are examples of how courts often view policy interpretations:

- The meaning of a plan of benefits is determined by the member's reasonable expectations of coverage.
- Uncertain wording that could be subject to more than one interpretation will usually be resolved against the plan and in favor of the member.
- When two equally believable interpretations may be made, the one that gives the greatest amount of protection to the member will prevail.

There are two types of damages that a court may award: compensatory damages and punitive damages.

Compensatory damages are designed to compensate an insured for all of the actual losses or damages to make that person whole again. For example, if a person has not been able to pay his or her home mortgage or car payment because of not receiving a monthly disability check and, therefore, the person's home and car are repossessed, he or she may be able to recover equity in the home and car as well as attorney fees and also possible damages for emotional stress.

Punitive damages are often the larger of the two awards and are intended primarily to punish a wrongdoing defendant and set them up as an example to help deter such actions in the future. Unlike compensatory damages, punitive damages are not automatically recoverable if bad faith is found. In addition to bad faith, a plan member in California, for example, must prove the plan to be guilty of oppression, fraud, or malice.

Bad Faith Awards

The dollar amount of a bad faith award is based on two concepts: (1) the degree of wrongfulness and (2) the wealth of the defendant.

All lawsuits are expensive not only in the dollar cost of the damages, but in other costs as well. These costs remain even if the case is settled out of court. If the case is settled out of court, the plaintiff's attorney's costs, miscellaneous costs, the attorney costs for the plan, and the benefit not originally paid must be paid and, finally, substantial "pain and suffering" costs may be included.

The value of the claim usually has no correlation to the amount of restitution (award) sought.

Part of the reason for the continuing escalation of premium costs is the necessity to be prepared for lawsuits, because whether the case is settled in court or out of court, the monetary damage to the plan is usually significant and often preventable.

In light of the foregoing information, it is important that every claim be handled quickly, correctly, and fairly. This responsibility falls on each and every claims examiner. To fulfill this responsibility, the following four guidelines should be incorporated into the routine handling and processing of claims:

1. Every customer and claimant is entitled to courteous, fair and just treatment. An acknowledgment of all communications with respect to a claim or bill should be received with reasonable promptness.
2. Customers and claimants should be treated equally and without outside considerations other than those dictated by the office policy or plan provisions.
3. Every claim is entitled to prompt investigation of all pertinent facts and objective evaluation in the fair and equitable settlement of the claim as soon as the liability has become clear.
4. Recognize the obligation to pay all just claims promptly.

Legal Definitions

Following are definitions of words that are often used concerning legal damages:

Fraud—Intentional misrepresentation of a fact with the intent to deprive a person of property or legal rights.

Malice—Intentional conduct to cause injury or conduct that is carried on with the conscious disregard of the rights of others.

Oppression—Putting a person through cruel and unjust hardships with conscious disregard of rights.

Medical Ethics

Ethics is defined as the rules or standards governing the conduct of members of a profession. In general, medical ethics defines a right and proper way of treating patients.

The American Medical Association has created a set of standards that all physicians are expected to uphold. These standards include the following:

- Providing competent service with compassion and respect for the patients
- Dealing honestly with people
- Being a law-abiding citizen, but also working to change those laws that may not be in the best interests of the patient
- Respecting the rights of others
- Continuing to study and upgrade skills with the latest in medical advancement
- Providing emergency medical treatment to anyone who is in need
- Working to improve the community

Although the medical biller may not have sworn an oath to uphold these principles, that person should realize that the physician he or she works with upholds this oath. As an adjunct to the physician, the medical biller should do the best also to uphold these standards and to assist the physician in doing so.

Summary

The medical biller needs to be aware of numerous legal and ethical issues. These include being aware of what it means to file a fraudulent claim, knowing the possible damages that could be assessed, understanding the

Right to Privacy Act, and agreeing to abide by the basic principles of medical ethics.

Assignments

Complete the Questions for Review.

Questions for Review

Directions: Answer the following questions without looking back into the material just covered. Write your answers in the space provided.

1. What are the two concepts that a court will usually look at to determine whether a plan has met the obligation of good faith and fair dealing?
   a. ________________
   b. ________________
2. When two equally believable interpretations may be made, the one that gives ________________ ________________ will prevail.
3. Name and explain the two types of damages that may be awarded in bad faith actions.
   a. ________________
   ____
   b. ________________
   ____
4. ________________ is intentional misrepresentation of a fact with the intent to deprive a person of legal rights.
5. ________________ is intentional conduct to cause injury or conduct that is carried on with the conscious disregard of the rights of others.
6. ________________ is to put a person through cruel and unjust hardships with conscious disregard of rights.
7. The dollar amount of a bad faith award is based on two concepts:
   a. ________________ and
   b. ________________
8. The diagnosis or disclosure of an illness should never be made to the patient even if he or she asks for this information. (True or False) ________________
9. If you are attempting to collect on a bill, is it legal to call the person names or to make derogatory comments regarding them, their sex, race, or ethnic background? ________________
10. What information are you allowed to give if you call a debtor and speak instead with a roommate or other family member? ________________
    ____

If you were unable to answer any of the questions, refer back to the section and then fill in the answers.

3

Medicare

In this chapter you will learn:

- To understand the two types of Medicare and the benefits and eligibility requirements for each type.
- To understand basic billing of Medicare claims.

Medicare is the Federal Health Insurance Benefit Plan for the Aged and Disabled, Title XVIII of Public Law 89-97 of the Social Security Act. This program is for persons 65 years of age or older and certain persons who are totally disabled.

Social Security Administration offices throughout the United States take applications for Medicare, determine eligibility, and provide general information about the program. The actual processing of the claims is administered by many different insurance companies, usually one or two within each state. Consequently, there may be a diversity in the application or denial of benefits and in the explanation of benefits forms.

TEFRA/DEFRA

When the TEFRA/DEFRA federal program was first introduced, it was determined that Medicare would be the primary payor for individuals as of their 65th birthday, regardless of employment status. The Tax Equity and Fiscal Responsibility Act of 1982 (TEFRA) (and amendments to it) has redirected the financial responsibility for medical coverage of active employees age 65 years and older and their spouses age 65 years and older.

Initially, TEFRA regulations did not apply to spouses over age 65 of active employees who were under age 65. The Deficit Reduction Act of 1984 (DEFRA), effective January 1, 1985, amended TEFRA so that now spouses, age 65 years and older, of active employees who are under 65 can elect their primary coverage, either Medicare or the private group plan. These regulations apply only to those employees who become eligible for coverage after their 65th birthday, not those who are covered and then reach 65.

The employers affected by these Acts are those who regularly employ 20 or more employees for each working day in at least 20 weeks of the current or preceding calendar year. Employees of such employers must be offered coverage under the group plan on the same basis as other employees. An election form choosing the primary plan must be completed and signed by each employee who is or becomes affected.

If coverage is chosen under the employer's group plan, the group plan will be the primary payor on all medical services. Medicare will provide the secondary coverage. If coverage under the group plan is rejected and thus Medicare is chosen, the employee or spouse, by law, can be covered only by Medicare. The group plan will not pay secondary.

Obviously, employers with fewer than 20 employees are exempt from the TEFRA/DEFRA regulations, and Medicare is the primary carrier for their active employees and spouses age 65 years of age or older. Medicare is also primary on all retired employees and on active employees and their spouses under age 65 who are totally disabled with conditions other than end-stage renal disease. (See Medicare Eligibility section.)

After it has been determined that the group plan is subject to TEFRA/DEFRA, it becomes necessary to determine the person's eligibility for Medicare.

Medicare Eligibility

Following are some of the guidelines governing Medicare eligibility.

Based on Age

An individual is eligible for Medicare coverage on the first day of the month in which he or she reaches age 65 years. Persons born on the first day of the month are eligible on the first day of the month preceding their birth date.

Example:
Birth date: June 15, eligible for Medicare on June 1
Birth date: June 1, eligible for Medicare on May 1

Based on Disability

Medicare coverage for totally disabled persons begins on the first of the 25th month from the date approved for Social Security Disability or Railroad Retirement benefits. Those covered include disabled workers of any age, disabled widows between the ages of 50 and 65, disabled beneficiaries age 18 and over who receive

Social Security benefits because of disability prior to age 22, the blind, and Railroad Retirement annuitants.

Based on ESRD

End-stage renal disease (ESRD) occurs when a person's kidneys fail to function. As a result, the patient must begin dialysis treatments. (Refer to Chapter 17 for a review of this type of service.) Because of the multiple problems associated with this disease, patients are considered to be totally disabled, even though some individuals with this disease continue to work. As a result, the following special rules apply to ESRD patients.

The employer's group health plan is the primary payor for the first 18 months after a patient (under age 65) with ESRD becomes eligible for Medicare. This 18-month period begins based on the earlier of (1) the month in which a regular course of renal dialysis is initiated or (2) the month the patient is hospitalized for a kidney transplantation.

Medicare is the secondary payor during this 18-month period but will revert to the primary status beginning with the 19th month. As a general rule, all services under a dialysis program are Medicare-assigned (defined later in this section).

Providers of Service

Providers of services and medical equipment suppliers under Medicare must meet all licensing requirements of the state in which they are located. To be a participating provider under the Medicare program, providers must meet additional Medicare requirements before payments can be made for their services. Medicare will not pay for the following 12 types of care received in nonparticipating facilities:

1. Hospital care
2. Skilled nursing facility
3. Home health agency
4. Hospice
5. Outpatient rehabilitation
6. Dialysis facilities
7. Ambulatory surgical centers
8. Independent physical therapists
9. Independent occupational therapists
10. Clinical laboratories
11. Portable x-ray suppliers
12. Rural health clinics

The Two Parts of Medicare

There are two parts to the Medicare program: Parts A and B. The services covered under the two parts of Medicare are as follows:

1. Part A is considered the basic plan or hospital insurance. This part covers facility charges for acute inpatient hospital care, skilled nursing, home health care, and hospice care.
2. Part B is the medical (supplementary, voluntary) insurance that covers physician services, outpatient hospital services, home health care, outpatient speech and physical therapy, and durable medical equipment.

Part A

The two parts have somewhat different eligibility requirements. Part A is automatic upon enrollment for the following individuals:

- All persons age 65 and over, if entitled to (a) monthly Social Security benefits, or (b) pensions under the Railroad Retirement Act
- All persons who reached age 65 prior to 1968, whether or not under the Social Security or Railroad Retirement Programs
- Workers who reach 65 in 1975, or subsequently, need 20 quarters of Social Security work credits if female, or 24 quarters of Social Security work credits if male, to be fully insured.

Effective July 1, 1973, all persons age 65 years and over who are not otherwise eligible for Part A may enroll by paying the full cost of such coverage, provided they also enroll in Part B.

There are certain exclusions such as those who are members of subversive organizations and aliens who have not been permanent US residents for 5 years.

Benefits

Part A is the hospital insurance portion of Medicare. There is a deductible amount that is deducted from the first admission. If the patient is out of the hospital for at least 60 consecutive days (including the day of discharge), a new benefit period begins and another inpatient deductible would be taken if the patient is readmitted. (This is known as the period of renewal.) For 1994, the Part A deductible is $696.00.

If a member remains in the hospital for an extended period of time, additional copayments are required. Medicare deducts the copay amount from the billed amount and then pays the amount in excess of the copay.

The 1994 inpatient hospital copayments are as follows:

- 1st day—60th day = Deductible only, no additional copayment
- 61st day—90th day = $174.00/day
- 91st day—150th day = $348.00. These days are known as the 60-day Lifetime Reserve. These copayments are not renewable. Once used, they are gone.

For skilled nursing facilities (SNF), there is a separate copayment schedule and requirement. To be eligible for this benefit, a doctor must certify the necessity of skilled nursing and rehabilitative care on a daily basis. Custodial care is not covered nor is occasional rehabilitative care. In addition, the Medicare intermediary approves the stay.

The 1994 SNF copayments are as follows:

- 1st day—20th day = No copayment. Since admission is usually from an acute care facility, during which time the deductible was met, 100% of the allowable is generally paid by Medicare.
- 21st day—100th day = $87.00 Coinsurance/copay per day

Multiple admissions can occur during a calendar year. However, the maximum number of allowable days is 100 per benefit period.

These deductibles and copayments are adjusted upward each calendar year, based on inflation.

Psychiatric inpatient hospital care is covered for a maximum of 190 days per lifetime of the member. These days do not renew. The only applicable deductible is the inpatient hospital deductible of $696.00 for 1994. There are no other copayments. Also, the facility must be a participating Medicare provider in order to be covered.

Foreign facilities are generally not covered. However, some qualified Canadian or Mexican hospitals may be covered during emergency situations. All such bills should be submitted to Medicare for consideration.

Part-time Home Health Care may be covered under the following four circumstances:

1. The care needed includes intermittent skilled nursing care, physical therapy or speech therapy.
2. The patient is confined to the home.
3. A doctor prescribes the care and sets up a home health plan.
4. The home health agency is a participating provider.

Medicare will not cover the following services:

- Full-time nursing care in the home
- Drugs and biologicals
- Meals delivered to the home
- Homemaker services
- Blood transfusions

Hospice care may be covered under the following three circumstances:

1. A doctor certifies that the patient is terminal.
2. The patient chooses to receive care from a hospice instead of receiving standard Medicare benefits (inpatient).
3. Care is provided by a Medicare-certified hospice program.

Special benefit periods and payments apply to this benefit. If additional clarification is required, refer to a Medicare handbook.

Part A insurance does not cover the following services:

- The replacement fees for the first three pints of blood
- Personal convenience items
- Private duty nurses (while inpatient)
- Private room difference, unless it is determined to be medically necessary

Part B

Part B is the supplementary medical insurance, which covers physician and outpatient hospital services. It is considered a supplemental plan because each participant must pay a stipulated amount each month for the benefits. The monthly premium is adjusted each year based on inflation.

The rules, limits, and maximums under this coverage are subject to change every year. In addition, certain types of services are covered under some circumstances but not under others. Therefore, it is less confusing to have a general idea of the most common benefits without becoming overly concerned with the details. Normally, you will not be concerned with Medicare except if it is the primary payor. In such circumstances, you will have to have the explanation of benefits to process the claim. The following briefly summarizes some of the more common benefits. For more particulars, refer to a Medicare booklet or carrier.

Benefits

The 1994 yearly deductible is $100.00, which has a 3-month carryover provision. After the deductible has been satisfied, generally 80% of the approved charge will be paid.

The following services are covered by Part B:

- Manual manipulation of the spine for subluxation demonstrated by x-rays
- Nonroutine podiatric care
- Dental care for surgery of the jaw-related structures and fractures of facial bones
- Some nonroutine optometry services
- Outpatient hospital services
- Outpatient physical/speech therapy—$750.00 1994 maximum
- Independent clinical laboratory/x-ray services
- Ambulance transportation
- Some durable medical and prosthetic equipment
- Outpatient treatment of mental illness
- Home health care

The following physician services are not covered by Part B:

- Routine physical examinations and related DXL (diagnostic x-ray)
- Routine foot care
- Eye or hearing examinations for eyeglasses or hearing aids
- Immunizations (exceptions: some pneumococcal and hepatitis B)
- Cosmetic surgery (some exceptions)

Approved or Reasonable Charges

Medicare payments are based on what the law defines as "reasonable charges," which are the amounts approved by the Medicare carrier based on what is considered reasonable for the geographic area in which the doctor practices. Because of the way the approved amounts are determined and because of high rates of inflation in medical care prices, the approved amounts are often significantly less than the actual charges billed by providers. The charge approved by the carrier will be the lowest of either the charge billed by the provider or the prevailing charge (based on all the customary charges in the locality for each type of service) as determined by Medicare.

Participating providers must write off the amounts in excess of the approved amount.

Billing Medicare Services

When billing for a patient who is a Medicare recipient, always request the patient's red, white, and blue health insurance card. This card indicates whether the patient has both Part A (hospital) and Part B (medical) and when each became effective. A copy of this card should be made for your files.

The card also has a letter code indicating the recipient's status. The letter codes are as follows:

A—Wage earner
B—Husband's number
C—Disabled child
HDA—Disabled adult
J, K1, or J1—Special monthly benefits, never worked

under Social Security

T—Uninsured and entitled only to health insurance benefits

Railroad retirees are indicated by the following letters preceding the patient's Social Security number.

MA

A	with six additional digits
WA	with six additional digits
A	with nine additional digits
WA	with nine additional digits

The HCFA-1500 should be used to bill for Medicare recipients' services. Instructions on completion of the HCFA-1500 are covered in Chapter 18.

Unique Physician Identification Number

Medicare has established a Unique Physician Identification Number (UPIN) for identifying the physician ordering or referring services. This is a national number used to identify the physician. The following list of services requires the UPIN in box 17a of the HCFA-1500 and the name of the ordering or referring physician in box 17 of the HCFA-1500:

- Laboratory
- Consultation
- Diagnostic tests
- Renal
- Ambulance
- Ultrasound
- Radiology
- Durable medical equipment
- Parenteral nutrition
- Magnetic resonance imaging
- Computerized axial tomography (CT) scan
- Prosthetics and orthotics
- Physical therapy
- Chiropractic services

If a physician is self-referring, his or her own individual UPIN should be entered on the claim.

Posting Medicare Payments

Payments received from Medicare may be lower than the physician's billed charge. If the provider accepts Medicare's assignment, it is important that the medical biller know how to post payments to the patient's ledger and make adjustments.

Upon receipt of the Explanation of Medicare Benefits (EOMB), the patient(s) chart(s) indicated on the EOMB should be pulled. Post each payment individually to each patient ledger card and to the daily journal. Separate entries should be made for each patient on the daily journal and not in a lump sum.

If the Medicare allowed amount is lower than the billed charge, an adjustment or write-off will need to be made on the ledger card. After the payment has been posted, the next entry on the ledger card should be the adjustment to the charges. Enter the differences between the billed amount and the Medicare approved amount. This amount will be entered on the ledger card in the adjustment column and will be subtracted from the remaining balance. This entry will ensure that Medicare recipients are not being billed for charges that exceed Medicare's approved amount.

New Physician Limitations

New physicians rendering services to Medicare recipients used to be subject to payment limitations if they were in their first through fourth year of practice.

Medicare has revised the new physician payments for services rendered after January 1994, when the new physician limitation no longer applies.

Part B Claims Time Limit

Medicare has established time limits for filing claims covered under Medicare Part B. These time limits are established according to the date of service.

For services rendered between October 1, 1993 and September 30, 1994, claims must be submitted by December 31, 1995. For services rendered between October 1, 1994 and September 30, 1995, claims must be submitted by December 31, 1996.

However, if documentation is submitted that shows that the delay was due to an administrative error on the part of the Social Security Administration or the Medicare carrier, the time limit may be waived. Even if the claim is filed within the filing deadline, a 10% reduction in payment is assessed on claims received more than 12 months after the date of service.

Medi-Medi

When a patient is eligible for both Medicare and Medicaid, that patient is considered to be a Medi-Medi patient. If a patient is eligible for benefits to be paid under Medicaid, Medicare will automatically forward the claim to the appropriate department for coordination of benefits. Through the use of computer files, Medicare cross-references all claims to check for Medicaid eligibility. Medicaid will always be the secondary payor to Medicare.

HCPCS

When billing Medicare services, three levels of coding are used to identify services rendered. The development of HCFA Common Procedural Coding System (HCPCS) was intended by the government to enhance the existing coding system by offering more specific codes and uniformity in identifying services. The system allows consistent billing of services and simplifies communication between Medicare and other insurers.

HCPCS are based on the American Medical Association (AMA) Current Procedural Terminology (CPT-4) with additional codes and modifiers developed by HCFA. HCPCS is made up of three levels of codes.

1. Level 1: The first level contains only the CPT codes and modifiers.
   Maintenance of these codes is the responsibility of the AMA, and updates are expected to be done on a yearly basis.
2. Level 2: The second level includes the HCFA designated codes. These are nonphysician services such as Durable Medical Equipment (DME), Prostheses and Orthoses, and so on. A few physicians' services that were not found in the CPT codes were assigned HCFA codes, such as J codes for injection. HCFA codes are alphanumeric beginning with A0000 and continuing through V9999.
3. Level 3: The third level contains codes local to the individual Medicare carrier and are not already found in the first two levels. These codes are also alphanumeric, but are located in the ranges beginning with W, X, Y, and Z. Medicare requires that HCPCS be used for all services rendered to Medicare recipients. It is important to understand the HCPCS coding system to enable you to correctly code Medicare services. Some examples of HCPCS are listed in the Relative Value Study located in the student exercise manual.

New Code for Routine Venipuncture

Effective for services rendered on or after January 1, 1994 when coding for a specimen collection, the code 36415 will no longer be accepted by Medicare as a valid code for venipuncture. The HCPC code G0001 has been established for reporting this service.

Assignment of Benefits

The Medicare Assignment of Benefits has nothing to do with the provider to whom the claims examiner will make payment. To be a participating provider, the provider must agree to accept assignment on all Medicare claims. By doing this, the provider receives payment directly from Medicare, rather than the payment going to the member. In addition, the provider has agreed to accept the amount approved by the Medicare carrier for the services covered. The patient is not responsible for any amount in excess of the approved amount. In such a case, the secondary carrier is also not responsible for the amount in excess of the approved amount.

Physicians Who Accept Assignment

When a physician agrees to accept Medicare assignment for a bill, Medicare will pay the physician directly for that bill. The physician may bill the patient only for any deductibles or coinsurance that Medicare has deducted from the assigned bill. As a result, the total fee that physicians may receive from Medicare and from beneficiaries for an assigned bill is limited by what Medicare deems to be an appropriate fee for the particular service or procedure (the Medicare "allowance").

To encourage physicians to accept assignment, the

Medicare allowance is higher for physicians who agree to accept assignment for all bills for Medicare-eligible persons. These physicians are called "participating physicians." Thus, participating physicians agree not to practice "balance billing," ie, charging patients for more than Medicare allows.

The phrase "participating physician" can be confusing since physicians who sign these agreements are not the only ones who treat Medicare patients. Physicians who treat Medicare-eligible individuals but who decide whether to accept assignment on a case-by-case basis are called "nonparticipating physicians." In exchange for the freedom to make this choice for each patient, these nonparticipating physicians receive only 95% of the reimbursement that participating physicians receive from Medicare. For example, if the Medicare allowance for a procedure is $100 for participating physicians, the allowance for nonparticipating physicians would be $95.

Therefore, assuming that the patient's deductible had been paid, a participating physician would receive $80 from Medicare (80% of $100), and a nonparticipating physician would receive $76 from Medicare (80% of $95). While the participating physician is bound not to charge the Medicare patient more than the $20 copayment, the nonparticipating physician has no such restriction. However, if the nonparticipating physician agrees to accept assignment for that bill, he or she can bill the patient only for $19 ($95-$76).

New Procedural Requirement

The least significant of the new Medicare changes took effect on October 1, 1990. Since then, all physicians who treat Medicare patients—both participating and nonparticipating physicians—have been required to complete the paperwork on behalf of their patients. Medicare beneficiaries have welcomed this change. Previously, only participating physicians were responsible for filling out Medicare claim forms.

Physicians may not charge for filling out the forms. If they fail to file a claim form within 1 year after performing the service, they can be fined as much as $1000.

Restrictions on Balance Billing

Beginning on January 1, 1991, the most important Medicare changes took effect. As of that date, balance billing by nonparticipating physicians was strictly limited. (Limits had no effect in states such as Massachusetts, where balance billing is prohibited by law. In New York, the limits affected only office and home visits, since New York has limits on balance billing for all other services. Also, participating physicians are not affected since they were not allowed to balance bill Medicare patients for any services.)

Specifically, as of January 1, 1991, nonparticipating physicians were not allowed to charge Medicare patients more than 25% above Medicare allowance for a particular procedure or service. (OBRA '90 increased the limit for evaluation and management services from 25% to 40% for 1991 only.) In 1992, the limit was lowered to 20%. In 1993, balance billing was restricted to no more than 15% above what Medicare allows.

Following are two examples of how this rule affects the payment of claims:

Example 1. *Provider accepts assignment.*

Billed Charge	$42
Approved Amt	$35
Medicare Pays	$35 to ded = 0 pd
Member Pays	$35
Billed Charge	$90
Approved Amt	$75
Medicare Pays	$20 to ded, $55 @80% = $44 pd
Member Pays	$20+20% of $55 = $11 = $31
Billed Charge	$480
Approved Amt	$400
Medicare Pays	$400 @80% = $320
Member Pays	20% of $400 = $80

Example 2. *Provider does not accept assignment.*

Charge	$42
Approved Amt	$33.25
Medicare Pays	$33.25 to ded = 0
Member Pays	$42

Charge	$90
Approved Amt	$71.25
Medicare Pays	$20 to ded, $51.25 @80% = $41 pd
Member Pays	$20+20% of $51.25 = $10.25+$18.75 = $49

Charge	$480
Approved Amt	$380
Medicare Pays	$380 @80% = $304.00
Member Pays	20% of $380.00 = 76+$100.00 = $176.00

Medicare Supplement

Supplements are separate plans written exclusively for Medicare participants. A supplement plan may be written with any optional benefits the policyholder wants. Three common options are:

1. Physicians' services—Covers Part B deductible and 20% coinsurance for reasonable charges.
2. Hospital services—Covers Part A deductible and may or may not cover the various copays not covered by Medicare.
3. Nursing care, prescriptions, and the nonreplaced fees on the first three pints of blood.

With the changes in Medicare, supplemental plans have become much more flexible. Therefore, the benefits can be very complex and comprehensive or very basic.

Estimating Medicare Coverage

Sometimes, a member is entitled to Medicare but has not enrolled. In these circumstances, some plans estimate what Medicare would have paid had the person been enrolled properly. Benefits may then be reduced by the estimated amount.

In this situation, the medical biller should contact the patient and inform him or her that a balance is due on their bill. The patient then must pay the balance due. The medical biller should suggest that the patient apply for Medicare coverage to prevent the situation from being repeated.

Diagnosis-Related Group Billing

Effective October 1, 1983, Medicare instituted Diagnosis-Related Group (DRG) payments for inpatient hospital claims.

Under DRG, a flat-rate payment is made based on the patient's diagnosis instead of the hospital's itemized billing. If the hospital can treat the patient for less, it keeps the savings. If treatment costs more, the hospital must absorb the loss. Neither Medicare nor the patient is responsible for the excess amount.

Provisions have been made for cases atypically expensive (based on the diagnosis) because of complications or an abnormally long confinement. Known as Outliers, these cases will be reimbursed on an itemized or cost-percentage basis instead of DRG. The bill from the hospital must indicate that it is an Outlier.

Excluded from DRG are long-term care, children's care, and psychiatric and rehabilitative hospitals. Also excluded are hospitals located in the states of Maryland, Massachusetts, New Jersey, and New York. These states have obtained waivers from DRG.

DRG Benefit Payment Calculations

As shown in the following examples, the maximum liability under a plan are only the expenses that are covered by the plan and that the insured is legally obligated to pay.

Example 1. *Itemized hospital bill exceeds Medicare DRG allowance.*

Hospital Bill	$8,700.00
DRG Allowance	$7,000.00
Medicare Payment	$6,324.00 (DRG minus $676 ded)
Patient's Responsibility	$676.00
Hospital Write-off	$1,700.00

Although the Medicare DRG allowance is less than the itemized hospital bill, the insured is legally obligated to pay only the $676.00 Part A deductible.

Example 2. *Medicare DRG allowance exceeds itemized billed amount.*

Hospital Bill	$ 8,700.00
DRG Allowance	$10,000.00
Medicare Payment	$9,324.00
Patient's Responsibility	$676.00

Even though the Medicare payment exceeds the itemized hospital bill, the insured is legally obligated to pay the $676.00 Part A deductible.

Summary

Medicare billing guidelines are changed by HCFA several times a year. The medical biller must keep abreast of all the changes that occur.

Medicare intermediaries send out bulletins on a regular basis. The medical biller should read through these bulletins as soon as possible to become familiar with any updates or changes in the billing procedures.

Assignments

Complete the Questions for Review.
Complete Medicare Exercise 3-1.

Questions for Review

Directions: Answer the following questions without looking back into the material just covered. Write your answers in the space provided.

1. What is Medicare? ______________________________
2. What three criteria is Medicare eligibility based on?
   a. ______________________________
   b. ______________________________
   c. ______________________________
3. Medicare ____________ is considered the basic plan or hospital insurance.
4. Medicare ____________ is the medical insurance that covers physician services.
5. What does it mean if a provider accepts assignment of benefits in regard to Medicare? ______________________________

____

____

If you were unable to answer any of the questions, refer back to the section, and then fill in the answers.

Exercise 3-1

Directions: Complete all the forms and steps necessary up to the claim submission. Post payments to the ledger and daily journal making any adjustments needed.

1. The following charges were billed to Medicare for Edward Edmunds.

   Date of Service 10/21/9x

   99205—Initial Comprehensive Exam

   81000—Urinalysis

You have received an Explanation of Medicare Benefits for Edward Edmunds indicating the following:

Date	Proc	Charge	Approved	Payment
10/21/9x	99215	110.00	70.13	56.10
10/21/9x	81000	10.00	4.72	4.72

2. The following charges were billed to Medicare for Edward Edmunds.

   Date of Service 11/17/9x (in office)

   99211—Minimal Exam

   G0001—Venipuncture

   81000—Urinalysis

You have received an Explanation of Medicare Benefits for Edward Edmunds indicating the following:

Date	Proc	Charge	Approved	Payment
11/17/9x	99211	35.00	20.00	16.00
11/17/9x	G0001	15.00	6.38	6.38
11/17/9x	81000	10.00	4.72	4.72

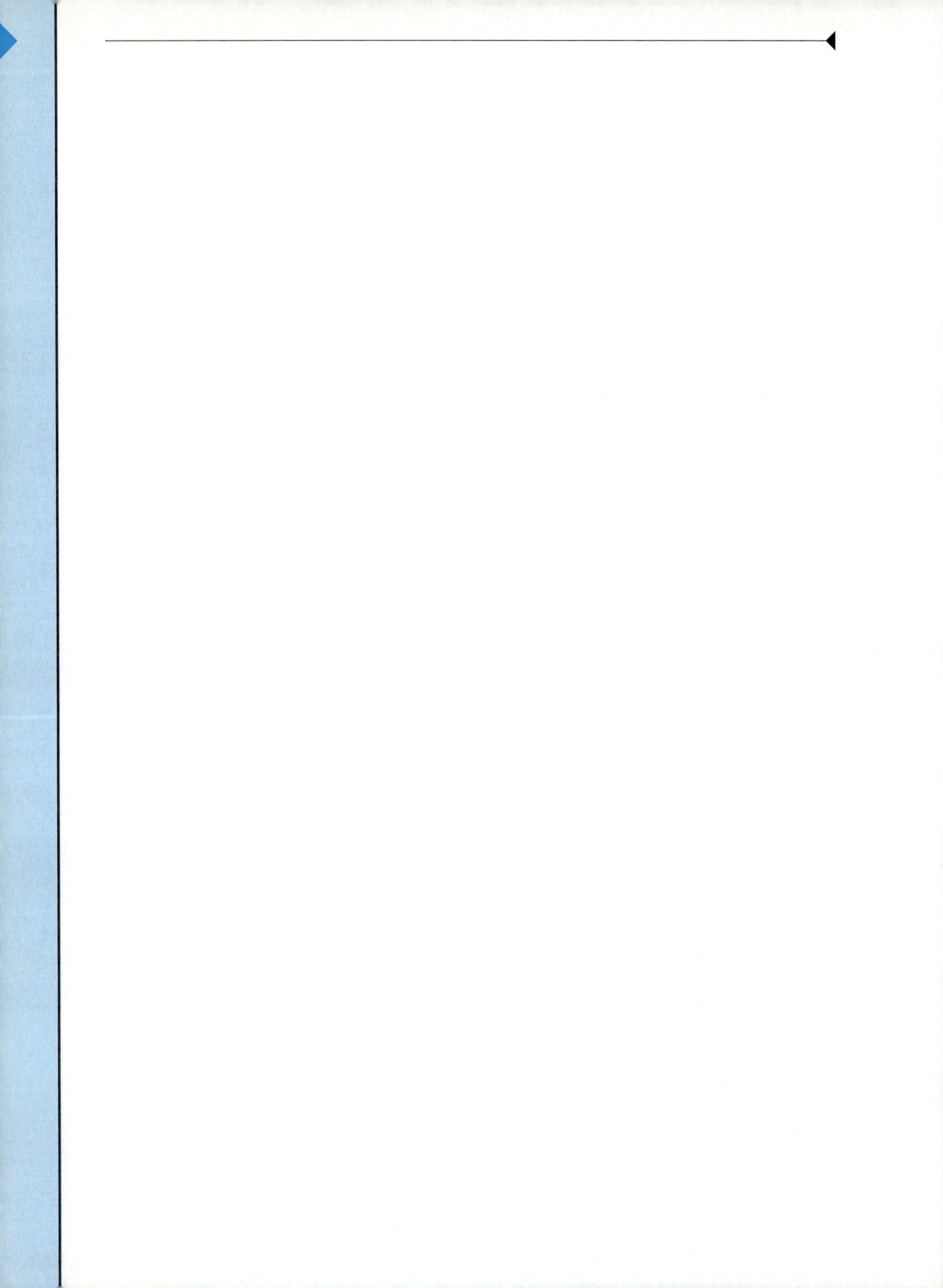

4

Medicaid

In this chapter you will learn:

- To understand Medicaid benefits and eligibility requirements.
- To understand basic billing of Medicaid claims.

Medicaid is not a health insurance program. The Federal Medicaid program was established under Title XIX of the Social Security Act of 1965. The purpose of this program is to provide the needy with access to medical care.

By law, Medicaid is always secondary to private group health care plans. If Medicaid inadvertently pays primary, it will exercise its right of recovery and seek reimbursement from the private plan. Once again, by law, the private plan is required to process Medicaid's request for reimbursement and pay back Medicaid the monies it paid the provider of services. The recovery process will be explained in greater detail later in this section.

The regulations governing eligibility under this program are extremely complex. Individuals may be entitled to coverage due to medical, family, or fiscal situations. The fact that the individual has private insurance does not preclude him or her from being eligible for Medicaid benefits.

The Medicaid program does not process its own claims. Medicaid contracts with an organization to act as the fiscal intermediary, similar to that which occurs with Medicare. The intermediary processes the claims according to specifications set forth by the Medicaid program.

The rates under this program are based on the results of reimbursement studies conducted by the Department of Health Services. Reimbursement for hospital inpatient services are based on each facility's "reasonable cost" of services as determined from audit cost reports and annual limitations on reimbursable increases in cost.

Providers are not allowed to bill or submit a claim to the Medicaid beneficiary for any service included in the program's scope of benefits except to collect money from a patient's private health care coverage prior to billing Medicaid.

In the Medicaid program, a 3-year statute of limitations extends from the date of service for recovery. In addition, there is a 3-year subrogation right (recovery of monies for claims covered by a third party).

For a claimant's services to be covered under Medicaid, the claimant must be a Medicaid beneficiary and the provider must be an approved Medicaid provider. To be an approved provider, the provider of services must agree to accept Medicaid's determination of approved amounts as binding. That is, similar to Medicare's approved amount on assigned claims, the provider is not allowed to bill the patient for any amount not approved by Medicaid. In recent years, many providers have dropped out of the Medicaid program because their allowances and payments are extremely low, even lower than those provided by Medicare.

Medicaid Billing Procedures

Medicaid eligibility is determined monthly through the county welfare office. When billing for services for medicaid recipients, you must have a copy of the Medicaid eligibility card for the month the services are rendered. If the eligibility card has adhesive stickers, one of the stickers must be attached to the billing form for payment.

The following 9 services are covered benefits under Medicaid:

1. Inpatient hospital care
2. Outpatient hospital services
3. Physician services
4. Laboratory and x-ray services
5. Screening, diagnosis, and treatment of children under age 21
6. Immunizations
7. Home health care services
8. Family planning services
9. Outpatient hospital services

Additional benefits may be offered in various states.

The eligibility card can be either plastic or paper. The paper eligibility card has adhesive stickers. These stickers are used for payment when claims are billed to the Medicaid office. Medicaid eligibility is determined on a monthly basis. The paper eligibility cards are issued monthly. You must have a copy of the month when services are rendered to receive payment. The plastic cards are issued once and are to last throughout the participant's eligibility on Medicaid. Verification of coverage must be obtained from the state for each month when services are given. Most states have a telephone verification eligibility system, which requires responding to various questions asked by a computer by pressing numbers or symbols on the headset.

The plastic card eligibility can be determined through a PSN (Provider Service Network) system. The system requires the provider to maintain a machine that will read the magnetic strip on the back of the eligibility card. The machine resembles a credit card machine. The card is swiped through the PSN, and the computer network will verify the eligibility of the person seeking services. The PSN system is able to indicate what benefits are available to the recipient, any restrictions, any third-party coverage, or Medicare coverage.

Some Medicaid-covered services require the Medicaid beneficiary to pay a small fee for services, called a copayment. The services that require copayments vary from state to state.

Medicaid claims must be submitted within 60 days of the month when services were rendered. There are six exceptions to this rule (these services must be billed within 1 year of the date of service):

1. Dental bills
2. Obstetric care
3. Treatment plan completion
4. When the patient has other insurance coverage
5. Retroactive eligibility
6. In the event that the patient did not inform the provider that there was Medicaid coverage

Treatment Authorization Request

In many cases, prior authorization is required before services are rendered. A Treatment Authorization Request (TAR) form is completed to obtain authorization for specific services (see Figure 4-1). This form must be completed and sent to the appropriate agency for authorization to be given prior to services being rendered. Please check with your state's Medicaid fiscal intermediary for prior treatment authorization guidelines. Some of the services that require TARs are:

- Inpatient hospital services
- Home health agency services
- Hearing aids
- Chronic hemodialysis services
- Some surgical procedures

Instructions for Completing the Treatment Authorization Request

Field 1

Leave blank

Field 2

A Verbal Control Number is given when there is insufficient time to request a Treatment Authorization Number for the services provided. Once a Verbal Control Number is given, you must complete and submit a TAR immediately.

Type of Service Requested

Place an "X" in the appropriate box.

Request is Retroactive

Place an "X" in the appropriate box.

Is Patient Medicare Eligible?

Place an "X" in the appropriate box.

Provider Phone Number

Complete this field with the provider of services' area code and telephone number.

Field 3

This number is used for a hospitalization TAR. Do not enter the physician's provider number. Enter the nine-digit hospital provider number for the facility where the services will be performed.

Field 3A

Enter the provider's name and address.

Field 4

Enter the patient's last name, first name and middle initial. Enter the patient's address and telephone number.

Field 5

Enter the patient's Medicaid identification number as it appears on the eligibility label or ID card.

Field 6

Leave blank.

Field 7

Sex—Enter "M" for male, "F" for female.

Age—Enter the age of the patient.

Field 8

Enter the patient's date of birth in a 6-digit format, ie 00/00/00.

Field 8A

Patient Status—Enter an "X" in the appropriate box.

Field 8B

Diagnosis Description and Medical Justification: Enter the diagnosis and medical justification (attach

STATE USE ONLY

2

CONFIDENTIAL PATIENT INFORMATION

1 FOR CSC USE ONLY

CCN

CSC USE ONLY 40 41 42 43

TYPEWRITER ALIGNMENT Elite Pica

TREATMENT AUTHORIZATION REQUEST

STATE OF CALIFORNIA DEPARTMENT OF HEALTH SERVICES

TYPEWRITER ALIGNMENT Elite Pica

(PLEASE TYPE) FOR PROVIDER USE (PLEASE TYPE) | FOR STATE USE

VERBAL CONTROL NO. | TYPE OF SERVICE REQUESTED 2 DRUG OTHER | REQUEST IS RETROACTIVE? YES NO | IS PATIENT MEDICARE ELIGIBLE? YES NO | PROVIDER PHONE NO. ( ) AREA

PLEASE TYPE YOUR NAME AND ADDRESS HERE

PROVIDER NAME AND ADDRESS

3 PROVIDER NUMBER

NAME AND ADDRESS OF PATIENT

4 PATIENT NAME (LAST, FIRST, M.I.)

5 MEDI-CAL IDENTIFICATION NO. CHECK DIGIT 6 P

STREET ADDRESS

7 SEX AGE 8 DATE OF BIRTH MM DD YY

CITY, STATE, ZIP CODE

PATIENT STATUS: HOME BOARD & CARE SNF/ICF ACUTE HOSPITAL

PHONE NUMBER AREA ( )

DIAGNOSIS DESCRIPTION: ICD-9-CM DIAGNOSIS CODE

MEDICAL JUSTIFICATION:

33 PROVIDER; YOUR REQUEST IS:

1 APPROVED AS REQUESTED

2 APPROVED AS MODIFIED (ITEMS MARKED BELOW AS AUTHORIZED MAY BE CLAIMED)

3 DENIED

4 DEFERRED

By ______ MEDI-CAL CONSULTANT

34 I.D. # 35 DATE M M D D Y Y

Comments/Explanation

RETROACTIVE AUTHORIZATION GRANTED IN ACCORDANCE WITH SECTION 51003 (B)

36 1 2 3 4 5

LINE NO	AUTHORIZED YES	NO	APPROVED UNITS	SPECIFIC SERVICES REQUESTED	UNITS OF SERVICE	PROCEDURE OR DRUG CODE	QUANTITY	CHARGES
1	9 X	X	10			11	12	$
2	13 X	X	14			15	16	$
3	17 X	X	18			19	20	$
4	21 X	X	22			23	24	$
5	25 X	X	26			27	28	$
6	29 X	X	30			31	32	$

TO THE BEST OF MY KNOWLEDGE, THE ABOVE INFORMATION IS TRUE, ACCURATE AND COMPLETE AND THE REQUESTED SERVICES ARE MEDICALLY INDICATED AND NECESSARY TO THE HEALTH OF THE PATIENT.

SIGNATURE OF PHYSICIAN OR PROVIDER TITLE DATE

AUTHORIZATION IS VALID FOR SERVICES PROVIDED 37 FROM DATE M M D D Y Y 38 TO DATE M M D D Y Y

TAR CONTROL NUMBER

39 OFFICE SEQUENCE NUMBER PI

15072585

NOTE: AUTHORIZATION DOES NOT GUARANTEE PAYMENT. PAYMENT IS SUBJECT TO PATIENT'S ELIGIBILITY. BE SURE THE IDENTIFICATION CARD IS CURRENT BEFORE RENDERING SERVICE. SEND TO FIELD SERVICES - CSC COPY

50-1 12/82

Figure 4-1: Example of Treatment Authorization Request Form

consultation report or other medical documentation if necessary) for the Medicaid consultant to determine medical necessity. Enter the hospital name and address on the first line on the Medical Justification section. If the patient is inpatient in a SNF/ICF, enter the name and address of the facility in the Medical Justification section.

Field 9

Leave blank.

Field 10

Approved units—Leave blank.

Specified Services Requested—Enter the name of the procedure or service requested.

Field 11

Procedure or Drug Code—Enter the procedure code for the CPT-4. The code on the claim submitted and the TAR must be the same.

Field 12

Quantity—Enter the number of times the service or procedure is to be preformed.

Charges—Enter the usual and customary fee for the requested services.

Fields 13 through 32

Complete these fields if requesting authorization for additional items.

Signature of Physician or Provider—Signature of the provider of services or authorized representative must appear in this space. Enter the title of the person signing the TAR and the date.

Field 33

This section will be completed by the state agency reviewing the TAR.

Final Status of Request—Indicates if the services requested are approved, approved but modified, denied or deferred. If the TAR is approved but modified, denied or deferred, the consultant will give an explanation in the Comments/Explanation section of Field 33.

Medicaid Consultant Signature and Date—The reviewing consultant must sign and date the TAR or it is not valid.

Fields 34 and 35

These fields to be completed by the reviewing consultant.

Field 36

The consultant will indicate in the correct field if retroactive authorization was given.

Fields 37 and 38

If the TAR is for a hospitalization, the claim submitted cannot have a date of service earlier than the "From Date" on the TAR.

Field 39

The TAR control number is preprinted on the form at the time of production. The consultant will add a two-digit prefix and a one-digit suffix. This 11-digit number must be enter as the TAR control number on the claim when submitted to Medicaid.

Posting Medicaid Payments

As with Medicare, Medicaid payment will probably be lower than the actual billed charges. Because Medicaid recipients are not financially responsible for the balance, an adjustment will have to made and written off. When the explanation of benefits is received from Medicaid, each patient ledger will need to be pulled and the payments recorded. The adjustments should be made on the next corresponding entry line on the ledger card. The payment amount should be subtracted from the billed amount and the difference should be written off. If the patient's eligibility for Medicaid is terminated at the time services are rendered, the patient becomes financially responsible for the charges. At that time the patient should be billed directly.

Appeals

If a Medicaid claim payment is not satisfactory to the provider of services, the provider has the option to file an appeal. An appeal must be made to the fiscal intermediary within 90 days of the action causing the grievance. The appeal must be submitted in writing. Copies of the appeal letter, claim, and any additional documentation should be included with the submission.

Completing the Medicaid Claim Form

Medicaid Claim Forms are required to be filled out when submitting claims to Medicaid. The Medicaid Claim Form is created by each state and thus varies from state to state (see Figure 4-2). However, much of the information is the same as the information required on the standard claim forms.

For illustration purposes, we will give instructions on completion of the claim form used by the State of California. This form is read by computer, like many states' Medicaid forms, so it is important to complete it correctly.

General Guidelines

The following five guidelines should be followed in the completion of Medicaid Claim Forms:

1. If possible, type the claim rather than write it by hand.
2. Use capital letters only when typing claims.
3. Do not strike over to correct errors.
4. Do not use N/A; leave space blank.
5. Be as complete and accurate as possible.

Field Descriptions

Listed below are the fields of the Medicaid claim form and the appropriate information that should be entered into each field.

Field	Description
1	Leave blank.
1A	Type provider's name and address.
2	Type provider's nine-digit Medi-Cal/Medicaid provider number.
3	Leave blank.
4	Enter an "X" in the Medi-Cal box.
5	For patients who have Medicare and Medicaid enter an "X" in boxes 4 and 5.
6	Enter the five-digit zip code.
7A	Enter the provider's telephone number (this field is optional).
7B	Attach a Medi-Cal/Medicaid sticker for month of services. If a photocopy of the entire card is used, it must be a full size $8\frac{1}{2} \times 11$" sheet of paper.
8	Enter the patient's last name, first name, and middle initial and full address as it appears on the Medi-Cal/Medicaid card.
9	Leave blank on Medi-Cal claims. For Medi-Medi, enter the Medicare number as it appears on the Medicare ID card.
10	Enter the patient's sex: M for male, F for female.
11	Complete this field only for services associated with an accident; enter an "X" in the Yes or No box to show if the patient's condition is related to employment.
12	Enter the onset date of the patient's illness or date of last menstrual period using six digits for month, date, and year.
13	Enter the complete 11-digit TAR Control number. If a TAR is not required leave blank.
14	Enter the patient's Medi-Cal ID number exactly as it appears on the eligibility label. If the patient is a newborn, the mother's ID number may be used. Enter the infant's name, sex, and date of birth in the appropriate boxes. Enter "newborn" in the remarks section.
15	Enter the patient's date of birth in six digits.
16	Enter the patient's last name, account number, or record number. This information appears on the EOB and is helpful in the reconciliation of claims.
17 & 18	Enter the hospital admission and discharge dates if the services are related to a hospital confinement.
19	Leave this field blank unless billing for emergency services. Enter an "X" if an Emergency Certification Statement is attached.
20	Enter an "X" if the patient has other insurance coverage. Enter the name and address of the carrier.
21	Claims must be submitted within 2 months of the month the services are rendered. If there is an exception, the appropriate Exceptions to Billing Limitations code must be entered.

Reason Code	Description
1	Proof of eligibility unknown or unavailable.
2	Other coverage.

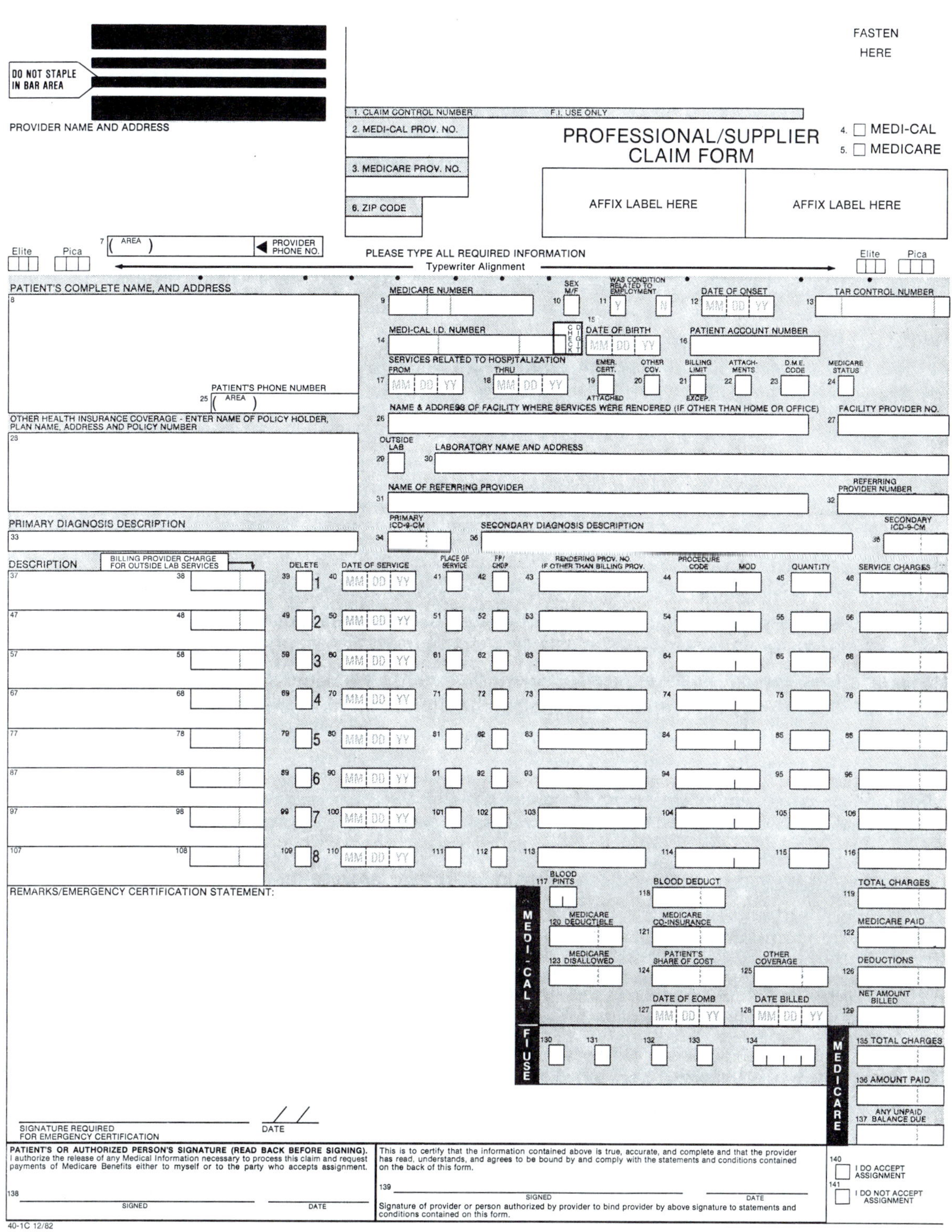

DO NOT STAPLE IN BAR AREA

PROVIDER NAME AND ADDRESS

FASTEN HERE

1. CLAIM CONTROL NUMBER | F.I. USE ONLY

2. MEDI-CAL PROV. NO.

3. MEDICARE PROV. NO.

6. ZIP CODE

PROFESSIONAL/SUPPLIER CLAIM FORM

4. ☐ MEDI-CAL
5. ☐ MEDICARE

AFFIX LABEL HERE | AFFIX LABEL HERE

7 (AREA) ◀ PROVIDER PHONE NO.

Elite Pica

PLEASE TYPE ALL REQUIRED INFORMATION

Typewriter Alignment

Elite Pica

PATIENT'S COMPLETE NAME, AND ADDRESS 8

9 MEDICARE NUMBER | 10 SEX M/F | 11 WAS CONDITION RELATED TO EMPLOYMENT Y N | 12 DATE OF ONSET MM DD YY | 13 TAR CONTROL NUMBER

14 MEDI-CAL I.D. NUMBER | 15 CHECK DIGIT | DATE OF BIRTH MM DD YY | 16 PATIENT ACCOUNT NUMBER

SERVICES RELATED TO HOSPITALIZATION FROM 17 MM DD YY THRU 18 MM DD YY | 19 EMER. CERT. ATTACHED | 20 OTHER COV. | 21 BILLING LIMIT EXCEP. | 22 ATTACH-MENTS | 23 D.M.E. CODE | 24 MEDICARE STATUS

25 PATIENT'S PHONE NUMBER (AREA)

26 NAME & ADDRESS OF FACILITY WHERE SERVICES WERE RENDERED (IF OTHER THAN HOME OR OFFICE) | 27 FACILITY PROVIDER NO.

OTHER HEALTH INSURANCE COVERAGE - ENTER NAME OF POLICY HOLDER, PLAN NAME, ADDRESS AND POLICY NUMBER 28

29 OUTSIDE LAB | 30 LABORATORY NAME AND ADDRESS

31 NAME OF REFERRING PROVIDER | 32 REFERRING PROVIDER NUMBER

PRIMARY DIAGNOSIS DESCRIPTION 33

34 PRIMARY ICD-9-CM | 35 SECONDARY DIAGNOSIS DESCRIPTION | 36 SECONDARY ICD-9-CM

DESCRIPTION	BILLING PROVIDER CHARGE FOR OUTSIDE LAB SERVICES	DELETE	DATE OF SERVICE	PLACE OF SERVICE	FP/CHDP	RENDERING PROV. NO. IF OTHER THAN BILLING PROV.	PROCEDURE CODE MOD	QUANTITY	SERVICE CHARGES
37	38	39 1	40 MM DD YY	41	42	43	44	45	46
47	48	49 2	50 MM DD YY	51	52	53	54	55	56
57	58	59 3	60 MM DD YY	61	62	63	64	65	66
67	68	69 4	70 MM DD YY	71	72	73	74	75	76
77	78	79 5	80 MM DD YY	81	82	83	84	85	86
87	88	89 6	90 MM DD YY	91	92	93	94	95	96
97	98	99 7	100 MM DD YY	101	102	103	104	105	106
107	108	109 8	110 MM DD YY	111	112	113	114	115	116

REMARKS/EMERGENCY CERTIFICATION STATEMENT:

SIGNATURE REQUIRED FOR EMERGENCY CERTIFICATION | / / DATE

MEDI-CAL

117 BLOOD PINTS | 118 BLOOD DEDUCT | 119 TOTAL CHARGES

120 MEDICARE DEDUCTIBLE | 121 MEDICARE CO-INSURANCE | 122 MEDICARE PAID

123 MEDICARE DISALLOWED | 124 PATIENT'S SHARE OF COST | 125 OTHER COVERAGE | 126 DEDUCTIONS

127 DATE OF EOMB MM DD YY | 128 DATE BILLED MM DD YY | 129 NET AMOUNT BILLED

FI USE

130 | 131 | 132 | 133 | 134

MEDICARE

135 TOTAL CHARGES

136 AMOUNT PAID

137 ANY UNPAID BALANCE DUE

PATIENT'S OR AUTHORIZED PERSON'S SIGNATURE (READ BACK BEFORE SIGNING). I authorize the release of any Medical Information necessary to process this claim and request payments of Medicare Benefits either to myself or to the party who accepts assignment.

138 SIGNED DATE

This is to certify that the information contained above is true, accurate, and complete and that the provider has read, understands, and agrees to be bound by and comply with the statements and conditions contained on the back of this form.

139 SIGNED DATE

Signature of provider or person authorized by provider to bind provider by above signature to statements and conditions contained on this form.

140 ☐ I DO ACCEPT ASSIGNMENT

141 ☐ I DO NOT ACCEPT ASSIGNMENT

40-1C 12/82

FORWARD TO APPROPRIATE F.I.

Figure 4-2: Front of a Medicaid Claim Form

IMPORTANT

MEDI-CAL PAYMENTS

The services listed on this form have been personally provided to the patient by the provider or, under his direction, by another person eligible under the Medi-Cal Program to provide such services, and such person(s) are designated on this form. The services were, to the best of the provider's knowledge, medically indicated and necessary to the health of the patient. The provider understands that the payment of this claim will be from Federal and/or State funds, and that falsification, or concealment of a material fact, may be prosecuted under Federal and/or State laws. The provider agrees to keep for a minimum period of three years from the date of service all records which are necessary to disclose fully the extent of services furnished to the patient. The provider agrees to furnish these records and any information regarding payment claimed for providing the services, on request, to California Department of Health Services; Medi-Cal Fraud Unit, California Department of Justice; Medical Audits Project, Office of the State Controller; US Department of Health and Human Services, or their duly authorized representatives.

Medical care services are offered and provided without discrimination based on race, religion, color, national or ethnic origin, sex, age, or physical or mental disability.

MEDICARE PAYMENTS

A patient's signature requests that payment be made and authorizes release of medical information necessary to pay the claim. If the "Other Health Insurance Coverage" block is completed, the patient's signature authorizes release of the information to the insurer or agency shown. In assigned cases, the physician agrees to accept the charge determination of the Medicare carrier as the full charge, and the patient is responsible only for the deductible, coinsurance, and noncovered services. Coinsurance and the deductible are based on the charge determination of the carrier, if this is less than the charge submitted.

> **SIGNATURE OF PHYSICIAN (OR SUPPLIER): I certify that the services shown on this form were medically indicated and necessary for the health of the patient and were personally rendered by me or were rendered incident to my professional service by my employee under immediate personal supervision, except as otherwise expressly permitted by Medicare regulations.**
>
> **For services to be considered as 'incident to' a physician's professional service, (1) they must be rendered under the physician's immediate personal supervision by his employee, (2) there was a covered physician's service rendered of which the other services are an integral, although incidental part, (3) they must be of kinds commonly furnished in physicians' offices, and (4) the services of nonphysicians must be included on the physicians' bill.**
>
> **NOTICE: Anyone who misrepresents or falsifies essential information to receive payment from federal funds requested by this form may upon conviction be subject to fine and imprisonment under applicable federal laws.**

Figure 4-2: Back of a Medicaid Claim Form

3 Authorization delays.
4 Delay by the department or fiscal intermediary in provider certification or in supplying billing forms.
5 Do not use.
6 Substantial damage by fire, flood, or disaster to provider records.
7 Theft, sabotage, or other willful acts by an employee.
8 Court decisions, fair hearing decisions, provider appeals, or other circumstances beyond the provider's control as determined by the department.
22 Enter "X" if attachments are included. If not leave blank.
23 Leave blank.
24 Leave blank if patient is Medicare recipient. If not, enter one of the codes below:

Code	Explanation
0	Under 65, does not have Medicare coverage.
1	Benefits exhausted.
2	Utilization committee denial or physician noncertification.
3	No prior hospital stay.
4	Facility denial.
5	Noneligible provider.
6	Noneligible recipient.
7	Medicare benefits denied or cut short by Medicare intermediary.
8	Noncovered services.
9	PSRO denial.

25 Optional.
26 Optional.
27 Enter the full nine-digit Medi-Cal provider number of the facility where the services were rendered.
28 If a claim submitted to a health insurer has not been paid within 90 days, the provider may then bill Medi-Cal using the Billing Limit Exception Reason code 2 and include a statement in the Remarks section or attach documentation that the other carrier has not paid.
29 Leave blank.
30 Leave blank.
31 Optional.
32 Enter the Medi-Cal number of the referring or prescribing physician.
33 Optional if an entry is made in field 34.
34 Enter all letters and numbers of the ICD-9 code.
35 Optional if an entry is made in field 36.
36 Enter all letters and numbers of the ICD-9 code, if applicable.
37 Optional, except when billing for unlisted procedures.
38 Leave blank.
39 If a mistake has been made, delete the entire line by typing an "X" in this space. Then enter the correct information on the next line.
40 Enter the date of service in six-digit format.
41 Enter the place of service code using the following codes:

Code	Place of Service
1	Office
2	Home
3	Inpatient hospital
4	Skilled nursing facility (SNF)
5	Outpatient hospital
6	Independent laboratory
7	Other (describe in Remarks section)
8	Independent kidney treatment center
9	Clinic
A	Surgery clinic
B	Emergency Room
C	Intermediate care facility (ICF)
D	Extended care facility (ECF)

42 Enter code 1 or 2 if the services are related to family planning.
43 Enter the Medi-Cal provider number or state license number of the provider only if it is different from the billing provider number or when billing under a group

number.

44 Enter the applicable code and modifiers from the CPT.

45 Enter the number of medical visits or surgical lesions.

46 Enter the usual and customary fee for the services.

47-116 Follow the same instructions for each claim line.

117 Leave blank.

118 Leave blank.

119 Enter the total amount of billed charges.

120 Leave blank.

121 Leave blank.

122 Leave blank.

123 Leave blank.

124 Leave blank.

125 Enter the amount of payment received from third party payor indicated in field 28.

126 Enter the amount paid by other insurance coverage. This amount is shown in field 125.

127 Leave blank unless billing for Medicare-denied or non-covered services.

128 Enter the date the claim is submitted to Medi-Cal in six-digit format.

129 Enter the difference between the Total Charges and Deductions (field 119–field 126 = field 129).

130-134 Leave blank.

135 Leave blank.

136 Leave blank.

137A Leave blank.

137B Use this area for any services requiring additional explanation or entering the Emergency Certification Statement.

138 Leave blank.

139 The claim must be signed and dated by the provider of services. Use of stamps and initials are not acceptable.

140 Leave blank.

141 Leave blank.

It is important to use the proper Medicaid billing form for your state in order to receive reimbursement from Medicaid. Without this form, Medicaid will refuse to pay.

Summary

Medicaid was established under Title XIX of the Social Security Act of 1965 to provide the needy with access to medical care. Medicaid eligibility is determined monthly, and each month a new Medicaid card is issued to the recipient. The information contained on this card must be used when billing for Medicaid services.

It is important to remember that providers who accept Medicaid patients are not allowed to bill the patient for any amounts that Medicaid does not cover. If the patient is covered by other insurance, the other insurance carrier is primary to Medicaid and should be billed first.

There are special Medicaid billing forms that vary from state to state. This special form must be used or Medicaid will not accept the claim for payment.

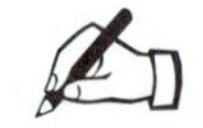

Assignments

Complete the Questions for Review.

Complete Medicaid Exercises 4-1 to 4-6. Medicaid claim forms can be found in Chapter 13 of the student exercise manual. Treatment Authorization Request forms are included in Chapter 1 of the student exercise manual.

Questions for Review

Directions: Answer the following questions without looking back into the material just covered. Write your answers in the space provided.

1. What is the purpose of the Medicaid program? ____________________

____

2. By law, Medicaid is always primary to private group health insurance plans. (True or False) __________
3. In what situation are providers allowed to bill or submit a claim to the Medicaid beneficiary? __________

____

4. The ____________ is a bill that lists the health care services paid by the Medicaid program on behalf of a person who has indicated that he or she has other health care coverage benefits available.
5. For a claimant's services to be covered under Medicaid, the claimant must be a ____________ and the provider must be an ____________.

If you were unable to answer any of the questions, refer back to the section and then fill in the answers.

Exercise 4-1

Directions: Post the charges and payments to the ledger of the following patient:

1. The following charges were billed to Medicaid for Daisy Doolittle.

   Date of Service 10/21/9x

   99205–Initial Comprehensive Exam

   81000–Urinalysis

You have received the following Medicare payments

Date	Proc	Charge	Approved	Payment
10/21/9x	99205	110.00	37.13	37.13
10/21/9x	81000	10.00	2.92	2.92

Exercise 4-2

Directions: Complete a Medicaid claim form using the following information:

Patient Medicaid Number: 33333000010-2
Patient Name: Daisy Doolittle
Address: (See Patient Information Sheet)

Date of Birth:
Relationship to Insured:
Marital Status:
Sex:
Insured Name:
Insured SSN:
Group Name:

Provider of Services: Dennis Doom, MD
Address: P.O. Box 4666
Denver, DE 90270
Employer ID number: 22-2867890
Medicaid Provider Number: EEE222000

Date of Service: June 11, 1994
Date First Seen: June 11, 1994

Initial consultation, expanded problem, straightforward visit performed at the office (CPT-4 Code = 99242) ($75.00).

Diagnosis: Upper Respiratory Infection ICD-9 Code = 465.9

Authorization to Release Information on File.
Provider Accepts Medicare Assignment.

Exercise 4-3

Directions: Complete a Medicaid claim form using the following information:

Patient Medicaid Number: 33333000010-2
Patient Name: Daisy Doolittle
Address: (See Patient Information Sheet)

Date of Birth:
Relationship to Insured:
Marital Status:
Sex:
Insured Name:
Insured SSN:
Group Name:

Provider of Services: Dennis Doom, MD
Address: P.O. Box 4666
Denver, DE 90270
Employer ID number: 22-2867890
Medicaid Provider Number: EEE222000

Date of Service: July 07, 1994
Date First Seen: June 11, 1994

Expanded problem, straightforward decision making visit performed at the office (CPT-4 Code = 99232) ($55.00).

Diagnosis: Tonsillitis, chronic ICD-9 Code = 474.0

Authorization to Release Information on File.
Provider Accepts Medicare Assignment.

Exercise 4-4

Directions: Complete a Medicaid claim form and a Treatment Authorization Request using the following information:

Patient Medicaid Number: 33333000010-2
Patient Name: Daisy Doolittle
Address: (See Patient Information Sheet)

Date of Birth:
Relationship to Insured:
Marital Status:
Sex:
Insured Name:
Insured SSN:
Group Name:

Provider of Services: Donald Danny, MD
Address: P.O. Box 1111
Denver, DE 90270
Employer ID number: 22-111222444
Medicaid Provider Number: DDD333000

Date of Service: July 09, 1994
Date First Seen: June 11, 1994

Initial consultation, problem-focused exam was performed by Dr. Doom in the office (CPT-4 Code = 99241) ($115.00).

Diagnosis: Tonsillitis, chronic ICD-9 Code = 474.0

Authorization to Release Information on File.
Provider Accepts Medicare Assignment.

Patient scheduled for tonsillectomy and adenoidectomy (CPT-4 Code = 42821) on July 11, 1994 at Daniel Community Hospital, P.O. Box 712, Denver, DE 90271. Surgery will be performed by Donald Danny, MD. Justification—Consultation on July 9, 1994. UCR = $1,650.00.

Exercise 4-5

Directions: Complete a Medicaid claim form using the following information:

Patient Medicaid Number: 33333000010-2
Patient Name: Daisy Doolittle
Address: (See Patient Information Sheet)

Date of Birth:
Relationship to Insured:
Marital Status:
Sex:
Insured Name:
Insured SSN:
Group Name:

Provider of Services: Dennis Danny, MD
Address: P.O. Box 1111
Denver, DE 90270
Employer ID number: 22-111222444
Medicaid Provider Number: DDD333000

Date of Service: July 11, 1994
Date First Seen: June 11, 1994
Hospitalized: July 11 through July 13, 1994

A tonsillectomy and adenoidectomy (CPT-4 Code = 42821) was performed at Daniel Community Hospital ($1500.00).

Diagnosis: Tonsillitis, chronic ICD-9 Code = 474.0

Authorization to Release Information on File.
Provider Accepts Medicare Assignment.

Exercise 4-6

Directions: Complete a Medicaid claim form using the following information:

Patient Medicaid Number: 33333000010-2
Patient Name: Daisy Doolittle
Address: (See Patient Information Sheet)

Date of Birth:
Relationship to Insured:
Marital Status:
Sex:
Insured Name:
Insured SSN:
Group Name:

Provider of Services: Debra Dankey, MD
Address: P.O. Box 22222
Denver, DE 90270
Employer ID number: 22-1333445555
Medicaid Provider Number: DDD555000

Date of Service: August 23, 1994
Date First Seen: August 23, 1994

Comprehensive, moderate complexity exam (CPT-4 code = 99204) was performed by Dr. Debra Dankey ($100.00) in the office.

Diagnosis: Gastroenteritis ICD-9 Code = 558.9

Authorization to Release Information on File.
Provider Accepts Medicare Assignment.

5

Miscellaneous Billing Procedures

In this chapter you will learn:

- To understand eligibility and basic benefits of worker's compensation and CHAMPUS.
- To understand Coordination of Benefits (COB) and order of benefit determination rules.

In this chapter we will discuss several other types of claims that will require special handling when they are encountered in the medical office. They are Workers' Compensation, Coordination of Benefits, and CHAMPUS. Following is a brief discussion of their benefits and billing procedures.

Workers' Compensation

Workers' Compensation (WC) is a separate medical and disability reimbursement program, which provides 100% coverage for job-related injury, illness, or conditions arising out of and in the course of employment. The employer, by law, is responsible for the benefits due an employee for work-related injuries and illnesses.

Each state's Workers' Compensation Appeals Board (WC Board) has the sole authority to oversee the rights and benefits of an injured or ill worker. It is through this Appeals Board that an applicant (employee) will file his or her WC application.

As a general limitation, most WC plans specify that the claimant will not be entitled to payment for "... bodily injury or disease resulting from and arising out of any employment or occupation for compensation or profit."

Most plans investigate and then provide benefits for medical care if they suspect that a claim(s) is work-related. A WC questionnaire should be sent out in such situations to determine whether or not the claim is work-related. Because the resolution of a WC case usually takes 1 to 2 years, private plans are obligated to pay the benefits for which the member is entitled and then file a lien with the member and the WC board to recover their losses when the case is settled.

After the WC carrier has accepted liability for the claim(s), the plan will discontinue providing benefits for medical care. At that point, the claim would be denied on the basis that it is work-related.

Employee Activities

This section contains some general guidelines as to what constitutes an injury or illness recognized by a WC Board in most states based on the type of activity, not injury.

Company Activities

Company activities can be defined as the following:

- Injury sustained while attending an activity sponsored by an employer for the purpose of obtaining some business gain (eg, company party for morale purposes; sporting activity for which the employee is provided transportation or the company gains advertisement by virtue of having the employee wear a company "athletic shirt").
- Injury sustained by an employee for which the company provides remuneration.
- Injury sustained while in the course of the employee's occupation.

Use of Company Vehicles

Most WC laws provide coverage for an injury sustained while an employee is driving a company vehicle that is provided with authorization in the course of his or her occupation or is provided as a part of the employee's benefits to use to and from work.

In addition, any person who is an authorized passenger in a company vehicle while in the course of company business is normally covered by the WC law if he or she sustained any injury while in the car.

The law's interpretation of "in the course of employment" is very different from the interpretation of most laymen. For instance, someone injured while eating lunch at a company-sponsored event may be considered covered by WC. Therefore, always do investigations and let the WC Board handle the final determination.

Business Trips

Most WC laws provide 24-hour coverage for a person who is on a business trip. This coverage is applicable to the entire trip, as long as the person is performing routine activities. Of course, there are always exceptions to this rule.

Company Parking Lot

Most WC laws provide that if an employee is injured on a parking lot that is owned or maintained by his or her employer and furnished to the employee free of charge, that employee may be covered under WC. In addition, coverage would extend, in some instances, to an injury sustained by the employee while on neutral ground between the parking lot and the place of employment. An exception would be if such incidents were specifically excluded in the WC law or if the injuries were sustained from willful or negligent actions on the part of the employee.

Usually, WC is not liable for injuries sustained on a parking lot that is owned by the employer and for which a rental fee is charged for a parking space. In such instances, the employee has a free choice to park elsewhere, which would relieve the employer of any and all responsibility.

Occupational Disease

Most of the time, coverage extends to employees who contract a disease that develops from working within a certain industry. For instance, most states provide compensation for persons who have worked with asbestos material over a period of years and then develop asbestosis or silicosis. Likewise, persons can develop dermatitis from working with certain chemicals, such as in the exterminating industry.

Sometimes, a claimant may have an occupational illness that is submitted to the WC Board, and a concurrent nonoccupational illness for which he or she may be reimbursed under the plan.

In such instances, a separate billing should be completed by the provider of service, indicating those charges that were solely for the treatment of the nonoccupational disability.

Types of Claims

There are three types of Workers' Compensation claims: nondisability claims, temporary disability claims, and permanent disability claims.

Nondisability claims are for minor injuries that will not require the patient to be kept from his or her job. The patient is able to continue working throughout the extent of the injury. On the patient's first visit to the physician, the physician should complete a "Doctor's First Report" of occupational injury or illness (Figure 5-1 shows the form used in California). This form and a copy of the bill should be submitted to the WC carrier.

Temporary disability claims are made when the patient is not able to perform the job requirements until he or she recovers from the injury involved. When a physician sees a patient in this situation, a First Report is submitted and ongoing reports are issued every 2 to 3 weeks until the patient is discharged to return to work.

Permanent disability usually commences after temporary disability when it is determined that the patient will not be able to return to work. The physician prepares a discharge report stating that the patient is "permanent and stationary." This means that nothing more can be done and that the patient will have the disability for the rest of his life. The case will be reviewed by the WC Board and, if the disability is determined to be permanent, a compromise and release are issued. This is a settlement from the insurance company for a lump sum of money to the injured party.

Liens

In permanent disability, a compromise and release are issued by the insurance carrier for the injuries to the patient. If the physician has been seeing the patient since the disability commenced, a lien should be filed for payment of services rendered. A lien is a legal document that expresses claim on the property of another for payment of a debt (see Figure 5-2). A lien is completed and submitted to the attorney representing the injured party to be paid upon monetary settlement of the WC claim.

A lien will be sent along with the initial visit. Whenever additional services are rendered, a copy of the bill should be submitted to the attorney so that all concurrent care will be included in the lien. All services must be for the care of the injury to be covered under the WC claim. (A sample copy of a lien letter is shown in Figure 5-3.)

Coordination of Benefits

Coordination of benefits (COB) is a process that occurs when two or more group plans provide coverage on the same person (see definition in next section). Coordination between the two plans is necessary to allow for payment of 100% of the allowable expenses but no more.

This process was developed in response to a growing problem of overinsurance. Overinsurance occurs

DOCTOR'S FIRST REPORT OF OCCUPATIONAL INJURY OR ILLNESS

STATE OF CALIFORNIA
AGRICULTURE AND SERVICES AGENCY
DEPARTMENT OF INDUSTRIAL RELATIONS
DIVISION OF LABOR STATISTICS AND RESEARCH

Immediately after first examination mail one copy **directly** to the Division of Labor Statistics and Research. Failure to file a report with the Division is a misdemeanor. (Labor Code Section 6413.5) Answer all questions fully.

A. INSURANCE CARRIER ....

Do not write in this space

1. EMPLOYER ....
2. Address (No., St. & City) ....
3. Business (Manufacturing shoes, building construction, retailing men's clothes, etc.) ....

4. EMPLOYEE (First name, middle initial, last name) .... Soc. Sec. No. ....
5. Address (No., St. & City) ....
6. Occupation .... Age .... Sex ....
7. Date injured .... Hour .... M. Date last worked ....
8. Injured at (No., St. & City) .... County ....
9. Date of your first examination .... Hour .... M. Who engaged your services? ....
10. Name other doctors who treated employee for this injury ....

11. ACCIDENT OR EXPOSURE: Did employee notify employer of this injury? .... Employee's statement of cause of injury or illness:

12. NATURE AND EXTENT OF INJURY OR DISEASE (Include all objective findings, subjective complaints, and diagnoses. If occupational disease state date of onset, occupational history, and exposures.)

13. X-rays: By whom taken? (State if none) ....
Findings:

14. Treatment:

15. Kind of case (Office, home or hospital) .... If hospitalized, date .... Estimated stay ....
Name and address of hospital ....
16. Further treatment (Estimated frequency and duration) ....
17. Estimated period of disability for: Regular work .... Modified work ....
18. Describe any permanent disability or disfigurement expected (State if none) ....
19. If death ensued, give date
20. REMARKS (Note any pre-existing injuries or diseases, need for special examination or laboratory tests, other pertinent information.)

Name .... (Type or print) Degree .... PERSONAL SIGNATURE OF DOCTOR ....

Date of report .... Address (No., St. & City) ....

Form 114

D OSP

Figure 5-1: Example of a Doctor's First Report

Workers' Compensation Appeals Board

STATE OF CALIFORNIA

Case No.__________________

NOTICE AND REQUEST FOR ALLOWANCE OF LIEN

LIEN CLAIMANT — ADDRESS

vs.

EMPLOYEE — ADDRESS

EMPLOYER — ADDRESS

INSURANCE CARRIER — ADDRESS

The undersigned hereby requests the Workers' Compensation Appeals Board to determine and allow as a lien the sum of ____________________ dollars ($ ________) against any amount now due or which may hereafter become payable as compensation to ________________ (EMPLOYEE) on account of injury sustained by him on __________ (DATE).

This request and claim for lien is for: (Mark appropriate box)

- ❑ The reasonable expense incurred by or on behalf of said employee for medical treatment to cure or relieve from the effects of said injury; or
- ❑ The reasonable medical expense incurred to prove a contested claim; or
- ❑ The reasonable value of living expenses of said employee or of his dependents, subsequent to the injury, or
- ❑ The reasonable living expenses of the wife or minor children, or both, of said employee, subsequent to the date of injury, where such employee has deserted or is neglecting his family; or
- ❑ The reasonable fee for interpreter's services performed on ________________ (DATE).
- ❑
- ❑

NOTE: ITEMIZED STATEMENTS MUST BE ATTACHED

The undersigned declares that he delivered or mailed a copy of this lien claim to each of the above-named parties on

ATTORNEY FOR LIEN CLAIMANT — DATE

ADDRESS OF ATTORNEY FOR LIEN CLAIMANT — LIEN CLAIMANT

EMPLOYEE'S CONSENT TO ALLOWANCE OF LIEN

I consent to the requested allowance of a lien against my compensation.

ATTORNEY FOR EMPLOYEE — EMPLOYEE

DEPARTMENT OF INDUSTRIAL RELATIONS
DIVISION OF INDUSTRIAL ACCIDENTS

Figure 5-2: Example of a Lien

TO: Attorney ______________________________

____

______________________________, California

RE: Medical Reports and Doctor's Lien

FOR ______________________________

I do hereby authorize the above doctor to furnish you, my attorney, with a full report of his or her examination, diagnosis, treatment, prognosis, etc, of myself in regard to the accident in which I was involved.

I hereby authorize and direct you, my attorney, to pay directly to said doctor such sums as may be due and owing him or her for medical service rendered me both by reason of this accident and by reason of any other bills that are due his or her office and to withhold such sums from any settlement, judgment or verdict as may be necessary to adequately protect said doctor. And I hereby further give a lien on my case to said doctor against any and all proceeds of any settlement, judgment or verdict that may be paid to you, my attorney, or myself as the result of the injuries for which I have been treated or injuries in connection therewith.

I fully understand that I am directly and fully responsible to said doctor for all medical bills submitted by him or her for service rendered and that this agreement is made solely for said doctor's additional protection and in consideration of his or her awaiting payment. And I further understand that such payment is not contingent on any settlement, judgment or verdict by which I may eventually recover said fee.

Dated: ______________________________ Patient's Signature: ______________________________

The undersigned being attorney of record for the above patient does hereby agree to observe all the terms of the above and agrees to withhold such sums from any settlement, judgment, or verdict as may be necessary to adequately protect said doctor named above.

Dated: ______________________________ Attorney's Signature: ______________________________

Attorney: Please sign, date, and return one copy to doctor's office at once.

Keep one copy for your records.

Figure 5-3: **Example of a Lien Letter**

when a person is covered under two or more policies and is eligible to collect an accumulation of benefits that will actually exceed the amount charged by the provider. The purpose of COB is to allow coverage and usually payment of 100% of allowable expenses without allowing the covered member(s) to "make" money over and above the total costs for care.

In response to the diversity of handling procedures used by various carriers and administrators in coordinating coverages, the National Association of Insurance Commissioners (NAIC) developed a standardized model for COB administration. The majority of benefit plans follow this model, but it is not mandatory.

Definitions

The following definitions are used when dealing with coordination of benefits.

Allowable Expense—Any necessary, reasonable, and customary item of medical or dental expense, at least partly covered under at least one of the plans covering the patient. Items excluded by the secondary plan, such as dental services and vision care services, would not be considered allowable. Conversely, amounts limited under the secondary plan would be considered allowable (the entire charge). For example:

- Each plan provides a limit of $35.00 per visit for outpatient psychiatric care. The psychiatrist charges $50.00 per visit. As long as the $50.00 is within the UCR guidelines of one of the two plans, the entire $50.00 would be considered an allowable expense under COB.
- Based on the primary plan's UCR guidelines, the amount allowed for a surgery is $1200. The secondary plan's UCR for the same surgery is $1000. When coordinating, the secondary plan would allow the greatest amount allowed by at least one of the plans. Therefore, the allowable amount when coordinating would be $1200.

Claim Determination Period—Usually means a calendar year. It does not include any part of a year before the effective date of duplicate coverage under the secondary plan. It does include any remaining amount during a calendar year occurring after the termination date of the primary plan. As long as the secondary plan is not terminated, COB continues to be performed even though there are no longer multiple coverages.

EOB—Explanation of Benefits is a letter from a payor indicating how a member's benefits have been applied in response to the submission of a claim for services. The EOB indicate deductibles, coinsurance amounts, nonallowed amounts, UCR limitations, and so on. An EOB is required by law to be generated on each claim submission showing the disposition of the claim (how it was paid, denied, pended for additional information).

Group Plan—A form of coverage with which coordination of benefits is allowed. A plan may include:

- Group, blanket, or franchise insurance policy or plan if not individually underwritten
- Health maintenance organization or hospital or medical service prepayment policy available through an employer, union, or association
- Trusteed policy or plan, union welfare policy or plan, multiple employer policy or plan, or employee benefit policy or plan
- Governmental programs (Medicare) or policies or plans required by a statute, except Medicaid
- "No fault" auto policy or plan. (Applies to some plans only. The plan must specify whether or not this is applicable.)

Primary Plan—Benefit plan that determines and pays its benefits first without regard to the existence of any other coverage.

Secondary Plan—Plan that pays after the primary plan has paid its benefits. The benefits of the secondary plan take into consideration the benefits of the primary plan and may reduce its payment so that only 100% of allowable expenses are paid.

Order of Benefit Determination

Before standardized coordination rules were adopted by the benefits industry, a person covered under two policies could collect full benefits from both. Thus, the individual would actually make a profit by being sick.

Since each plan would prefer to pay as the secondary payor, it became necessary to develop rules to determine when a plan should pay as primary, secondary, and so on.

The 13 rules determining the order of payment are referred to as the Order of Benefit Determinations (OBD):

1. The plan without a COB provision will be primary to a plan with a COB provision.
2. The plan that does not have these OBD rules and, as a result, the plans do not agree on the OBD, will determine the order of payment.
3. The plan that covers a person as an employee will be primary to a plan that covers that person as a dependent.
4. If the person is an employee under two plans, the primary plan is defined as the one that has been in effect the longest.
5. If an employee is an active employee under one plan and a retiree (or laid off) under another, the active plan will pay as primary.

   The parent birthday rule, explained in rules 6 and 7, affects the OBD for dependent children of parents who are living together and married (not divorced or legally separated).
6. The plan of the parent whose birthday (based on month and day only) occurs first in the calendar year is the primary plan.
7. When both parents' birthdays are the same (based on month and day), the benefits of the plan that covered one parent the longest is the primary plan.

   For dependents of legally separated or divorced parents and those whose parents have remarried, the order of benefits determination will be based on the following rules:
8. If there is a court-approved divorce decree, the plan of the parent specified as having legal responsibility for the health care expense of the child is the primary plan.

If there is no court decree:

9. The plan of the parent with custody is prime.
10. The plan of the step-parent with whom the child resides is secondary.
11. The plan of the natural parent without custody is tertiary.
12. The step-parent (if any) who does not reside with the child has no legal right to declare dependency of the child and, therefore, no coordination should be performed, since the child is (probably) not an eligible dependent under the plan.
13. For joint custody, with no additional responsibility designation, the plan of the parent whose coverage has been in effect the longest would be the primary payor.

Right of Recovery

If the amount of the payments made by the plan is more than should have been paid under the COB provision, the plan may recover the excess from one or more of the following:

- The persons it has paid or the person(s) it has paid on behalf of
- Other insurers/plans
- Other organizations

The "amount of the payments made" includes the reasonable cash value of any benefits provided in the form of services.

When billing for patients who have dual coverage, determine the primary carrier to be billed first. After payment is received from the primary carrier, post the payment to the patient's ledger card to determine the balance. When billing the secondary carrier, always attach a copy of the primary carrier's explanation of benefits to the claim being submitted. The secondary carrier will not process the claim without this information. Upon receipt of the secondary carrier's payment, post the payment to the patient's ledger card. Any balance remaining after all adjustments should be billed to the patient.

COB with Health Maintenance Organizations

A health maintenance organization (HMO) is a type of prepayment plan in which providers agree to charge members for their services in accordance with a fixed schedule of rates. The HMO member (insured) may pay a specified copayment at the time the service is rendered or may not be required to pay anything. The patient and the doctor are never involved in having to complete claim forms for submission to a payor. Instead, the HMO is billed directly or the HMO pays a monthly retainer fee to the physician for membership plus other specified fees.

If the required medical services are available through the HMO but the insured does not go to an HMO provider for the treatment, he or she may be held entirely responsible for all of the expenses.

Prepayment plans are included in the definition of the type of policies to which COB provisions apply. However, many HMOs do not have COB provisions, although more are now starting to incorporate this concept since the spiraling costs of medical care are affecting them, also.

An example of an HMO is Kaiser Permanente. Kaiser provides a prepayment policy for hospital and professional medical services at no cost or at a small fee, as long as the member goes to a Kaiser facility. Subsequently, they provide the member with a "reasonable cost statement," which represents what would have been charged to a nonmember. If the HMO does not have a COB provision, they would be considered the primary payor. To coordinate benefits, a request must be made for receipts or statements showing the actual out-of-pocket expense. The secondary plan would pay no more than the amount that would be considered the allowable expense. If the HMO does have a COB provision, the regular OBD determination rules should be applied.

Civilian Health and Medical Programs of the Uniformed Services

The Civilian Health and Medical Programs of the Uniformed Services, also known as CHAMPUS, provides a comprehensive program of health care benefits for active-duty and retired services personnel, their dependents, and the dependents of deceased military personnel. Persons eligible for CHAMPUS will be enrolled in the Defense Enrollment Eligibility Reporting System (DEERS). This is a computer data base used to verify CHAMPUS eligibility.

CHAMPUS is secondary to all other insurance or health policies except Medicaid and CHAMPUS supplemental insurance. However, because many services are provided free of charge or at a minimal fee at veterans' administrative clinics and facilities, many medical billers will never have to bill CHAMPUS.

Uniformed Services Identification and Privilege cards are assigned to all dependents of CHAMPUS beneficiaries 10 years of age and older. Dependents under age 10 are covered under the parent's card.

CHAMPUS claims can be submitted on a HCFA-1500. Copy the Uniformed Services Identification and Privilege card to obtain the needed information for billing. Complete the HCFA-1500 and submit to the fiscal intermediary for the state. Claims for CHAMPUS must be submitted no later than the last day of the calendar year following the year in which the services were rendered.

Summary

Three types of billing require special handling: Workers' Compensation, CHAMPUS, and Coordination of Benefits. It is important for the medical biller to understand the basic benefits provided by Workers' Compensation and CHAMPUS and to know how to coordinate benefits when there is more than one payor who may cover payment for a patient. This will allow the provider to recover the maximum amount possible from the various payors, leaving less of a balance for the patient to pay or for the physician to write off.

Assignments

Complete the Questions for Review.

Questions for Review

Directions: Answer the following questions without looking back into the material just covered. Write your answers in the space provided.

1. What does COB stand for? ______________________________
2. What is the purpose of COB? ______________________________
____
3. The ____________________ is the benefit plan that determines and pays its benefits first without regard to the existence of any other coverage.
4. The ____________________ is the plan that pays after the primary plan has paid its benefits.
5. What does CHAMPUS stand for? ______________________________
____
6. What is Workers' Compensation? ______________________________
____
____
7. What is a lien? ______________________________
8. Define temporary disability? ______________________________
9. Define permanent disability? ______________________________
10. Which form is used to bill CHAMPUS services? ______________________________

If you were unable to answer any of the questions, refer back to the section and then fill in the answers.

Exercise 5-1

Directions: Assume that all of the adults in the following questions have active coverage. For each example, indicate which party would be primary, secondary, tertiary, etc., by writing 1, 2, 3, etc., in the blank space next to the person. If the person is not responsible for the dependent(s) at all, indicate NA.

1. A remarried mother has custody of her children six months of the year. Her coverage was effective 6/1/89 and her date of birth (DOB) is 10/15/49. The natural father's coverage was effective 5/1/90 and his date of birth is 8/10/50. The mother's husband's coverage was effective 5/1/79 and his date of birth is 9/1/46. The father's wife's coverage was effective 6/15/89 and her date of birth is 7/4/53.

_______ Mother _______ Father _______ Stepmother _______ Stepfather

2. A remarried mother has custody of her children. However, by court decree, the father has financial responsibility for their health care costs. The mother's DOB is 4/1/53 and her coverage was effective 2/15/90. The father's DOB is 3/15/50 and his coverage was effective 3/1/87. The stepfather's DOB is 12/15/50 and his coverage was effective 3/1/86. The stepmother's DOB is 8/17/54 and her coverage was effective 6/1/89.

_______ Mother _______ Father _______ Stepmother _______ Stepfather

3. Two natural parents are married. The mother's date of birth is 7/1/52. The father's date of birth is 7/1/51. The mother's effective date of coverage is 6/1/88. The father's effective date of coverage is 6/1/89.

_______ Mother _______ Father

4. Two natural parents are married. The mother's date of birth is 7/1/52. The father's date of birth is 7/1/51. The mother's effective date of coverage is 6/1/88. The father's effective date of coverage is 6/1/89. The mother's plan has no COB provision.

_______ Mother _______ Father

5. Two natural parents are divorced and neither has remarried. By court decree, the grandparents have legal custody of the children. Also by decree, the father has financial responsibility for their medical care. The mother's DOB is 4/1/53 and her coverage was effective 2/15/90. The father's DOB is 3/15/50 and his coverage was effective 3/1/87. The grandmother's DOB is 12/15/27 and her coverage was effective 3/15/76. The grandfather's DOB is 8/17/22 and his coverage was effective 6/1/79.

_______ Mother _______ Father _______ Grandmother _______ Grandfather

6

General Office Procedures

In this chapter you will learn:

- To understand basic office procedures.
- To understand the proper use and operation of basic office equipment.

A number of basic procedures need to be followed to help an office run smoothly and to facilitate the organized management of services. Without organization, precious time is lost searching for information or other items. In addition, an unorganized office creates difficulty for clients. An unorganized office and unskilled personnel add to the stress level of the client, which requires that person to wait longer to receive services. The client will worry that your lack of concern for the office is also reflective of a lack of concern for the client.

Mail

Mail can be separated into two types: incoming mail and outgoing mail. Each type has its own set of procedures.

Incoming Mail

In any office, it is imperative that the mail be handled properly and routed to the correct person. Generally, one person is designated to handle the incoming mail. Most offices prefer to have the mail sorted according to the department or person to whom it is addressed. Of course, every office has its own preferences, so check with your supervisor to see what handling procedures have been established for the company where you are employed. The following are eight general guidelines:

1. Separate the mail according to the department or person to whom it is addressed. While separating, take note of any mail that was delivered incorrectly to your address. Separating the mail before opening allows you to return incorrectly delivered mail in the same condition in which it arrived.
2. If your company or organization prefers to have the mail opened before it is distributed, you should slit the envelope neatly across the top or down one side. Do not tear or otherwise destroy the envelope. In this way you can best preserve any needed information that the envelope contains. This information may include the date of postmark, a return address, or the city from which the envelope was mailed.

   Some companies and organizations prefer to have the envelope saved with its enclosed correspondence. Either way, the pieces of correspondence that are to be distributed should have the pages of each piece of correspondence paper-clipped together. This allows the recipient to easily see all pieces of paper that were included in a single correspondence.
3. Prior to discarding the envelope, double check that everything has been removed from the envelope. Often small items such as a business card become detached and slide to the bottom of the envelope.
4. Many companies date-stamp their mail upon receipt. If this is the procedure of your company or organization, there are seven steps that you should follow.

   a. First, change the date on the stamper to the correct date. This date can be very important when certain pieces of correspondence need to arrive in a timely manner. The correct date is especially important for the billing department when interest or late fees are charged on overdue accounts.

   b. Next, stamp the date stamper on a piece of scratch paper to ensure that it has enough ink and that the impression is coming out clearly. (Stamping on a sheet of scratch paper allows you to check that you moved the dates or other numbers into the correct position.) If the impression is faint, stamp the ink pad several more times (if it is used) or stamp the date stamper on a piece of paper (if the stamp is self-inking). This will start the ink flowing again. If the impression is still too light, add ink or get a new ink pad.

   c. When you stamp a piece of correspondence, place the date in an area where the impression will not cover any of the writing. This is important so that there will be no question about the date the correspondence was received or the information that is on the document.

   d. Stamp down once, firmly and securely. Do not

hold the stamp down and wiggle it back and forth as this causes an unclear impression.

e. Many companies prefer to have only the first page date-stamped, whereas other companies like each piece stamped individually. Stamping each page individually allows the recipient to know when the correspondence was received even if the pages become separated.

f. Do not stamp checks, business cards, legal documents, or order forms unless your company or organization specifically requests you to do so. Date stamping such items can result in difficulty in processing a check, in ordering, or in complying with legal requirements.

g. If you have a choice of ink colors, black is best. Other colors are more difficult to photocopy or may cause a negative impression. This is especially true of red, since most people associate red ink with a warning. If a piece of correspondence is date-stamped in red, it gives the subtle impression that the correspondence arrived later than it was expected.

5. If you receive checks in the mail, securely attach them to any additional papers (eg, invoices, statements) that are included. Often these additional papers are the only clue to finding out to which account the check should be credited. Many companies prefer that the person who opens the mail immediately write the account number on the check. This ensures that the check will be credited to the proper account even if it is separated from its attached documentation.

   If no documentation is attached, check the envelope for additional clues. If the name and address on the check do not match the name and address on the envelope, attach the envelope to the check. This may assist the billing department in locating the correct account number.

   In most companies, the person who first opens the checks is requested to make an adding machine tape and provide a total of the day's receipts. Always run the tape twice, ensuring that you get the same amount both times. Then, take an extra minute to double check your figures. Often numbers become transposed, and once a number is in your mind, it is easy for the transposition to occur a second time.

6. When distributing the mail, put urgent-looking correspondence on the top of the stack. Also, put the mail in a place where the recipient is sure to see it, not where it will be buried. Likewise, don't set it on the extreme edge of a desk or shelf, because it may fall off and become scattered.
7. For correspondence marked "Personal and Confidential," leave the envelope sealed and deliver it to the intended recipient unopened.
8. If you receive any document in a "next day" or "urgent" mail envelope, deliver it immediately. This type of document should never sit on your desk for more than 5 minutes.

Although handling mail may seem like a minor task, it is important to do it properly and efficiently. Mail is the lifeblood of many companies. Without it, checks and revenues are lost, clients are not served, and communication breaks down.

Signing for Mail

Some incoming mail requires a signature upon delivery. Before signing, know exactly what you are signing for. Most shipping companies include a notation in fine print stating that your signature is verification that the package was received in good condition and that the contents were not damaged. Also, note the number of packages you are signing for. Your signature across four lines of the receipt column states that you received four packages. Be sure that the order is complete before signing for it; otherwise you or your company may be held liable for any unreceived merchandise or shipments.

It is impossible to tell whether the contents of a package are undamaged without opening the box. Take the time to look at the boxes before signing. If any damage is indicated on the box, insist on opening it and checking the contents before signing. The delivery person will attempt to have you sign immediately so that he or she can get on to the next delivery, but if you do sign, the damaged goods may not be replaced or paid for by the shipper.

If the contents of the package appear to be damaged, note this on the receipt next to your signature.

Be sure you are authorized to sign for a package. In many companies, the right to sign for packages is limited to a few people, not to any employee in the office.

Returned Mailings

In any company, there will be mail returned due to improper addressing, lack of postage, or the inability of the Postal Service to locate the intended recipient.

If a piece of mail is returned for lack of postage, place a postage tape with the correct postage amount over any writing in the upper right-hand corner. If postage tape is not available, place the mail in a new envelope and post it.

Mail will be forwarded for only 1 year from the date of the recipient's move. After that time, a sticker will be placed on the envelope indicating the new address, and the article will be returned to the sender. If a piece of mail was returned because a forwarding address had expired and the Postal Service has indicated the new address, the mail should be placed in a new envelope, addressed with the new address and remailed. Keep the old envelope so that you can update your records.

If a piece of mail is returned with no forwarding address indicated, delete the name and address from your records. If there is an outstanding balance on an account that has had mail returned, be sure that the patient's records are also updated. If an outstanding balance or a current patient history does not exist, do not delete the record. Take the time to contact the patient by phone and attempt to locate his or her new address.

Outgoing Mail

The condition of your outgoing mail is a direct reflection on you and your company. Therefore, it is imperative that your mail be handled properly. You can imagine the response of a client who receives a letter bearing bad news, which has also been stamped by the Postal Service "Postage Due."

The first thing is to make sure that the mail has been packaged properly. Be sure the envelope is of adequate size for the material. If there are more than five pages in a document, a #10 (standard sized) envelope should not be used. The thickness of the pages can cause the envelope to become jammed in the Postal Service's automated equipment. This results in tearing and loss of the contents. To ensure that envelopes mailed in larger packages arrive in good condition, place a thin sheet of cardboard in the envelope to add resilience.

When packing boxes, use boxes in good condition and do not overload them. Boxes should never bulge out at the sides. Before sealing the box, place a letter or other item inside, that lists the company's and the recipient's address. This will allow the package to be delivered even if the address shown on the outside tears off or becomes obliterated.

Boxes should be sealed with strong packing tape—not string—and there should never be any kind of paper wrapping on the outside of the box.

Your company's address (the return address) should be clearly placed in the upper left-hand corner of the package or letter. The recipient's address should be placed in the center of the document. Stamps, meter stamps, or postage tapes should be placed in the upper right-hand corner of the package.

All shipping companies, including the US Postal Service, have weight and size limits for the packages they ship. Most have a weight limit of 70 pounds per box. The combined length and girth should not exceed 108 inches. To determine the measurement, wrap a tape measure once around the box, then add to the resulting measurement the length of the box. Before shipping, contact the carrier and be sure that you know the exact weight and measurement limits that they allow.

Special Shipping Services

Most companies offer numerous shipping services. These include certification (proof of delivery), return receipt requested, COD (payment upon receipt), insurance, overnight delivery, and 2- or 3-day delivery and courier services. Additional charges, above and beyond the normal shipping charges, are added for each of these services. Keep any receipts issued to you by the shipper. Without these documents, it is impossible to trace lost articles or to make a claim for services not delivered.

Certified mail is a package or envelope that must be signed for upon delivery. This provides you with a record of when the item was delivered and the name of the person who signed for it. To send an envelope by certified mail, fill out the certified mail slip provided by the shipping company. The basic information requested is the name and address of the recipient. This tag is attached to the envelope or package to the right of the return address. The tag has a tracking number printed on it. The top portion of the tag is torn off at the perforation and kept as a receipt. If the envelope or package does not arrive, a tracer can be put on it by using this number.

With return receipt requested, upon delivery, a receipt is issued and mailed back to the sender of the package. This allows the sender to have proof of the delivery and the name of the person who signed for it. This procedure is usually used with certified mail. The recipient's name and address are placed on one side of the card. The sender's name and address are placed on the reverse of the card. The card is then attached to the envelope or package on the front, or, if there is not sufficient room, on the back. When the article is delivered, the recipient signs the card and the date of delivery is listed. If requested (and an additional fee is paid), the recipient's address will be provided. The sender may also choose to restrict delivery only to the person or persons to whom the article is addressed.

When mailing a shipment of merchandise that the recipient must pay for, COD is often requested. This means that the shipper will collect payment for the item at the time of delivery. When shipping COD, you must specify whether cash, check or either is acceptable and the amount to be collected. Add any shipping charges to the amount if the recipient is to pay for shipping.

You may wish to purchase insurance for the items being shipped. This insurance will pay for lost or damaged items. With many shippers, the first $100 of insurance is included in the cost of shipping a package. Any amount over this must be requested and paid for prior to shipping. The fee is usually nominal, between $.50 and $.75 for every $100 of insurance.

If you need an envelope or package to arrive overnight, it is possible to request this service. Articles can be scheduled for either an afternoon delivery or, for an additional charge, a morning delivery. The delivery area is limited, usually to within the continental United States. In addition, articles must be picked up or delivered to the shipper prior to a specified time to qualify for next-day delivery. This time varies according to your location and the shipper. You must also complete special address labels that request the sender's and receiver's name, address, and phone number, as well as the specific services requested. Many carriers require you to use special packaging and generally provide this packaging free of charge upon request.

Like overnight delivery, there is a special charge for 2- or 3-day delivery, and it is usually limited to the continental United States. There are also similar labels and packaging requirements. Check with your shipper for specifics.

In large cities, it is possible to have an envelope or letter delivered by courier or messenger. The courier service comes to your office, picks up the article, and hand delivers it to the recipient. These services are generally expensive and are used only for important documents.

Ordering Supplies

Every office needs a certain amount of supplies to run efficiently and smoothly. These supplies may include minor items like paper and pens, or major purchases such as office equipment and machinery.

Often the medical biller is required to order supplies, if not for the company, then at least for his or her own use. Therefore, it is important to know basic ordering guidelines. Although many companies have their own procedures, the following are 11 general guidelines to follow:

1. Know what you need before you need it. It doesn't help to order supplies 2 days after you have already run out of things. This means going

through your desk and any supply cupboards and looking to see what is needed. If you are running low on something, put it on the order list. It is far better to have a little extra than to run completely out of something. However, do not order more than you can use in 3 or 4 months. Having money tied up in supplies decreases the amount available to the company for other operating costs or emergencies.

2. Order everything at once. Numerous small orders are much more difficult to handle and keep track of than one large order. Also, many supply companies offer volume discounts or free delivery or gifts if your order exceeds a certain amount. Be aware of what these levels are. For example, you could save your company money if you were to order $5.00 more in supplies rather than pay a $20.00 shipping charge.
3. Know the company from which you order office supplies. Many companies have dealt exclusively with one office supplier for years. The company has established a rapport with the supplier and will purchase only that supplier's products, regardless of whether another company offers the same supplies at a lower rate. At times an alternative relationship is set up where you support the supplier's business and they support yours. At other times it is merely a matter of personal loyalty to a supplier that has treated your company well in the past. Regardless of the reason, it is best to purchase all supplies from the supplier your company has chosen.
4. Be sure you know the payment procedures before ordering. Some companies bill you and allow payment within 30 days. Others demand payment upon receipt. You don't want to have to unexpectedly come up with a check when no one is around to sign it and the supplies were sent COD.
5. Fill out the order form completely and accurately. Print or type the information requested, using black ink. Double check all figures and all order numbers. Proofread the form before sending it out. You don't want to end up with 200 of the wrong item and go through the hassle of sending it back and trying to get the right item.
6. Before sending in an order, make a copy of it for your records. This allows you to check your order against the items you receive when the order arrives.
7. If you are ordering by phone, write out the order before you place the call. This helps to keep everything accurate and helps the ordering process to run smoothly. It also gives you a permanent record of what you did order so that you can compare it to the packing slip and the invoice when they arrive.
8. Check the shipment and the packing slip as soon as an order comes in. Make sure that everything is either in the box or is listed on the packing slip as a back-ordered item. If an error occurs in the shipment, first double check your order form. Was the mistake your fault or the supplier's? Then, call the office supplier immediately. If the error was your fault, admit it and resolve the problem. Most suppliers have no problem with exchanging an item. If the fault was theirs, be understanding. Mistakes occur and no one is perfect. If you receive supplies that you did not order, do not open them. Once an item has been opened, many suppliers will not accept a return on it.
9. If the entire shipment is received correctly, make a brief note to that effect on the packing slip and initial it. Then, put the supplies in their appropriate place.
10. Often the invoice arrives at a later time than the order. When the invoice arrives, check it against the packing slip and the original order. If there are any discrepancies, contact the company immediately. If not, turn it over to the person who pays the bills.
11. Finally, if you are aware that finances are a consideration for your company and that a different company offers supplies of the same quality at a lower price, do your homework first. Order catalogs from both companies and compare the costs on the items that you purchase the most. Read

the fine print and compare items of the same quality. Also, consider payment options and credit interest rates. If the savings is substantial enough that your company might change, talk to a supervisor and show him or her the differences. It is your supervisor's job to approach the company leaders with a possible change.

Office Machines

In every office, you will use a number of machines nearly every day. These include the telephone, fax machine, computer, calculator, and copy machine. The use of the computer and the calculator are covered in Chapters 8 and 10.

The Telephone

Virtually every company in existence has a telephone and uses it extensively during the working day. The telephone is often more important than the mail in communicating with customers and helping with the running of the office. Therefore, it is important that you understand how to properly use the telephone.

Most companies have multi-line phones. This means that there is more than one telephone line into the office. However, the number of these phone lines is limited. If all of the lines are being used, the customer or caller will hear a busy signal and the call will not be connected. For this reason you should keep your calls as brief as possible.

Multi-line phones often work the same as do single-line phones, with a few exceptions. Most multi-line phones have a single number (ie, 555-1234) with each additional line numerically increased by one (ie, line two is 555-1235; line three is 555-1236). The caller needs only to dial the original number (555-1234) and, if that line is busy, the call will automatically roll over to the first available line.

When placing an outgoing call on a multi-line phone, many times you will need to choose a line by pushing a button. Prior to picking up a line, make sure that it is available. Usually, a small lighted button indicates whether the line is currently in use.

Multi-line phones often give you the option of placing callers on hold by depressing a hold button. When transferring a call, speaking with a co-worker, or interrupting a conversation for any reason, it is best to put the caller on hold rather than to hold your hand over the mouthpiece or set the phone down.

Different types of phones and phone systems have different ways of transferring calls and returning to a held call. These procedures will need to be described to you by someone who is familiar with the phone or system. It is important to know these procedures prior to needing them so that you don't delay or disconnect a caller.

For further information regarding phone etiquette, please see Chapter 7.

The Facsimile Machine

The facsimile machine (more commonly referred to as the fax machine) is a machine that transmits pictures over the phone lines by transmitting a series of dot messages. This allows for nearly instantaneous transmission of a letter, picture, or other document from one place to another, even when the participants are halfway around the world from each other.

The invention of the fax machine has made life easier in offices and has taken some of the stress out of having to mail documents early so that they can be received on time. Although the fax machine is a wonderful invention, it is not perfect. Documents can be lost in transmission and they are generally not as clear as printed material. The special paper used in many fax machines is thinner than normal paper and also bruises or leaves an imprint if it is pressed on. For these reasons, it is important that you always follow up a fax with a hard copy of the document sent through the mail.

The ease of transmitting using the fax machine has often led to using it for nonessential situations. Always remember that a fax transmission is not as clear, and therefore not as professional looking as something that is directly from a typewriter or printer. Also, remember that when transmitting long distances, you are using a phone line. Therefore, a charge will appear on the telephone bill the same as if you had spoken over the phone.

If the company you are faxing to has several different departments, it will be difficult to direct the fax to the correct person without a fax cover sheet. There may be one fax machine used by the entire company or several fax machines throughout the company. To ensure that the information will be routed to the correct person, it is important that a cover sheet accompany the material being faxed. A cover sheet should include the following:

- The date and time the fax is being sent.
- The name and telephone number of the person sending the fax.
- The name of the person to whom the fax is directed and his/her department or company.
- The number of pages being sent.
- Sufficient space for messages to be conveyed to the receiver.

The Copy Machine

The copy machine is one of the most widely used office machines. There are always numerous reasons for needing a second copy of a document.

Copy machines can be one of the easiest machines to operate if you understand the basic principles. The first item of importance is the placement of the original. The original should be placed face down on the glass. The exact placement is usually indicated by markings running along the left-hand side of the glass or the bottom. The cover should be closed before making a copy.

To begin the copy process, push the button marked "start." Do not lift the cover or remove the original until the copying is complete. To do so will cause a blurred or darkened image on the copy.

Many copiers have special features, such as reduction or enlargement of the original, special paper sizes or types, and collation of the copies. These special features are usually selected by the push of a button.

Since copiers vary according to style and brand name, it is important that you be shown the exact features and the correct operating procedures for the copier that your company uses.

Other Office Machines

A number of other machines may be used in a medical office setting. These can include the postage meter machine, postage scale, binding machines, folding machines, coffee makers, and vending machines.

Binding machines bind several pages of a document together, often with a strip down the left-hand side of the document. There are numerous types of binding machines, and numerous brands for each type. Generally, the bindings fall into one of three categories: comb binders (have a plastic strip with projecting teeth), spiral binders (have a curved plastic strip with rounded teeth forming an enclosed circle), and spiral wire binders (have a single continuous piece of wire wound through successive holes from top to bottom of the document).

Folding machines are used to fold numerous pieces of paper. The folding guides can be adjusted to various lengths to handle different sizes of paper and different folds. Due to the strength and speed of most folding machines, care should be taken that jewelry, loose clothing, and long hair are not allowed to enter the machine.

Many offices provide free or low-cost cups of coffee to their employees. However, the responsibility often falls to one or more of the employees to keep the pots filled. All coffee machines require the addition of fresh coffee grounds, and some require the addition of water. Care should be taken to keep the pots cleaned on a regular basis. Also, never set an empty or near-empty glass pot on a heated burner. The glass will shatter.

Vending machines are available in many offices. Most are stocked and serviced by outside vending companies that are also in charge of handling the monies received. Many vending companies return a portion of the proceeds to the company that has allowed space for the machine, and the vending company should be called if the machine is allowed to run out of items or if service is needed.

Time Management

To become an efficient claims examiner, managing your time is a high priority. Most companies have production and quality standards for claims handling personnel. To maintain these standards, it is of the utmost importance to manage your time effectively.

Without time management, assigned tasks cannot be completed and things back up, causing stress in our lives.

Following are six time management guidelines:

1. Make a daily list of "Things To Do." List daily goals and set priorities to ensure that unimportant trivial tasks are not being attempted when there are items that are near their deadlines.
2. Determine what the best use of your time is right now. Are you currently working on something that is best done by someone else? If so and if you can, delegate the task to that person. Focus energies on the task at hand. Decide what you want from your time, determine how you will use it, and use it wisely.
3. Use your calendar as a follow-up system. Make notations on calendar days to indicate when follow-up calls are to be made, when follow-up letters are to be sent, and when deadlines are approaching.
4. Begin and end each day. That is, begin each day with the above "Things To Do" list, prioritizing the most important items at the top of the list and eliminating or putting trivial tasks at the bottom of the list. End your day by going over your list to determine what tasks were not accomplished. Those tasks should be put at the top of the list for the next day, unless they are trivial. Make a rule to move trivial items only a maximum of 3 days. On the third day it must be completed. By doing this, you prevent turning trivial matters into urgent tasks.
5. Organize calls. Determine which calls should be made first and at what time they should be made. Take into consideration the area of the country you are calling. If you are calling from the West Coast to the East Coast, making a call after 1:00 PM is probably a waste of time since most businesses close around 4:00 PM.
6. Organize your work area. Place frequently used items within arms' reach to eliminate time wasted looking for them.

Use of the previous guidelines helps to effectively and efficiently manage your valuable time and to reach all goals and maintain all standards set before you as a medical biller or claims examiner.

Summary

Although each office has its own procedures to follow, it is important to understand the basic procedures that govern incoming mail, outgoing mail, special shipping services, ordering supplies, and dealing with office machines.

Without basic knowledge of the equipment and how to use it, it is impossible for the health claims examiner or the medical biller to do their jobs properly.

Assignments

Complete the Questions for Review.

Questions for Review

Directions: Answer the following questions without looking back into the material just covered. Write your answers in the space provided.

1. What is the best ink color to use when date stamping incoming mail? ______
2. When signing for receipt of a package, your signature certifies that the contents were received undamaged and in good condition. (True or False) ______
3. Name five special shipping services that you can purchase.
   a. ______
   b. ______
   c. ______
   d. ______
   e. ______
4. When dialing out on a multi-line phone, what is the first thing you should check before picking up the phone?
   ______
5. What are the six guidelines of time management?
   a. ______
   b. ______
   c. ______
   d. ______
   e. ______
   f. ______

If you were unable to answer any of the questions, refer back to the section and then fill in the answers.

7

Customer Service

In this chapter you will learn:

- To understand communications in order to enhance the claims examiner's effectiveness in a customer service role.
- To build skills that will enhance your rapport with customers.
- The best ways to solve customer concerns.
- To give customers prompt, accurate and courteous responses to their inquiries.
- To enhance your professionalism and improve your customer service performance with experience.
- The six basic steps of resolving customer problems or concerns.
- Six ways to be in control of a call.
- The terms empathy, stroking and attitude.
- Ways to use the telephone more effectively.
- Knowledge of ethical behavior and the importance of professionalism in the business sector.

Customer service is one of the most vital functions any company can provide. Without it, the company soon loses customers. Without customers, the company ceases to exist.

Whenever you speak with a customer, either on the phone or in person, or write to a customer, you are performing a customer service function. Many times the claims examiner or medical biller is the only contact the client or claimant will have with the company. Therefore, to that client, you are the company. The image you convey will be what the customer believes is the company's attitude toward him or her. Accounts have been won and lost based solely on a client's experience with customer service personnel. Even a single encounter can be enough to win or lose a customer.

This chapter is designed to assist the claims examiner and medical biller in developing a more professional and positive approach to client/customer relationships.

Understanding Needs

To respond appropriately to the needs of your customers, you must be able to look beneath the surface of the behavior they exhibit to examine the factors that motivate their actions.

An individual's ability to tolerate problems, disappointments, or frustrations is influenced by the many needs he or she experiences. Those needs include such things as sleep, food, comfort, love, self-esteem, and achievement. All behavior grows out of need and is directed toward the meeting of those needs. Needs that have not been met can alter normal behavior.

When experiencing negative emotions such as pain, anxiety, frustration, discomfort, fear, guilt, concern, or worry, the customer's behavior can be difficult to deal with. What would usually be perceived as an insignificant or minor problem can be an important issue to a customer whose needs have not been met.

When dealing with customers, bear in mind that their primary concern is meeting their needs. If you assist them in doing so in a pleasant and friendly way, their opinion of you, and thus of the company, will be greatly enhanced. Likewise, if you allow their reaction to a situation to influence you in a negative manner, their opinion of the company will be a negative one.

Attitudes and Feelings

The dictionary defines attitude as "the manner of acting, feeling or thinking that shows one's disposition or opinion." Therefore, an attitude is the way you think and your view of the world. You may not always be able to choose your situation, but you can always choose your attitude about the situation. The way you think shapes what you become and how your environment is formed. To assist you in understanding your current attitude, complete the Exercises 7-1 and 7-2.

Feelings come into play whenever people interact. Like our attitudes, our feelings strongly influence our actions, if we let them. However, in customer service, the only acceptable attitude is a positive one. Therefore, it is important to ensure that only positive feelings and attitudes influence your actions.

Every time you have contact with someone, you are in effect recognizing this person. This recognition can be verbal or nonverbal (such as nodding and smiling at someone).

Recognition can be either negative or positive. When someone compliments you on the way you did something, that is positive recognition. When someone says your idea is stupid, that is negative recognition. If you imply, through your tone of voice, that your customer's question is stupid, that is negative recognition. If you provide the information in a cheerful way, that is positive recognition.

In other words, negative recognition makes us feel terrible and positive recognition makes us feel good. Both kinds of recognition influence whether or not we do things again, as well as the attitude we adopt toward that act. Consequently, if the amount of positive recognition is increased and the amount of negative recognition is decreased, future behavior is influenced positively.

The following are some examples of positive and negative recognition.

Examples of Positive Recognition

- A smile!
- Returning calls as promised.
- Direct eye contact with a person.
- Greeting those you work with daily.
- Speaking in a pleasant tone of voice.
- "Good afternoon, Mrs. Smith."
- "May I place you on hold while I check that for you?"
- "You're well organized."
- "Thank you!" (with a smile)
- "How do you feel about it?"
- "That was very thoughtful of you."
- "You're always so reliable."

Examples of Negative Recognition

- Not greeting someone you know.
- Ignoring a customer or co-worker.
- Grumbling and complaining.
- Looking grouchy.
- Sounding bored.
- Refusing to hurry.
- Not speaking to someone.
- "Stupid. Don't you ever listen?"
- "That idea is ridiculous."
- "Another area handles that type of problem."
- "Don't complain to me."
- "That's not my job."

The way someone receives recognition from others can be positive and negative, too! We are all familiar with the person who has a difficult time accepting a compliment. Instead of saying, "thank you," the response is a belittling or contradicting of the compliment. This is negative recognition. How do you respond when someone gives you recognition?

First Impressions and Image

First impressions are a vital part of creating how a customer feels about a person, company, or organization. This impression is usually formed within 4 minutes of the first meeting. Four minutes is not a long time, but it is long enough for someone to form an impression that may remain with him or her throughout the life of the relationship.

The kind of first impression a person makes on another person is often made without anyone recognizing it. Everything communicates something. For example, the first thing people use to form an impression about you is your appearance. This consists not only of your clothing and general appearance, but also of your posture, gestures, facial expressions, and the way you move.

The next largest impact is made by your vocal communication. This includes the tone of your voice, its volume and pitch, and the rate of speed at which you speak.

Last comes your verbal communication. This includes not only the words you speak, but the terminology you use and the way you speak. Because of this, it is important to use terminology that will be understood by the person to whom you are speaking and to speak distinctly and clearly.

Characteristics of Customer Relations

It is vital to keep customer relations a high priority in any business. The personnel who deal with customers and clients must possess highly disciplined personality characteristics. The following characteristics should be demonstrated in each and every customer and client interaction in order to be effective as a customer service representative:

- Thorough job knowledge
- Good telephone techniques
- Knowledge of privacy guidelines and their importance
- Positive attitude
- Ability to listen well
- Knowledge of the business and its practices (in this case medical billing and claims processing work flow)

Customer Service Job Functions

In the health claims examining and medical billing arena, a customer representative's primary functions usually include, but may not be limited to the following eight responsibilities:

1. Utilizing computerized or manual claim files to take care of inquiries from claimants, client representatives or attorneys, providers of service, other insurers or benefit plans, and federal, state or local agencies. These inquiries may include myriads of topics, including the dispensation of a claim, contractual interpretations, and benefit determinations. The claims examiner must be knowledgeable about the account(s) they handle.
2. Promoting positive client relationships through client interaction.
3. Handling written correspondence. Strong letter-writing skills are required to articulate the company's position regarding claims, benefit determinations, and company policies and handling procedures.
4. Determining benefit payment amounts, including adjusting or approving benefit payment adjustments.
5. Meeting with walk-in customers and handling their questions concerning services and costs or coverages and benefits.
6. Detecting and handling the initial investigation of potentially fraudulent claim submissions.
7. Advising supervisors of adverse trends or issues noted through contact with clients, client representatives, and others, and maintain an accurate activity log that documents these trends or issues.
8. Recording comments and reactions (both positive and negative) of customers relative to the services provided.

The Art of Listening

Listening is one of the most important skills a person can learn, especially in the customer service arena. Listening is defined as making an effort to hear. Without effort, true listening does not occur. This means that your entire focus should be on what the person is saying, not on any errands you may have to run, other items you may have to get done, or people you would rather be with. The following 10 ideas should be learned and practiced:

1. Limit your own talking. It is impossible to talk and listen at the same time.
2. Try to put yourself in the customer's place. The customers' problems and needs are important to them and should therefore be important to you. You can understand and retain the concerns of the customer better if you listen to the customer's point of view.
3. Ask questions. If you don't understand something or if you need clarification, there is nothing wrong with asking questions. In fact, asking relevant questions helps the customer to feel you are listening closely.
4. Don't interrupt. A pause doesn't always mean the customer is finished. Very often people pause when they are trying to formulate a sentence in their mind. Don't rush them. If you allow a pause of at least 5 seconds between sentences, it will give the customer time to add any other points they wish to make.
5. Concentrate. Focus your mind on the conversation, shutting out all outside distractions. If you find your mind wandering, put it back on track.
6. Take notes. This will help you remember important points in the conversation. However, don't try to write down every word. Note only key words that are relevant to the problem and will help you to remember the issues at a later time.
7. Interjections. An occasional, "Yes," "I see," or "I understand," shows the customer that you are still tuning in to their words. Just be careful not to overdo it. Too many interjections will make the customer feel you are constantly interrupting.
8. Keep your words and thoughts concise. Personal concerns and stories of what happened to you or someone else waste time and confuse the customer. In addition, it does not help to move the

conversation forward, toward resolution of the customer's problem.

9. React to the problem or concern not to the person. Don't allow yourself to become irritated at things the customer says or the way in which he or she says them.
10. Don't jump to conclusions. Don't assume that you know what the customer is about to say. Also, don't finish his or her sentences, either mentally or verbally. Let the customer finish completely before you offer a solution or suggestion.

Listening with Empathy

Empathy means being able to participate in another person's feelings or perceptions and to try to sense and understand how another person is feeling or what he or she is experiencing. In customer service, this is a critical part of the listening process.

Empathetic listening, on its own, may resolve your customer's problem. Often giving people a chance to verbally walk through their problem may clarify their understanding of the situation. It also often provides emotional release and allows them to gain a more logical point of view. Since it gives customers a chance to voice their opinions, it can reduce tension and hostility. When people feel you are truly interested in them as well as their problems, thoughts, and opinions, they respect you and are more willing to cooperate with you toward a resolution of problems. Thus, empathetic listening promotes communication, which is essential in the business world. Often communication breaks down because neither party has learned to listen.

Problem Resolution

Listening skills are used throughout the entire problem resolution process. However, there are also specific steps that will bring you and the customer to the resolution of a problem or concern. The six basic steps in this process are:

1. Greeting the customer.
2. Acknowledgment of the problem.
3. Questioning the customer to determine the best way to proceed toward resolution of the problem.
4. Verifying the information received from the customer and any agreed-upon further actions.
5. Counseling the customer regarding the steps he or she will need to take toward resolution of the problem.
6. Closing the conversation.

Greeting the Customer

The way you greet the customer and begin the conversation sets the tone for the entire encounter. This depends not so much on the words you say, but on the tone of your voice and the way you say them. A pleasant greeting can defuse an angry customer and improve the outlook of a concerned customer. Your voice should communicate pleasantness, caring, and concern from the first word.

Practice greeting customers in a pleasant and happy voice. Then, before you answer the phone or turn toward a customer, take a moment for a quick breath and a smile. Focus your attention on the customer, not on the task in front of you or any other thoughts. If your mind is not focused, the customer will hear your distraction in the tone of your voice.

When a customer enters the office, it is important to greet the customer as soon as you see him or her. If you are on the phone or are unable to give your full attention, smile and say, "I'll be with you in just a moment." Then get to them as quickly as you can.

Acknowledging the Problem

Acknowledging your customer's concern or problem opens the line of communication and lets the customer know that you are interested in helping to find a solution. It also tells the customer that he or she is important, that you empathize with the concern, and that you want to resolve the problem or prevent it from occurring again. For instance:

Representative: "This is John Doe. How may I help you?"

Customer: "I just got a notice from my doctor's office that you refused to pay my bill. The last claim I sent in you only paid a little bit. What are we paying premiums for if you're not going to cover the bills?"

Representative: "I can understand why you might

be upset, Sir. If I can ask you a few questions, we can resolve this quickly for you."

Notice that the response should not be an apology or an admission of error. It also should not accuse or place the blame on the customer. Your primary goal is to acknowledge that a problem or situation exists and that you are willing to work with the customer to find a solution. Your voice should remain soft and slow, not allowing the customer's anger to seep into your own voice.

In the following exercise, choose the statement that best reflects complete acknowledgment:

1. It's no problem to issue you a new card. Let me get your policy number and address so I can send it right out.
2. I can understand your concern. I'll issue you a new card immediately. That way you'll have it when you go in for surgery.
3. Certainly, I can issue you another card. If you ever misplace it again, just give us a call.

Questioning the Customer

Questioning is a learned skill. It is used to clarify the reason for the call and to gain information needed to work toward a resolution of the customer's concern. There are two kinds of questions: open-ended and closed-ended.

Open-ended questions are questions that cannot be answered with a yes, no, or other brief response. These questions encourage customers to respond freely. They usually begin with words such as "tell me," "why," or "what." Examples of open-ended questions include:

- "Why were the tests performed?"
- "What kind of coverage are you interested in?"
- "What happened that makes you feel that way?"

Closed-ended questions limit or restrict the customer's response, usually to a yes or no answer or other brief response. These types of questions usually begin with words like "who," "are," "did," "what," and "which." Therefore, a closed question is closed-ended and brings about a specific, narrow response.

Closed-ended questions should be used when you need specific information, need to take more control of the conversation, or need to confirm or verify your understanding of the situation. Examples of closed questions include:

- "What is your plan number?"
- "Are you enrolled as a dependent under your husband's policy?"
- "Which physician did you visit?"

Both types of questions usually are necessary in a conversation. This will allow you to resolve the problem quickly while retaining the best possible interrelationship. If too many closed-ended questions are used, the customer may feel as if he or she is being interrogated. Too many open-ended questions allow the conversation to wander.

Regardless of the type of questions used, listen carefully for the answer in order to resolve the situation. Think through the meaning of the answer before you consider what your next step or your next question should be.

Verifying the Information

Verification means repeating the information and asking if you have understood it correctly. It is important to ensure that you have understood the customer's concerns and the answers to your questions, especially when you are speaking to someone with an accent. Minor mispronunciations in language can lead to big misunderstandings. For example, consider the ramifications of misunderstanding the following two sentences: "Call me tonight" and "Kill me tonight." As you can see, a mispronounced vowel can change a lot.

By using verification, you can ensure that you and your customer are saying the same thing and have the same understanding of the situation. Verification also builds a stronger rapport with the customer, since the customer realizes you are trying to understand and are truly listening to what he or she is saying. Verification sentences often begin with phrases such as:

- "If I'm understanding you correctly..."
- "May I repeat this back to you to make sure I understand?"
- "So you mean..."
- "Then you want us to..."

If you believe the customer may not understand, question him or her to find out what is unclear.

For example:

- "You seem unsure, Mr. Brown; what concerns you?"
- "Specifically, what part is unclear to you, Mrs. Hall?"
- "Is there anything that you would like explained again, sir?"

When repeating information for a second time, it is often better to rephrase it than to repeat it word for word. If there still seems to be a problem, use examples such as:

- "For example, if you had gone to your primary physician before seeing the specialist, the services might have been covered differently."
- "For example, if this was your first visit to the doctor he would want to discuss your history before the surgery.

It might also be helpful to offer any resource material that is available. This may include pamphlets, copies of policy documents, or other resource material.

Counseling the Customer

Now you are ready to move on to the counseling step. Counseling may not be necessary in all encounters. When a short or simple answer is required, simply answer the question and conclude the conversation. For example:

- "Yes, Mrs. Minor, we have your appointment listed at 2 o'clock on Tuesday."
- "Yes, Mr. Sampson, the check for that claim was mailed Monday."

However, counseling can be an invaluable skill when the response is lengthy or complex. For example:

- "According to our records we never received a claim from Dr. Jordan. May I suggest you talk with Dr. Jordan's office and find out when the claim was submitted. If it has been longer than 2 weeks, ask them to resubmit the claim and we will process it."

Counseling is also helpful when the response requires that you take further action. For example:

- "I need to check our records to see if that claim has been processed. Are you able to hold a moment while I pull up the file?"

Finally, counseling assists when the response requires a delay before the problem can be resolved.

- "I need to contact the doctor's office for a copy of the medical records. It will probably take a few days. When I receive it, I'll call you back. You should hear from us by Monday, Mr. Smith."

Counseling entails explaining the situation and then explaining both what the customer should do next and what you will do next. In the previous examples:

- The customer was expected to contact the doctor's office and you would wait for the claim form.
- You would check the records and the customer would hold.
- You would contact the doctor's office and the customer would expect your call before Monday.

Counseling allows a clear picture of the situation and the actions to be taken. In this way each party is clear about what the next step should be in helping to bring the situation to a successful resolution.

Closing the Conversation

Once a plan of action has been agreed upon or the client's questions have been answered, it is time to close the call. The important thing to bear in mind is that the encounter should not be considered finished until the customer is as satisfied as possible.

When you feel the customer is satisfied, use the following two steps to close the call:

1. Summarize the outcomes. A summary is a brief statement reminding the customer what you have agreed on together and how it will help or solve his or her concern. It needs to be clear and concise, and stated in a positive way. For example:
   - "Good, then I'll send that claim form right away, Mrs. Phillips, and if you have any questions about it, just give me a call."
   - "So, you'll call Medicare with the toll-free number I just gave you and find out why they've rejected the claim. You'll also ask them what they need to review the claim. If you still have a concern after you've talked to them, just give us a call. Thank you for calling. Goodbye, Mr. Smith."

2. Thanking the customer. Don't forget to thank the customer. If customers feel unappreciated they may take their business elsewhere. The two words "thank you" may be the easiest and one of the most important ways to keep your job.

Occasionally, a customer may want to continue to chat after a resolution has been reached. In such a case, summarizing the agreed-upon actions in a succinct way will send the message that the conversation is concluding. With determined customers, it may be necessary to firmly but kindly let them know that you have other matters to attend to and, although you would love to chat, you need to get back to work.

The use of the six basic steps in problem resolution will bring positive results and will help your customers to feel important and appreciated. That's what customer service is all about.

To help assess your strengths and weaknesses in the areas just discussed, complete Exercise 7-3 at the back of this chapter.

Handling Difficult Customers

Occasionally, you will receive a call from or be forced to meet with a customer who is irate, tearful, or unprepared, or who can't seem to figure out what to say. The following suggestions will help you to handle customers who generally pose the greatest problem for customer service personnel.

Irate Customers

Most people you deal with will be polite, kind, and courteous. Occasionally, however, you will have to deal with a customer who is irate and has no qualms about taking out his or her anger on you. Remember that your behavior influences the behavior of others. Instead of becoming irate yourself, consider this type of customer a challenge. See how long it takes you to get this customer calmed down and the problem resolved.

Most irate customers perceive themselves as victims who have been wronged by the provider or company. By providing a listening, sympathetic ear, you can let this customer know that he or she is important to your business and that these concerns do matter to you. Remember that the customer may have a legitimate complaint that needs to be resolved, even if it wasn't your fault.

Start by listening to what the customer has to say. Let the customer vent anger for a bit and finish what he or she has to say without being interrupted. Try to understand the customer's point of view.

If the customer uses offensive or abusive language, ignore it. Always try to remember that the customer is angry at the company and the circumstances, not at you. Ignore the hurt the words cause. If you can't do this, you've lost the situation. If it happens often, you may lose your job.

If the customer continues with abusive language, try asking if you have done something to personally offend him or her. Often this helps to calm the customer and begin moving the situation toward a resolution.

If you are dealing with an abusive caller and this approach doesn't work, (and if your employer allows you the option of terminating such calls) interrupt the caller and firmly but politely say, "Excuse me, but I prefer not to hear such language. If you don't stop, I'm going to have to end this conversation." Say this two times, the second time a little more forcefully than the first. If the language or abuse continues, say, "I'm sorry but I need to terminate this call. Please call back when we can discuss this problem." Then hang up immediately. On terminating such a call, inform your supervisor immediately. This type of caller nearly always calls back. Most of the time the caller is apologetic and you can work toward resolving the problem. If the caller is still irate and abusive, the call should be transferred to your supervisor.

If a phone customer is a screamer, let him or her vent to allow release of pent-up emotions that you don't want to have to deal with later. However, if the customer is facing you in person, especially if other customers are around, you need to try to calm the customer down as soon as possible.

With either type of customer (on the phone or in person), try not to interrupt. This will make the customer more angry. Your voice and actions should show that you understand and accept the customer's feelings, regardless of whether or not you agree with them. Use statements such as "I can see why you are upset" or "I understand that you're angry. Let's see what we can do to resolve the problem." Usually, letting the customer know you understand and care and offering to work with him or her to resolve the problem will defuse the anger. Then try to resolve any problems without transferring the customer (if a phone call) or referring him or her to another person or agency. If you cannot help the customer and you need to transfer or refer him or her, be sure to explain why and give all the information that the customer needs to get hold of the person to whom you are referring.

Don't make excuses. It doesn't help to resolve the situation or help the customer feel better. If errors have been made, apologize for them without placing blame. Promise to do what you can to resolve the situation, and then do it.

If the caller insists on speaking with your supervisor, put him or her on hold and briefly explain the situation so that the customer will not need to repeat everything a second time. Before transferring the call, inform the caller of your supervisor's name and that you have briefed him or her on the situation.

If your supervisor is unavailable, tell the customer this, and attempt to handle the problem. If you cannot, take down the customer's name and telephone number and let him or her know that you will have the supervisor return the call as soon as possible. This delay often allows the customer to "cool down" and be able to discuss the situation more calmly when the supervisor returns the call.

Remember the following 11 guidelines in dealing with irate or angry customers:

1. Remain calm. Remember that the customer is angry with the situation, not at you. If you take it personally and become upset, the discussion will become an argument.
2. Never argue. Listen! Don't try to match wits with the customer. Allow the customer time to vent feelings.
3. Ask questions. Direct, open-ended questions help to define the problem. However, questions that begin with "Why" are best avoided since they can sometimes be construed as threatening.
4. Listen carefully to what the customer is saying. Even angry customers will give you valuable information by what they say and how they say it. Let the customer know you are listening and are interested by saying "I see" or "Yes, sir." If you are speaking with the person face to face, maintain good eye contact, nod, and keep an attentive facial expression and an open body position.
5. Be prepared. Be well informed regarding your company and your department. If a customer is upset about a policy that cannot be changed, explain how the policy was designed to protect the customer, you, or the company.
6. Avoid giving customers a runaround or transferring them to someone else.
7. Accept criticism without becoming angry. People who are angry are often looking for a fight to justify their anger. Your pleasant demeanor can be disarming to an angry customer.
8. Agree. Find something in the customer's remarks with which you can agree. This will help the customer to feel you are an ally rather than an enemy. However, never agree to anything that can be misconstrued as a promise of what you or the company will do. Don't place blame. You don't want the customer to like you and dislike the company.
9. Avoid defensive behavior. Don't make excuses such as "We're short-staffed," "I'm new here," or "It's not my job."
10. Offer choices. Whenever possible, allow the customer to choose a plan of action by offering several options. Or ask the customer how he or she would like you to resolve the problem. This way, the customer feels in control of the situation and will take responsibility for the outcome.
11. Be personal. Introduce yourself and learn the customer's name. Say the name as often as it is appropriate during the conversation.

Remember that the more friendly, pleasant, and helpful you are, the more helpful, responsive, and satisfied your customer will be.

Unprepared Customers

An unprepared customer may not have sufficient information for you to answer questions. Sometimes the customer has not taken the time to formulate thoughts, and it may be difficult to determine exactly what the question is. Be patient. Explain what information you need and why you need it. Assure the customer that you will be happy to be of assistance when the information is provided.

Customer service means serving the customer. However, don't allow yourself to be taken advantage of or talked into performing functions that are not the responsibility of you or your company (eg, filling out the customer's forms). Once a customer begins taking advantage of you, it usually continues, leaving you little time to accomplish your assigned tasks.

Long-winded or Tearful Customers

Long-winded or tearful customers attempt to make you feel sorry for them in an attempt to get their way. Sometimes they call or come in simply because they are lonely and want someone to talk to or because they need reassurance. Both types of customers have a tendency to try to continue the conversation after their questions have been satisfied.

It is important with these types of customers to maintain a professional attitude. Show your concern, but don't allow yourself to become overly sympathetic.

Question the customer to be sure that he or she is satisfied with your answers. Verify that there are no further questions, then try to terminate the conversation by politely but firmly explaining that there are other matters that require your attention.

Professionalism

In customer service, it is vitally important to use language that conveys a professional attitude. Slang, rudeness, and other discourteous ways of speaking should not be allowed to creep into your vocabulary. Eleven comparisons between professional and unprofessional language follow:

1. Use courtesy rather than rudeness or sarcasm: "Do you have/need a copy of your contract to refer to?" rather than "Haven't you read your contract?"
2. Use patience rather than rushing the customer: "I can explain that for you," rather than "Will you let me answer your question?"
3. Use a calm and composed voice rather than reacting personally: "Yes, an error was made," rather than "Don't take it out on me. I didn't do it."
4. Sound concerned rather than bored or bothered: "How can I be of help?" rather than "What do you want me to do about it?"
5. Be reassuring rather than uncaring: "That's okay. In your situation it doesn't matter," rather than "I don't care about that. It doesn't mean anything."
6. Use acceptance rather than implying blame:
   - (internally) "It was processed incorrectly," rather than "The Claims Department processed it wrong."
   - (externally) "Our record shows no accident date indicated at the time of your claim processing, but I can check," rather than "Your doctor's office didn't put an accident date on your claim."
7. Suggest rather than demand: "You might want to..." rather than "You have to..." or "We need from you..." rather than "You have to send..." or "May I suggest..." rather than "You must..."
8. Restrict your conversation to business rather than discussing personal experiences or opinions: "I can understand this must be an inconvenience for you," rather than "I know someone with that problem who saw a lawyer..."
9. Use business-like language rather than slang or nicknames: "Ma'am/sir" rather than "Honey/Dear/Sweetie" or "That is correct," rather than "You got it. You bet." "Your file is complicated," rather than "Your file is screwed up." "I'm doing my best," rather than "Get off my case." "It might not be best..." rather than "You're getting ripped off." "Request prompt attention," rather than "Get them on the stick."
10. Try to sound knowledgeable and logical rather

than confused or uninformed: "I don't have an immediate answer to your question but let me find out for you," rather than "I have no idea."

11. Respect the customer rather than imply that you have superior knowledge. "The figure on your form, located in the fourth column indicates the amount," rather than "I don't see why you don't understand—it's right there on your EOB form."

To practice, complete Exercise 7-4 at the end of this chapter.

Telephone Techniques

Medical billers have approximately half of their customer contact in person and half over the phone. However, health claims examiners have over 90% of their customer contact by phone. Therefore, proper telephone etiquette is very important.

Answer Promptly

When your telephone rings, make a point of answering it before the third ring, whenever possible. Prompt answering helps avoid irritation and builds a reputation for efficiency.

Identify Yourself

Let the caller know whom he or she is speaking with. It establishes a rapport and lets the caller know that you are a person and are willing to work to resolve the problem or concern.

Be Friendly

Your tone of voice conveys your willingness to help and to make the client feel that the problem is important to you. Make your voice pleasant and control the speed at which you speak. Make the client, insured, or provider feel that you are eager to be of assistance. To accomplish this:

- Be a good listener so that the caller will not have to repeat things.
- Indicate that you are interested. Use the caller's name when possible (but use the last name, not the first name; you are not personal friends).
- Be sincere and genuine, and let this come through in your voice.
- Give your full attention to the caller. Discussions with others while a customer is waiting on the line is inconsiderate and irritating.
- Avoid interrupting the caller.

Returning to the Line

When you must leave the line to get information, be courteous. Ask if the caller is able to hold or if it would be more convenient for you to call back. Don't automatically assume that the caller has the time or inclination to wait on the line. Here are some suggestions:

- If the caller agrees to hold, use the hold button. If this is unavailable on your phone, set the phone down gently. Bear in mind that the customer can overhear conversation when the phone is not placed on hold. Be careful not to say anything that might be overheard or misunderstood.
- If it takes longer than anticipated to obtain the information, update the caller on your progress. If it is going to be more than a couple of minutes, tell the caller that you will contact him or her as soon as you can get the information. Give the caller an estimate of how long it will take, then stand by your promise to call back.
- When you return to the line, let the caller know you have returned. For example, say, "Thank you for waiting."

Transferring Calls

Try to take care of the caller's concern by yourself. It is irritating for the caller to constantly be transferred from one person to another with no one wanting to assist. If the caller has a simple problem that is not your responsibility (eg, change of address, request for claim forms or material), take the information down and give it to the person who is responsible for that function. When it is necessary to transfer a call, take the following four steps:

1. Explain why you need to transfer the call ("I'm unable to assist you with that. However, Mr. Gonzales can help you. May I transfer you?").

2. Wait for the caller's answer. If the person does not wish to be transferred, write down the name and phone number and tell the caller that someone will call back ("I'll have Ms. Smith call you back with the information.").
3. If the caller agrees to be transferred, be careful not to disconnect the call. To be safe, always give the caller the name of the person you are transferring to and their extension or phone number. Then if the worst happens, he or she can call that person directly.
4. Finally, briefly explain the situation or problem to the person to whom you are transferring the call, along with the caller's name. Be concise, but convey enough information that the caller will not need to repeat everything a second time.

Closing the Call

Summarize the conversation to be sure that it is closed and to note any follow-up action required of either party. Try your best to say good-bye in a way that will leave the caller feeling satisfied that his or her problem will be handled correctly. Hang up quietly, or better yet, let the calling party hang up first.

Telephone Tips

In addition to the previous points, here are 14 more suggestions that will help:

1. If your call is going to be lengthy, make an appointment with the customer for a date and time for the extended call. In this way, your call will have a better chance of being answered, and your customer will have a better chance of having the time needed to resolve the situation.
2. Outline the topics you need to discuss before placing the call; then stick to the list of topics.
3. Just before placing the call, try to picture the other person in your mind, and smile at that person. This will put you in a friendly frame of mind.
4. Be kind to whomever answers the phone, even if it is not the person with whom you wish to speak. This person may be your only link to the person you want.
5. If you are unable to reach the person you need, leave a message and make sure the messenger also takes down your phone number. This increases the chances for your call to be returned.
6. Make sure the person has a few minutes to speak to you. A simple, "Do you have a moment to speak with me?" can help a lot. If the answer is no, ask when the best time would be for you to call back.
7. Most callers find it unnerving to be asked what their call is about. If you are unable to answer your own phone, instruct those who answer for you not to ask this question.
8. Avoid doing something else (eg, writing or typing) while on the phone.
9. Complex information is best handled in person or in writing, especially if it contains critical information or details.
10. Make sure that your caller is satisfied and fully understands before closing a conversation. You can't see a confused expression over the phone, so listen for it in the caller's voice.
11. If you are taking a message for someone else, do not tell the caller when they can expect a call back. If the caller is unable to reach the person at that time, he or she will become upset.
12. Never slam down the receiver, no matter how upset you may be with the caller.
13. Don't eat, drink, chew, or smoke while on the phone. The telephone receiver can magnify these sounds, and they can be very annoying to the caller.
14. Always terminate a call pleasantly and politely.

Placing Outgoing Calls

When placing outgoing calls, a few items of etiquette should always be practiced.

- Place your own calls: You save time and money by placing your own calls rather than using the operator. Whenever possible, use toll-free numbers or WATTS lines.
- Allow sufficient time to answer: Give the person

you're calling at least 10 rings to answer the phone.

- Identify yourself: Give your name and the name of the company you are calling from before any other information. Don't expect anyone to recognize your voice even if they are expecting your call.
- Remember time differences for different areas: When calling long distance, don't forget the four time zones in the United States. Call at an appropriate time for business in the time zone you are calling. A detailed map showing these zones is usually included in the introductory pages of your local telephone directory.

Phone Usage

The following are general guidelines regarding phone usage. Since these guidelines may vary from company to company or even between departments in a company, be sure you understand the policies.

- Collect call policy: Some companies accept collect calls from clients or insureds regarding their policy or the handling of specific services. Often collect calls are not accepted from a provider of service because this is considered part of their cost of doing business. If you are going to be handling inquiry calls, it is important that you know your company's policies prior to getting a call, not after.
- Long distance: Long distance calls to clients, insureds/claimants, and providers are usually permitted if the information requested in the call is necessary for the completion of a claim. You should organize your thoughts and write down your questions prior to making the call so that you can spend as little time on the call as possible. This will drastically reduce the overhead costs of the company.
- Telephone system: Telephone systems can vary greatly from one company to another. Be sure you know how to answer a call, transfer a call, and put a caller on hold properly. Nothing is more irritating to a caller than to be disconnected after being on hold for 5 minutes.

Telephone Etiquette

It is important to use proper etiquette on the telephone. The word etiquette is defined as the practices and forms prescribed by convention or by authority. In essence, etiquette is manners.

While using the telephone, etiquette includes your tone of voice, some basic telephone manners, speaking on the level of the caller, controlling the conversation, and making the appropriate verbal responses.

Tone of Voice

Your tone of voice is the single most important factor in conveying your willingness to help a customer. Be pleasant and professional. If you pay attention to the other person and respond to his or her questions in a sincere manner, the caller will be more willing to work with you toward a resolution of the problem. If you smile while on the phone, this smile will usually come across in your voice.

Working in a customer service area can be very demanding, frustrating work. Many callers are angry, irritated, or tired. But the difference between a good customer service person and a poor one is that a good customer service person is always pleasant and kind to each customer, no matter how the customer feels. You cannot allow the customer's feelings to influence your own.

Be natural and use simple straightforward language. Use a normal volume that can be heard easily, but isn't too loud. Talk at a moderate rate, neither too fast nor too slow.

In many geographic areas, there are high concentrations of non-English-speaking or English-as-a-second-language-speaking persons. If you do not speak the caller's language and they do not speak English well, it is important to speak slowly and to pronounce words correctly. Do not yell. These callers are not deaf, they just have difficulty with the language. If possible, find someone in your office who speaks the caller's language. If that is not possible, take the time to work with the caller. If necessary, spell out words. Many people have a higher understanding of written language than of spoken language. Above all else, be patient and don't try to rush the situation.

Telephone Manners

Use the caller's name as often as is appropriate. It makes the caller feel more connected to you. However, address the person by the last name, not by the first name. Speak to the person at the other end of the line, not to the telephone.

Every call is important to the caller and should be treated as such by the customer service representative. When the caller feels that you are giving individual attention to the call, rather than routine consideration, he or she will have more confidence in you and the company.

Be tactful. When you must refuse a request because of company policy, give a full and sympathetic explanation. Avoid expressions such as "you must" or "you have to." A comment such as "If you will submit your request in writing, we will be glad to give it consideration" sounds more tactful than, "you have to send it to us in writing to get an answer."

Apologize for errors or delays, even if they are not your fault. Things may not always go right, but a little courtesy can help defuse much anger. However, be sure your apologies are sincere; otherwise they will sound phony.

Take time to be helpful. It only takes a little more effort to make your phone contacts pleasant, and it can brighten your day as well as the caller's. Remember that it is better to spend a few minutes trying to keep a customer happy than months trying to regain his or her business.

If you are having a bad day and all your customers seem to be angry or defensive, consider that the problem might be you. People respond to what they think they hear in your voice. If there is irritation, it makes them irritated and begins a downward spiral. Break the chain by changing the way you're talking or your tone of voice. This simple change may turn your day around.

Speak on the Caller's Level

As a customer service representative, you will receive calls from people with varying degrees of education and knowledge. Listen to the way the caller pronounces words and the type of words. Then use words on a similar level that the caller can understand. Regardless of the level of the caller, you should avoid the use of technical words and insurance jargon such as EOB, COB, primary carrier, secondary carrier, TPL, OOPS, or coinsurance. You cannot expect any caller to understand these terms.

Controlling the Conversation

Your primary goal should be to give the customer complete satisfaction in the least amount of time. The following six suggestions can help you accomplish this:

1. Find out as soon as possible what the question or problem is. Have the caller tell you exactly what he or she wants to know. Don't try to guess. You may guess wrong and provide unwanted or incorrect information or you could bring up questions the caller may not have thought of.
2. Obtain specific information immediately. This may include information such as:
   - What is the ID number of the member?
   - What is the policy number?
   - What is the name of the patient on this claim?
   - What was the date of service and the billed amount?
   - What is the name of the provider of service?
3. Answer all questions and be sure the caller understands the issues. Before closing the call, ask whether there are other questions.
4. Don't bring up issues or claims unrelated to the caller's question(s).
5. Don't chit-chat with the caller. Be polite, but keep the conversation centered on the business at hand.
6. Choose your words and tone of voice carefully. If the caller becomes angry or irritated, the call will take longer.

After the caller's questions have been answered or the requested information has been given, politely close the conversation.

Appropriate Verbal Responses

If a question requires a simple "yes" or "no," it is appropriate to answer as such. However, be aware of questions with which disclaimers should be used. These can involve questions such as, "Does the doctor perform this type of surgery?" or "Does my insurance provide surgical coverage?" Answers to these questions should include disclaimers such as, "Yes, for most patients who aren't at high risk" or "Yes, with certain restrictions. Cosmetic surgery is not covered, or a second opinion may be needed to verify the need for some surgeries." Explain that without the proper information from the doctor or medical documentation, you cannot tell the caller whether his or her particular procedure will be performed or covered and whether other conditions might need to be taken into consideration.

Coverage of certain services falls into a "gray area." These services can include nursing services, speech therapy, experimental procedures, and possibly cosmetic surgery. When the caller is inquiring about these types of services, the health claims examiner should be very careful of the language used because most controversies (and lawsuits) arise from these types of services. Your answer should always include disclaimers and should indicate that you cannot provide a definite answer without complete medical documentation of the situation.

Many insurance companies have a "preauthorization process," which allows the provider of service to submit documentation regarding the case and suggested procedures prior to the performance of these procedures. This information is reviewed and a qualified approval may be given. This is similar to obtaining an estimate before car repair work is done, but here the estimate covers not how much it will cost, but how much the insurance carrier will cover. If the procedure falls into the gray area, health claims examiners and medical billers should suggest that a preauthorization review be performed prior to the services.

If a customer requests a specific dollar amount of coverage, suggest that the provider submit documentation for a preauthorization review. This is the only way for benefits to be calculated.

If the caller is presenting a hypothetical question, the variables may range too widely to give an answer. Without documented facts, it is difficult to make a decision regarding any situation. If the caller insists that you give an answer, explain that your reply is based on the information given and that the answer could vary greatly when the written documentation is received.

If you are unsure about the answer to a question, do not guess. Always play it safe and remember that you may be making statements that the provider or carrier can be held responsible for at a later date. Tell the caller that you are not sure but that you will find out the answer and call him or her back.

When verifying benefits, all facts of coverage should be checked. This includes the diagnosis, the eligibility status, current coverage, dependent eligibility, age limits, and others (these terms will make more sense when you begin processing claims in this course). Here again, tell the caller that you are basing your answer on the facts supplied and that the answer could change based on other factors involved in the processing of a claim.

Most calls can be handled using your knowledge, common sense, and patience. Remember never to make any promises you can't guarantee. Actually, the only promise you should ever make is to follow through in handling the situation.

Summary

Customer service is one of the most vital functions that health claims examiners or medical billers can perform. Without good customer relations, customers go elsewhere. Although it takes hard work, patience, and a good disposition to perform good customer service functions, it is well worth the time and effort.

The following are the most important topics discussed in this chapter, which should always be kept in mind when dealing with your customers:

- Greet the customer promptly.
- Identify yourself by giving your name and title.
- Write down the customer's name and ID number as soon as identification is provided.

- Be professional in voice and choice of words.
- Listen to what the customer has to say. If the customer is angry, let him or her get the anger out.
- Don't react to a customer's hostility with hostility of your own.
- Give out accurate information. If you don't know the answer to a question, take the caller's name and phone number and tell him or her that you will find out and call back.
- Stay informed concerning all policies and procedures and know the procedures of the company you work for.
- Be patient with the customer. He or she might not be familiar with procedures.
- Always be supportive of your peers and your company. Acknowledge when a mistake has been made but don't make any derogatory remarks about other personnel or company policies or procedures.
- Be empathetic. Many customers are experiencing serious illness, death of a family member, or financial problems.
- Use appropriate disclaimers when quoting benefits.

Assignments

Complete the Questions for Review.

Complete Customer Service Exercises 7-5 to 7-8.

Questions for Review

Directions: Answer the following questions without looking back into the material just covered. Write your answers in the space provided.

1. What is an attitude? ______________________________

____

2. What is positive reinforcement? ______________________________

____

3. A person's positive or negative impressions about another person or an organization are formed within 2 minutes. (True or False) ______________________________
4. Define empathy. ______________________________
5. What are the six basic steps that will bring you and the customer to the resolution of a problem or concern?
   a. ______________________________
   b. ______________________________
   c. ______________________________
   d. ______________________________
   e. ______________________________
   f. ______________________________

If you were unable to answer any of the questions, refer back to the section and then fill in the answers.

Exercise 7-1

Directions: Identify the statements that are positive recognition by placing a "P" in the space indicated. Place an "N" if the response is negative.

1. _______ "That idea is ridiculous!"
2. _______ "Don't complain to me."
3. _______ "May I place you on hold while I check that for you?"
4. _______ "Another area handles that type of problem."
5. _______ "That was very thoughtful of you."
6. _______ Not speaking to someone.
7. _______ A smile!
8. _______ Direct eye contact with a person.
9. _______ Sounding bored.
10. _______ "Stupid, don't you ever listen?"

Exercise 7-2

Directions: Rate the following statements as to how often you say or feel that way. 5 = Always, 4 = Often, 3 = Sometimes, 2 = Seldom, 1 = Never.

1. ________ I can't remember people's names.
2. ________ I'm not good on the telephone.
3. ________ I have very little control over my moods.
4. ________ I often think of my job as a chore.
5. ________ What's the use. Nobody cares!
6. ________ I don't seem to have much patience.
7. ________ These customers drive me nuts!
8. ________ If my boss were more understanding, I wouldn't be so upset all the time.
9. ________ I just can't seem to get going in the morning.
10. ________ I don't have as much energy as I used to.

What other statements do you often make or think about yourself?

1. ____
____
2. ____
____
3. ____
____
4. ____
____
5. ____
____

Exercise 7-3

Directions: Ask three people who know you well or who are around you often to rate you on the following statements. 5 = Always, 4 = Often, 3 = Sometimes, 2 = Seldom, 1 = Never.

1. _______ He/she can't remember people's names.
2. _______ He/she isn't good on the telephone.
3. _______ He/she has very little control over his/her moods.
4. _______ He/she often thinks of his/her job as a chore.
5. _______ He/she often says or gives the impression that he/she feels "What's the use. Nobody cares!"
6. _______ He/she doesn't seem to have much patience.
7. _______ Customers drive him/her nuts!
8. _______ If his/her boss were more understanding, he/she wouldn't be so upset all the time.
9. _______ He/she just can't seem to get going in the morning.
10. _______ He/she doesn't have much energy.

What other statements does this person often make or seem to think about him/herself?

1. ____
____
2. ____
____
3. ____
____
4. ____
____
5. ____
____

Exercise 7-4

Directions: Fill out the following in the space provided.

1. Of the six steps just covered in The Art of Listening, which is your strongest?

____

____

____

2. Which of these steps needs more attention? List all that apply.

____

____

____

3. Specifically, list three actions that you can take to improve the techniques you listed in the previous question.

   a. ____

   b. ____

   c. ____

Exercise 7-5

Directions: Review the following statements and write an improvement in the space provided.

1. "He's on break." ______

2. "She's busy. Call back." ______

3. "Sorry. We're getting ready to close." ______

4. "I don't know where your file is." ______

5. "I can't do that for you now. Come back later." ______

Exercise 7-6

My Customer Service Quotient

Directions: This is a self-assessment quiz designed to determine your current skills in customer service. Take a few minutes to read the statements and rate yourself on how you feel you handle customers. Be honest. This is the only way you can recognize your strengths and weaknesses and work toward improving the weaknesses.

Use the following numbers to answer the questions: 5 = Always, 4 = Often, 3 = Sometimes, 2 = Seldom, 1 = Never.

1. _______ I want the service I provide to leave an excellent impression, so I constantly look for ways to improve it.
2. _______ I put the customer's needs first since (s)he is my ultimate boss.
3. _______ I accept people without judging them.
4. _______ I am aware that my attitudes and moods affect the way I respond to customers.
5. _______ I show patience and courtesy regardless of the customer's behavior.
6. _______ I don't allow myself to become irritated or lose my composure when dealing with angry customers.
7. _______ I have developed the habit of following up on all complaints that are brought to my attention.
8. _______ I understand the customer and see his/her problem as most important, and I do all I can to resolve it.
9. _______ I treat all customers equally, regardless of their position, rank, color, clothes, accent or other distinguishing features.
10. _______ I recognize that it is perceptions that count when dealing with customers, so I don't allow my frustrations or irritations to show.
11. _______ If something the customer says offends me, I focus on what the customer's feeling, not on getting even.
12. _______ I use professional language in my dealings with customers.
13. _______ I use proper telephone techniques and always identify myself to the caller.
14. _______ I make sure the customer is satisfied before terminating the conversation.
15. _______ I do not transfer a call unless it is absolutely necessary to resolve the customer's problem.

_______ Total

Scoring: Add the total for each question and then compute your score. The following scale gives an analysis of your customer service quotient.

68-75	Excellent! Your behavior and attitudes set examples for others to follow.
59-67	Good. You have a high awareness of how important your role is in customer service.
50-58	Moderate. You may be allowing your own biases and feelings to affect customer service.
41-49	Needs definite improvement. Time to get in touch with the obstacles between you and the quality service you should be providing.
Below 40	Poor. You need to make a concentrated effort to turn your attitudes and values around. Change may be slow.

Exercise 7-7

Directions: Choose the statement that best reflects customer service in the following situations:

1. Mrs. Smith has lost the statement of her account. ________
   A. "It's no problem to issue you a new statement of your account. Let me get your account number and address so I can send it right out."
   B. "Your next billing date is in 15 days, and you'll get a new statement of your account at that time."
   C. "I'm sorry, we issue only one statement per patient per month."

2. Mrs. Jones wants an appointment for her son immediately. The situation is not an emergency. ________
   A. "The next available appointment is 2 weeks from today. I'm sure your son can wait that long."
   B. "Since this doesn't seem to be an emergency, I will schedule you for the first available appointment, which is on Monday, 2 weeks from today. Would you like me to call you if there are any earlier cancellations?"
   C. "I'm sorry, but since it isn't a real emergency, your son will have to wait his turn."

3. Mr. Anderson is concerned about the cost of his proposed services. ________
   A. "Isn't your health worth more to you than money?"
   B. "I can understand how the cost might concern you. If you would like, we can set up an account so you can spread your payments out over several months."
   C. "Yes, it is expensive, but with the cost of overhead, malpractice insurance, and equipment, we just have to charge more."

Exercise 7-8

My Personal Action Plan

Successful people know their strengths as well as areas that need improvement. Please take a few moments to reflect on what you learned in this chapter.

1. Identify three strengths you currently possess that contribute to positive customer service.
   a. ____________________
   b. ____________________
   c. ____________________

2. Identify three areas in which you would like to grow to be more effective in customer service.
   a. ____________________
   b. ____________________
   c. ____________________

3. Specifically, what action steps can you take to improve in the previous three areas?
   a. ____________________
   b. ____________________
   c. ____________________

8

Calculator Basics

In this chapter you will learn:

- To understand the basic function and use of a calculator.
- To use the 10-key calculator by touch.
- To identify the different function keys and explain their purposes.
- To gain speed and accuracy in the use of a calculator.

A calculator is a machine that computes numbers. It is used to add, subtract, multiply, and divide numbers, as well as to compute percentages, square roots, and other mathematical calculations.

Whether you work as a health claims examiner or a medical biller, you will probably use a calculator every day. Often there are charges that need to be totaled and amounts that need to be figured. Doing each of these sums by hand would take countless extra hours. Therefore, it is vital that both health claims examiners and medical billers master the use of the calculator.

Key Descriptions

Following are the keys most commonly found on a calculator and a description of what these keys do.

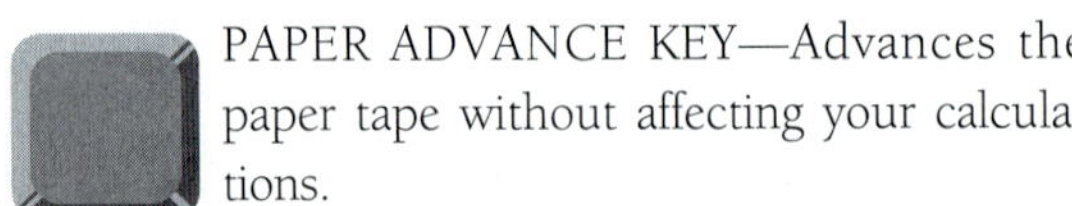

PAPER ADVANCE KEY—Advances the paper tape without affecting your calculations.

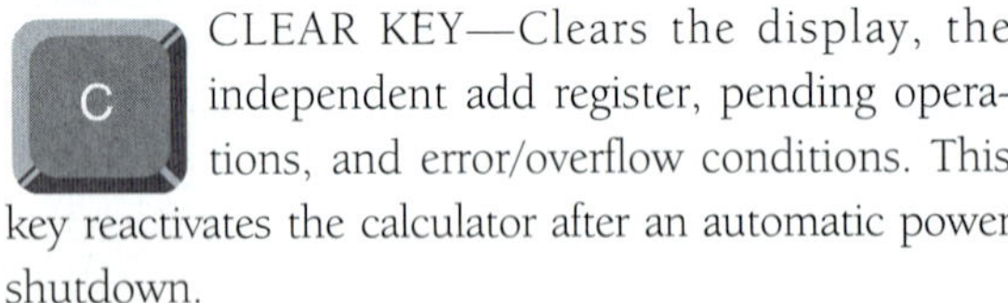

CLEAR KEY—Clears the display, the independent add register, pending operations, and error/overflow conditions. This key reactivates the calculator after an automatic power shutdown.

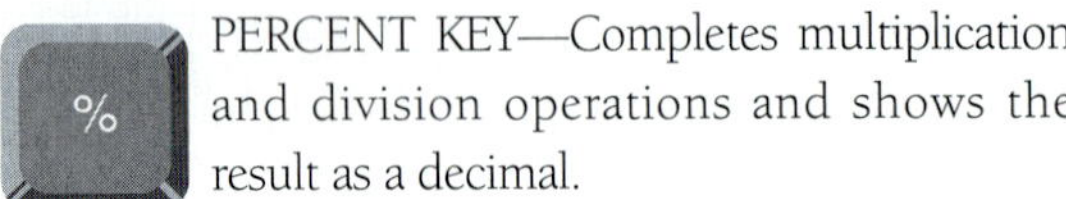

PERCENT KEY—Completes multiplication and division operations and shows the result as a decimal.

CE CLEAR ENTRY KEY—Clears the last entry only, enabling you to enter another number in its place without clearing all previously entered numbers.

÷ DIVIDE KEY—Instructs the calculator to divide the number in the display by the next value entered.

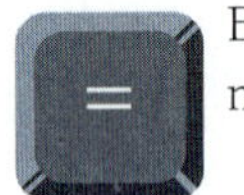

EQUAL KEY—Completes any pending multiplication or division operation.

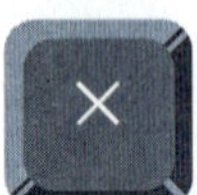

MULTIPLY KEY—Instructs the calculator to multiply the number in the display by the next value entered.

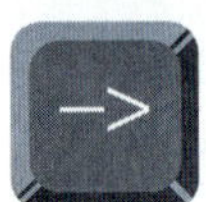

RIGHT SHIFT KEY—Deletes the right-most digit in the display and shifts the remaining digits one place to the right.

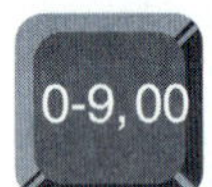

NUMBER KEYS—Enters numbers containing up to 10 digits. For numbers between 1 and -1, a zero automatically precedes the decimal, allowing a maximum of nine digits to the right of the decimal.

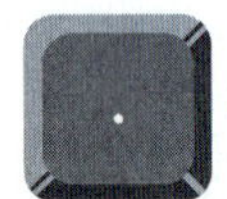

DECIMAL POINT KEY—Enters a decimal point. Most calculators have a floating decimal point that allows you to automatically set the decimal point at a given spot in the number.

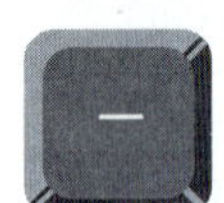

SUBTRACT KEY—Subtracts the number in the display from the independent add register.

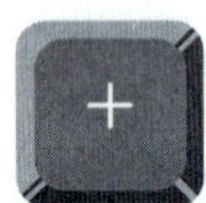

ADD KEY—Adds the number in the display to the independent add register.

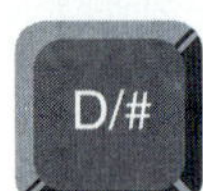

DATE/NON-ADD KEY—Prints a reference number or date without affecting calculations in progress.

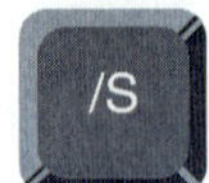

SUBTOTAL KEY—Displays and prints the subtotal in the independent add register. Pressing this key does not affect the contents of the add register.

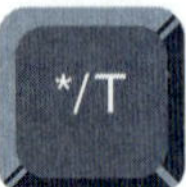

TOTAL KEY—Displays and prints the total in the independent add register, then clears the register.

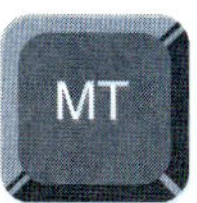

MEMORY TOTAL KEY—Displays and prints the value in memory, then clears the memory.

MEMORY SUBTOTAL KEY—Displays and prints the value in memory without clearing the memory.

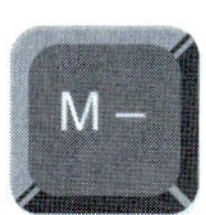

SUBTRACT FROM MEMORY KEY—Prints the number in the display and subtracts it from the value in memory. If a pending multiplication or division operation has been entered, this key completes the operation and subtracts the result from memory.

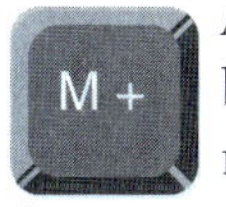

ADD TO MEMORY KEY—Prints the number in the display and adds it to the value in memory. If a pending multiplication or division operation has been entered, this key completes the operation and adds the result into memory.

Printer Tape Symbols

Multiple symbols may be printed on printer tapes during calculations. Usually, these symbols appear to the right of entries on the tape. Symbols not indicated below should be explained in the specific calculator manual in the section titled "Error/Overflow Conditions."

SYMBOL	MEANING OR EXPLANATION
+	Addition to the independent add register
–	Subtraction from the independent add register
<>	Subtotal of additions and subtractions in the independent add register
*	Total after =, %, or */T is pressed
×	Multiplication operation
÷	Division operation
=	Completion of a multiplication or division operation
%	Percentage
+ *	Percentage add-on
– *	Percentage discount
#	Reference number or date (printed in the center of the printer tape)
C	Clear key erases all entries
M *	Addition to memory
M –	Subtraction from memory
M <>	Memory subtotal
M *	Memory total
E	Error/overflow condition
IC	Item counter symbol. When the printer switch is in the IC position, the number of additions to and subtractions from the independent add register is printed above each total or subtotal. The item counter for the independent add register is reset when */T is pressed.

Summary

Proficient use of the calculator is essential for health claims examiners and medical billers. Learning the functions of each of the keys and how to use the calculator takes practice.

Assignments

Complete the Questions for Review.
Complete Calculator Basics Exercises 8-1 to 8-5.
Practice gaining speed and accuracy by repeating Exercises 8-1 and 8-2 until you have mastered the feel of the keys.

Questions for Review

Directions: Answer the following questions without looking back into the material just covered. Write your answers in the space provided.

1. The _______________ key completes multiplication and division operations and shows the results as a decimal.
2. What function does the divide key perform?_______________
3. The _______________ key completes any pending multiplication or division operations.
4. What is the function of the total key? _______________
5. The memory total key displays and prints the value currently in _______________, then clears the _______________.

If you were unable to answer any of the questions, refer back to the section and then fill in the answers.

Exercise 8-1

Directions: Add the following columns of numbers and total them. Then subtract the numbers from your total to arrive at zero. Clear the entries from your calculator and subtract the following columns of numbers and total, then add the numbers to your total to arrive at zero. Use the printer tape to check accuracy.

71459	12181	128.49	12.89
28695	57926	321.67	.92
13579	71349	014.89	7.16
58246	02763	906.76	18.21
69021	75396	741.08	267.93
54321	74185	529.63	1234.56
67891	29630	369.25	892.10
83214	36925	801.47	809.13
47986	80147	753.85	693.21
32694	42569	102.36	5679.32
15723	00147	564.12	137.14
38014	73528	321.65	432.78
98752	60413	498.70	6789.50
20361	13311	321.65	1090.17
13979	21769	789.93	578.15
02031	24989	456.89	692.00
11484	67400	999.01	780.29
25763	09121	847.03	566.17

Exercise 8-2

Directions: Add the following columns of numbers and total them. Then subtract the numbers from your total to arrive at zero. Clear the entries from your calculator and subtract the following columns of numbers and total, then add the numbers to your total to arrive at zero. Use the printer tape to check accuracy.

54659	46181	645.25	54.65
54165	35164	618.46	.12
41579	87319	614.79	2.76
45126	63453	641.76	78.11
56421	34150	123.08	457.12
20131	78455	469.61	3894.94
78991	23459	849.25	845.79
54164	89925	456.57	209.46
77986	24875	172.85	568.78
12094	23459	501.36	1056.23
12323	57847	841.43	347.51
71014	56748	051.65	351.91
71952	80893	540.71	6519.19
13671	10781	211.65	5056.20
24563	80974	549.93	645.51
63541	43729	635.45	345.48
0.168	89174	333.01	470.00
48567	39874	514.45	456.47

Exercise 8-3

Directions: Perform the function indicated for each list of numbers. Try not to watch your hands. Speed is not important at the beginning. It will come later as you become more familiar with the keys.

1. Add the following numbers.

A.	B.	C.	D.
12	65	44	334
24	70	69	781
67	49	26	456
41	52	73	241
92	100	84	908
34	99	35	528
72	34	21	803

E.	F.	G.	H.
295	4576	54	32.514
630	8493	835	8.123
816	90.56	046	61.54
902	3809	516	123.64
517	9238	943	543.55
703	12.98	.0015	999.83
491	540.5		

2. Enter the first number, then subtract the following numbers.

A.	B.	C.
9999	7654	4329
45	11	649
66	92	42
90	561	631
1504	341	42
3535	940	792
901	52	406

D.		E.		F.	
	1000.00		564.000		410014
	10.00		.630		.123
	.20		.920		654.456
	341.00		162.000		84.25
	1.78		.789		67.48
	.78		231.000		138.03
	592.00		501.000		486.381

Exercise 8-4

Directions: Perform the function indicated for each list of numbers. Try not to watch your hands. Speed is not important at the beginning. It will come later as you become more familiar with the keys.

1. Multiply the following.

A.		B.		C.		D.	
	231 × 42		5482 × 61		7602 × 201		891 × 23.61
E.	43.92 × .639	F.	24.51 × 70%	G.	903.45 × 85%	H.	2503.99 × 90%
I.	492.67 × 75%	J.	29.16 × 55%	K.	564465 × 21%	L.	654.21 × 75%

2. Divide the first number by the second number in the following equations.

A.		B.		C.		D.	
	5634 51		56348 543		999999 .99		3541 66
E.	1000 .01	F.	65430 125	G.	514623 1523	H.	5100 45

Exercise 8-5

Directions: Perform the function indicated for each list of numbers. Try not to watch your hands. Speed is not important at the beginning. It will come later as you become more familiar with the keys.

1. Perform the functions indicated in each problem.

   A. (234 × 32.40) – (432/4) =

   B. (4561/15) + (26.96 × .079) – 46.01 =

   C. (68459 + 541)/53 =

   D. (358416 – 64523) × 80% =

   E. (456.58 × 75%) + (54.87 × 80%) + (235.46 × 100%) =

   F. 56849 + (543.87 × 135%) =

   G. 317371 – (3697.89 × 75%) + 683.55 =

   H. (9999.99 – 999.99) × 338.01 + 2895.48 =

   I. (8361.64 × 85%) + 6415.23 – (68549 – 64589) =

   J. (8150/25) + (6895.46 × .50) =

   K. 20356.55 × 20% + (523.99 × 80%) =

   L. 6458.25/(6489.73/90%) =

9

Typing Skills

In this chapter you will learn:

- To understand the basic function and use of a typewriter.
- To understand the keys on the typewriter keyboard and which typewriter keys are struck with which fingers.
- To use the typewriter and know where the keys are.
- To gain accuracy and speed in the use of the typewriter.

Typing is a required skill for most health claims examiners and medical billers. Often correspondence, reports, and numerous other items need to be typed to make them look neat and professional.

Accuracy is the most important aspect of typing, followed by speed. Without accuracy, your documents look unprofessional and may even be unreadable. In this chapter, you will learn the parts of a typewriter and keyboard and how to type with speed and accuracy.

Learning the Keyboard

Learning the keyboard is the most important part of learning to type. After you have memorized the positioning of the keys and know which fingers are used for which keys, you will have the ability to type. At that point all you need to develop is speed and accuracy.

The keys for nearly all computers and typewriters are in a similar position. Some minor differences are based on brand, type, and model, and, in the case of computer keyboards, on the computer system. However, these differences are usually minimal. Look at your keyboard and compare it with Figure 9-1. This will help you to become familiar with the keyboard and the basic position of each key.

Types of Keys

First, let's discuss the uses of each of the keys.

Letter, Number, and Symbol or Character Keys: The 26 letter keys give you each individual letter of the alphabet. The number keys are the keys across the top line of the keyboard. These create numbers or symbols. The symbol keys are located along the right-hand side of the keyboard and across the bottom. These keys type punctuation characters and other symbols.

Each letter key, number key, and character key has the ability to type two items. In the case of the letter keys, the letter can be typed as either an upper case letter or a lower case letter. In the case of numbers and characters, the two items are shown on each key.

Shift Keys and Caps Lock: Upper case letters are accessed by pressing either the Shift keys or the Caps Lock key. The Caps Lock key locks the shift into place so that all letters become upper case letters. However, numbers and characters remain in the lower case position. To type the characters or symbols that appear above the lower symbol on a number or character key, hold the Shift key down while striking the key.

Space Bar: With all keyboards, one touch to the space bar moves you one space to the right. Pressing and holding down the space bar on both electric typewriters and computers gives you an indefinite number of spaces to the right (continuous as long as you hold

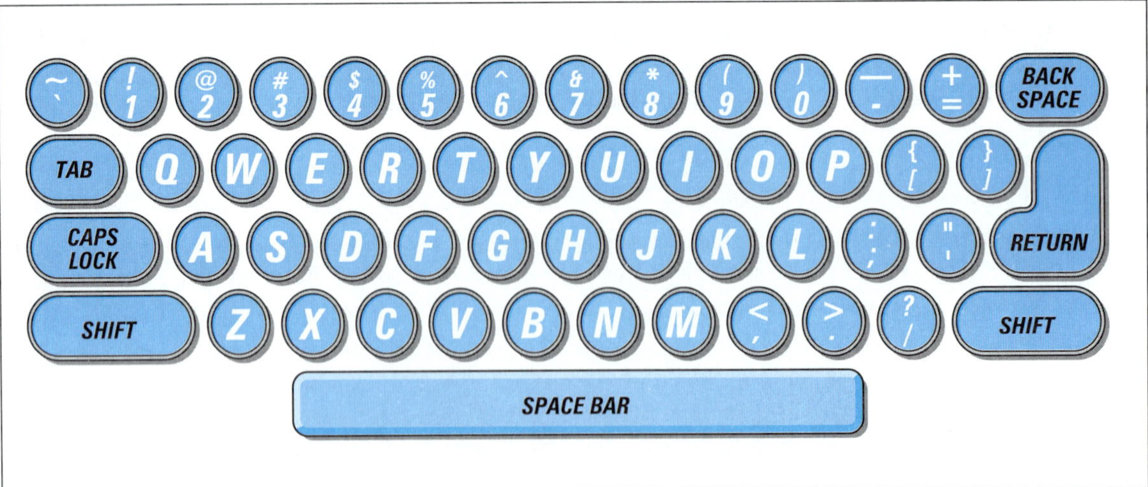

Figure 9-1: Typewriter Keyboard

down the space bar).

Back Space Key: The Back Space key moves you one space to the left if you press it once. On computers, this key also automatically erases any character or space it steps into. When pressed and held down, the Back Space key on electric typewriters will continue to move to the left. On computers, it will move you an indefinite amount of spaces to the left deleting or erasing any letters if may find on its way.

Return or Enter Key: This key is pressed with your right little finger when you want to start a new line or return to the left-hand margin. It will take you one space down and flush to the left margin when depressed. On typewriters, the Return key must be depressed at the end of each line or when your type reaches the right-hand margin. Computers and some electric typewriters have an automatic wrap-around feature. This means that when your type nears the right margin, it automatically drops to the next line and begins at the left margin. This characteristic is called Word Wrap.

If you wish to double space between lines or paragraphs, simply depress the Return or Enter key two times. For more spaces, press it as many times as spaces are needed.

Tab Key: The Tab key indents your type to a set location. It is possible to set the tab stops at any location you desire, and there is usually an unlimited number of tab stops that can be set per document. Each keyboard is different in the setting of tabs, but usually you move the cursor or type mechanism to the position desired and depress a key.

The Mechanics of Typing

When learning to type, carry out the motions properly from the very beginning. Otherwise, you may develop a habit that will eventually prevent you from gaining accuracy and speed. The six basic rules to follow include:

1. Sit in a comfortable chair with your back held straight and your feet flat on the floor. Elbows should be held at your sides and your lower arms should protrude perpendicular to your body. The keyboard should rest at an angle that allows your arms to be held at a 90° angle, not raised toward your chest or lowered to your lap. Your wrists should be held firm and straight, and your fingers should curve downward over the keyboard. Never rest your wrists or palms on the edge of the keyboard. Continual typing with your arms and hands in an incorrect position can cause muscle strain and damage.
2. Strike the keys swiftly and firmly, with just enough pressure to cause the key to depress and the character to appear. Striking the keys too lightly will cause errors because some of the keys will not appear. Striking the keys too hard can, over a period of time, cause tendinitis and damage to your fingers.
3. Strike the keys with the proper finger, regardless of how unnatural it may seem at first. With time, your fingers will grow accustomed to their positions. Type smoothly and evenly, with rhythm.
4. Never look at your fingers while typing. This can be an extremely difficult habit to break. It also causes a lack of speed and accuracy, since it is impossible to look at your fingers and the document from which you are typing from at the same time. When learning to type, place a picture of the keyboard nearby, but not in your direct line of vision. Then, if you forget the position of a key, refer to the illustration instead of looking down at your hands.
5. Keep your book or whatever original material from which you are typing at your right-hand side. If you have a typing stand, place it in front of your keyboard and slightly to the right.
6. Do not become discouraged. It takes time to correctly memorize all the keys and to train your fingers to remember where they are. The only way to gain speed and accuracy is by practicing for long periods of time. Remember that if typing were a skill that took only a few hours to learn, everyone would know how to type and it would cease to become a marketable skill.

Following these simple rules from the beginning will help you to gain accuracy and speed without causing possible harm or injury.

Home Keys

The keys A, S, D, F, J, K, L, and the character ; are considered the home keys. This means that these are the keys that your fingers normally rest on. Your fingers are placed on the home keys as follows:

Left little:	A
Left ring:	S
Left middle:	D
Left index:	F
Right index:	J
Right middle:	K
Right ring:	L
Right little:	;
Right thumb:	Space Bar
Left thumb free	

Memorizing the keys and training your fingers takes time and practice. There is no other way to learn how to type. After you have studied the above keys and the position of your fingers, type each of the following lines 3 times without looking at your fingers or the keyboard.

```
fff jjj fff jjj fff jjj fff jjj fff jjj
ddd kkk ddd kkk ddd kkk ddd kkk ddd kkk
sss lll sss lll sss lll sss lll sss lll
aaa ;;; aaa ;;; aaa ;;; aaa ;;; aaa ;;;
fdsa jkl; fdsa jkl; fdsa jkl; fdsa jkl;
fd sa jk l; fd sa jk l; fd sa jk l; fd
f d s a j k l ; f d s a j k l ; f d s a
aaa ;;; aaa ;;; aaa ;;; aaa ;;; aaa ;;;
sss lll sss lll sss lll sss lll sss lll
ddd kkk ddd kkk ddd kkk ddd kkk ddd kkk
fff jjj fff jjj fff jjj fff jjj fff jjj
asdf ;lkj asdf ;lkj asdf ;lkj asdf ;lkj
as df ;l kj as df ;l kj as df ;l kj as
a s d f ; l k j a s d f ; l k j a s d f
```

If you feel comfortable that you have mastered the placement of the home keys, continue to the next section. If not, practice the preceding letters. Move on only when you are comfortable. Trying to learn too much too soon only causes confusion and errors.

G and H

Next, place your fingers on the home keys and reach the G and H keys with the following fingers:

Left index:	G
Right index:	H

When you are reaching for a key, your hands should remain in position over the home keys. Only the finger you are reaching with should move.

To practice, type each of the following lines 3 times without looking at your fingers or the keyboard:

```
asdfg ;lkjh asdfg ;lkjh asdfg ;lkjh as
asg dfg g ;lh kjh h gh g h h g hg h g
g h a h g d g h f h g j g h k h g l g h
gfdsa hjkl; gfdsa hjkl; gfdsa hjkl; gfd
sag gad gas dag gag gla ga; gal gag gak
has sha ash hsg hal hla jah hsh ha; haf
```

R, T, U, and Y

Now place your fingers on the home keys and reach the R, T, U, and Y keys with the following fingers:

Left index:	R
Left index:	T
Right index:	U
Right index:	Y

To practice, type each of the following lines 3 times without looking at your fingers or the keyboard:

```
fff ffr frr rrr frf fff ffr frr rrr frf
fff fft ftt ttt ftf fff fft ftt ttt ftf
jjj jju juu uuu juj jjj jju juu uuu juj
jjj jjy jyy yyy jyj jjj jjy jyy yyy jyj
frf far jr; kar dra jar lar gra har ard
ftf fat jt; tag lat tal gat sat rat tar
juj jug dul suk ful tul usu sur aru rud
jyj jay day lay say ray yay yat suy fuy
```

V, B, M, and N

Now place your fingers on the home keys and reach the V, B, M, and N keys with the following fingers:

Left index:	V
Left index:	B
Right index:	M
Right index:	N

To practice, type each of the following lines 3 times without looking at your fingers or the keyboard:

```
fff ffv fvv vvv fvf fff ffv fvv vvv fvf
fff ffb fbb bbb fbf fff ffb fbb bbb fbf
jjj jjm jmm mmm jmj jjj jjm jmm mmm jmj
jjj jjn jnn nnn jnj jjj jjn jnn nnn jnj
fvf jav vul vak vs; vur uva gav vas tav
fbf bat but bar bla blu aba bad fab buk
jmj mat may mud mak tam sam ham mam yam
jnj jan nal ny; tan nul tun sun nan man
```

E, W, Q, I, O, and P

Place your fingers on the home keys and reach the E, W, Q, I, O, and P keys with the following fingers:

Left middle:	E
Left ring:	W
Left little:	Q
Right middle:	I
Right ring:	O
Right little:	P

Type each line 3 times without looking at your fingers or the keyboard. Remember to also keep your hands held over the home keys and reach up with your fingers, not with your whole hands.

```
ddd dde dee eee ded ddd dde dee eee ded
sss ssw sww www sws sss ssw sww www sws
aaa aaq aqq qqq aqa aaa aaq aqq qqq aqa
kkk kki kii iii kik kkk kki kii iii kik
lll llo loo ooo lol lll llo loo ooo lol
;;; ;;p ;pp ppp ;p; ;;; ;;p ;pp ppp ;p;
ded bed tre sel yen met set men ten des
sws saw law mew wed was wer ewe wev new
aqa qua meq kaq teq que naq quq laq gbq
kik sid hit qui ali imi qui tri sif kri
lol low ono dos boy quo oso dos lof mot
;p; ps; pro pep map pie gap pre pap pla
```

C, X, Z, Comma, Period, and /

Place your fingers on the home keys and reach the C, X, Z, ,, ., and / keys with the following fingers:

Left middle:	C
Left ring:	X
Left little:	Z
Right middle:	,
Right ring:	.
Right little:	/

To practice, type each of the following lines 3 times without looking at your fingers or the keyboard:

```
ddd ddc dcc ccc dcd ddd ddc dcc ccc dcd
sss ssx sxx xxx sxs sss ssx sxx xxx sxs
aaa aaz azz zzz aza aaa aaz azz zzz aza
kkk kk, k,, ,,, k,k kkk kk, k,, ,,, k,k
lll ll. l.. ... l.l lll ll. l.. ... l.l
;;; ;;/ ;// /// ;/; ;;; ;;/ ;// /// ;/;
dcd doc cab ice cat cut mic com mac cap
sxs sox pix rex tax tix xas six max tex
aza zap zig zoo zem zag zeb zip aze laz
k,k hi, is, as, me, no, he, a,e r,z fa,
l.l it. be. do. we. .a. ed. so. of. it.
;/; /a/ p/m w/m z/x w/o w/i a/m /p/ f/s
```

5, 4, 6, and 7

Now we will begin learning the number keys. Place your fingers on the home keys and reach the 5, 4, 6, and 7 keys as follows:

Left index:	5
Left index:	4
Right index:	6
Right index:	7

To practice, type each of the following lines 3 times without looking at your fingers or the keyboard:

```
fff ff5 f55 555 f5f fff ff5 f55 555 f5f
fff ff4 f44 444 f4f fff ff4 f44 444 f4f
jjj jj6 j66 666 j6j jjj jj6 j66 666 j6j
jjj jj7 j77 777 j7j jjj jj7 j77 777 j7j
f5f if5 s5e j5l 5m. 5m5 5,5 5ea 5am 5pm
f4f of4 4kw ,4. 4ol 4aa 4so 4or as4 be4
j6j mi6 d6s z6; p6w ba6 6m6 6pm 6gh w6q
j7j 7nu me7 v7b pa7 j7a 7k7 er7 nm7 7ju
```

3, 2, 1, 8, 9, and 0

Place your fingers on the home keys and reach the 3, 2, 1, 8, 9, and 0 keys as follows:

Left middle:	3
Left ring:	2
Left little:	1
Right middle:	8
Right ring:	9
Right little:	0

To practice, type each of the following lines 3 times

without looking at your fingers or the keyboard:

ddd dd3 d33 333 d3d ddd dd3 d33 333 d3d
sss ss2 s22 222 s2s sss ss2 s22 222 s2s
aaa aa1 a11 111 a1a aaa aa1 a11 111 a1a
kkk kk8 k88 888 k8k kkk kk8 k88 888 k8k
lll ll9 l99 999 l9l lll ll9 l99 999 l9l
;;; ;;0 ;00 000 ;0; ;;; ;;0 ;00 000 ;0;
d3d f.3 3,g 3ox p3a 3d; cd3 mr3 q3. 3o3
s2s so2 mr2 i2x li2 2sw 2mx 2i2 iu2 to2
a1a pa1 ,1. ic1 my1 1qa 1mp 1st 1e1 pc1
k8k k8d je8 oa8 8r; 8th i8i m8t 8b8 8w8
l9l ls9 im9 9g9 as9 9th 9.9 nw9 tp9 o9o
;0; e0; kw0 0v0 rb0 0b0 hs0 0w0 0ta 0ma

The Shift Keys

Place your fingers on the home keys and reach the left Shift key as follows:

Left little: Shift

To practice, type each of the following lines 3 times without looking at your fingers or the keyboard (note that : is the upper case of ;):

Hi: No, He: Is. Low: Hit How: Yes
Your Poll Mine Hunt Kilo Poet Much
Piles Halls House Jacks Liver Minor
Heroic Intern Joggle Knives Lagoon
Misery Needle Option Partly United
Yogurt Profit Indeed Kindly Manage

Now, place your fingers on the home keys and reach the right Shift key as follows:

Right little: Shift

To practice, type each of the following lines 3 times without looking at your fingers or the keyboard:

Bus Tea Dry Was Fit Cuts Said Quit
Rice Toys When Cars Exit Fire Sold
Quiet Zebra Bones Color Trash Drive
Accept Become Citrus Dreamy Eldest
Finder Goggle Quorum Rubber Sleepy
Tendon Vanity Warren Zodiac Symbol

Caps Lock Key

Your left little finger should tap the Lock or Caps Lock key once to type all capitals (do not hold it down). Tap it one more time to get lower case type. Put your fingers back to their normal position reaching and typing the necessary keys:

Place your fingers on the home keys and reach Lock or Caps Lock as follows:

Left little: Lock/Caps Lock

To practice, type each of the following lines 3 times without looking at your fingers or the keyboard:

DO NOT cross the street.
Judith Smith spelled LOVE.
Welcome to THE ZOO.
The band MONEY will perform at CITY PARK on December 1st.
The typist misspelled CHARACTERISTIC.
PLEASE RECYCLE.
1994 will be THE YEAR OF ACCOMPLISHMENTS.
DOWNTOWN HOSPITAL buys medical supplies at SUPPLIES UNLIMITED.
She wants to shop at BROADWAY STORE. Tell her to make a LEFT on 2nd Avenue and a RIGHT on Broadway Street.
Some students will attend CONTINENTAL SCHOOL in N.Y.

Symbols or Characters

Symbols or characters are included on every typewriter and computer. However, different keyboards may vary slightly in the types of symbols offered and the position of these symbols. When learning the following symbols, consult the illustration at the end of this chapter. If the symbols that your keyboard offers are different from the ones included here, replace the listed symbol with the one that appears in the same position on your keyboard.

It is important to practice the use of symbols. Although you may not use them as much as you will the other types of keys, you should know what symbols are available and where they are located.

Lower Case Symbols

Place your fingers on the home keys and reach the following keys: ‘ - = [ ] ’ as follows:

Left little: ‘

Right little: - = [ ] ’

To practice, type each of the following lines 3 times without looking at your fingers or the keyboard:

```
aaa aa` a`` ``` a`a aaa aa` a`` ``` a`a
;;; ;;- ;-- --- ;-; ;;; ;;- ;-- --- ;-;
;;; ;;= ;== === ;=; ;;; ;;= ;== === ;=;
;;; ;;[ ;[[ [[[ ;[; ;;; ;;[ ;[[ [[[ ;[;
;;; ;;] ;]] ]]] ;]; ;;; ;;] ;]] ]]] ;];
;;; ;;' ;'' ''' ;'; ;;; ;;' ;'' ''' ;';
a`a `d` fg` jo` `im p`l `e` ``s `cc z`n
;-; -w- if- c-c v-v be- -so o-o a-- h-g
a=b e=i o=m =k= w== x=z ==b e=g p=u
[a. [t; [if /[a [qu [i, [rr [be [or [my
he] or] .], ed] ]ol ]qu to] si] yu] no]
'i' 'k' km' re' m's to' 'x' 'sa 'tr 'si
```

Upper Case Symbols

Place your fingers on the home keys and reach the remaining symbol keys as follows. You will need to depress the opposing Shift key at the same time (hold the left Shift key with your left little finger when typing a character with your right hand, and vice versa). When the Caps Lock button is turned on, these keys still function on the lower case character unless the Shift key is held. In essence, it makes no difference whether or not the Caps Lock key is on. The finger positions are as follows:

Left index: %
Left index: $
Left middle: #
Left ring: @
Left little: !
Left little: ~
Right index: ^
Right index: &
Right middle: *
Right ring: (
Right little:)
Right little: _
Right little: +
Right little: {
Right little: }
Right little: "
Right middle: <
Right ring: >
Right little: ?

To practice, type each of the following lines 3 times without looking at your fingers or the keyboard:

```
AAA AA~ A~~ ~~~ A~A AAA AA~ A~~ ~~~ A~A
AAA AA! A!! !!! A!A AAA AA! A!! !!! A!A
SSS SS@ S@@ @@@ S@S SSS SS@ S@@ @@@ S@S
DDD DD# D## ### D#D DDD DD# D## ### D#D
FFF FF$ F$$ $$$ F$F FFF FF$ F$$ $$$ F$F
FFF FF% F%% %%% F%F FFF FF% F%% %%% F%F
JJJ JJ^ J^^ ^^^ J^J JJJ JJ^ J^^ ^^^ J^J
JJJ JJ& J&& &&& J&J JJJ JJ& J&& &&& J&J
KKK KK* K** *** K*K KKK KK* K** *** K*K
LLL LL( L(( ((( L(L LLL LL( L(( ((( L(L
::: ::) :)) ))) :): ::: ::) :)) ))) :):
::: ::_ :__ ___ :_: ::: ::_ :__ ___ :_:
::: ::+ :++ +++ :+: ::: ::+ :++ +++ :+:
::: ::{ :{{ {{{ :{: ::: ::{ :{{ {{{ :{:
::: ::} :}} }}} :}: ::: ::} :}} }}} :}:
::: ::" :"" """ :": ::: ::" :"" """ :":
KKK KK< K<< <<< K<K KKK KK< K<< <<< K<K
LLL LL> L>> >>> L>L LLL LL> L>> >>> L>L
::: ::? :?? ??? :?: ::: ::? :?? ??? :?:
```

When you have completed this section, you have learned all the keys. Practice is needed to learn to type with speed and accuracy.

Typing Speed

Typing speed is measured in words per minute (wpm). Most jobs for health claims examiners and medical billers require a typing speed of at least 50 wpm. To figure out the speed at which you type, you will need to take a timed test.

Most timed tests are based on a 5-minute test. To take a 5-minute timed test, you will need a manuscript of sufficient length to test your skills and a timer. Do not use a clock because you will be constantly looking at the clock rather than the manuscript, and the test will not be accurate.

Get all equipment ready to type. This includes putting paper in the typewriter or warming up the computer and making sure the keyboard, your chair, and the manuscript are all in the correct positions. Then place your name in the upper left-hand corner of the page. In the right-hand corner, place the words Typing Test. Directly below the words Typing Test, put the date and time of the test. This will allow you to place your tests in chronologic order and to chart your progress over a period of time.

When you are ready, start the timer and begin to type the manuscript. Keep your body in the proper position and remain focused on what you are doing. If you make a mistake, ignore it and continue. Do not try to fix it. You should attempt to copy the manuscript exactly. This means that you should strike the Enter key to return at the end of each line.

Continue typing until the timer goes off. When the time is up, immediately stop typing, even if you are in the middle of a word. Remove the paper from the typewriter or print the page if you are typing on a computer.

Read through the document you typed, comparing it with the original. Circle any errors, typographic mistakes, and misspelled or omitted words. Errors include any punctuation and upper or lower case differences from the original. Transposed letters (eg, teh for the) count as one error. However, if you make two mistakes in a single word, each mistake should be counted separately.

Now, count the words you typed. Each word counts as a single word, regardless of its length. Do not count any unfinished words at the end of the test. However, count any words that contained errors or misspellings. Next, subtract the total number of errors you made from the number of words you typed. This gives you your typing speed for a 5-minute run. To figure out your words per minute, you need to divide this number by five. Round your answer to the nearest whole number. This is your typing speed.

Do all your calculations on the paper where you can see it. This way you can plot not only the change in your typing speed, but the changes in the number of errors. Remember that accuracy is as important as speed, and reducing your errors will increase the resultant wpm figure.

Some companies use a 3-minute timed test or a 1-minute timed test. These shorter tests are not as accurate as a 5-minute timed test because you tend to start out typing quickly, then lose concentration and speed as more time passes.

Do not be discouraged if progress seems slow. It takes much time and practice to learn to type quickly and accurately.

Summary

Learning to type is one of the greatest skills you can have in the job world. It gives you a marketable skill, without which your services would be far less valuable. In learning to type, it is important to follow the basic rules and keep them in mind at all times.

When you have memorized the rules and the positions of the keys, practice alone will give you speed and accuracy. This can be achieved by typing many different types of letters, reports, and manuscripts.

To figure out your typing speed, subtract the total number of errors from the total number of words typed and divide by the number of minutes in the timed test.

Assignments

Complete the Questions for Review.
Complete Typing Exercises 9-1 to 9-3.
Continue typing on a regular basis until you have gained a speed of at least 50 wpm.

Questions for Review

Directions: Answer the following questions without looking back into the material just covered. Write your answers in the space provided.

1. What are the two most important aspects of typing?
   a. ______
   b. ______
2. Which are the Home Keys? ______
3. Which key will give you an indefinite amount of spaces to the right if you press it and hold it down? ______
4. What finger do you use for the RETURN or ENTER KEY? ______
5. What key do you tap to get upper case type? ______
6. Which two keys do you press at the same time to type the symbol * ? ______
7. Which finger do you use to type v and b? ______
8. Which finger do you use to press the SPACE BAR? ______
9. Can you use the Caps Lock key to access the symbols shown above the numbers? ______
10. How do you figure out your typing speed? ______

If you were unable to answer any of the questions, refer back to the section and then fill in the answers.

Exercise 9-1

Directions: Type each of the following at least 10 times. These sentences contain each of the letters of the alphabet.

1. Aa Bb Cc Dd Ee Ff Gg Hh Ii Jj Kk Ll Mm Nn Oo Pp Qq Rr Ss Tt Uu Vv Ww Xx Yy Zz
2. Frank's quaint, cozy garden had lamp boxes just to view.
3. Many joyous zoo giraffes quietly wept for they lacked a voice box.
4. Agatha, Buzzy, Jack, Fred and Vicky Wixcomb are quintuplets.
5. Jonquils, daisies, honeysuckle, ivy, box elder, and zinnias; what a pretty formal garden.
6. The quick yellow duck jumped into the bag to hide from seven lazy vixen.
7. Brown, gold, fuscia, honey and jade mixed crazy quilts look very pretty.
8. The yellow daisies grew quickly next to farmer Jezpon's bean vine.
9. Frederick Blimpton's quiet horse is known as The Crazy Jug Vox.
10. The lazy jack-in-the-box quickly grew defensive around the toy mop.

Exercise 9-2

Directions: Type each of the following at least 10 times. The sets contain numbers, characters and letters.

1. 1111000022229999333388884444777755556666

2. 2299338844770011992288338844773388229900

3. !!!!))))@@@@((((####****$$$$&&&&%%%%^^^^

4. @@((##**$$&&%%&&^^&&$$!!))@@(($$**^^))!!

5. ++!!__~~++##(($45*440#)$*@0920(39012$0@4

6. thei381982*e929*(73 *^82(0817(8j*we732qp

7. qplc,eiltight,zalpwi.b,keiltilcnakwi.ait

8. o3smco2qpm2858908cmws3u03mx,.xcm-1098477

9. 'qie0018c8fm,ml2k4ualj(8672347(964#6^7&t

10. thisisafunexercisetotypewehopeyouenjoyedit

Exercise 9-3

Directions: Type the following page without looking at your fingers or at the keyboard.

Customer service is one of the most vital functions that health claims examiners or medical billers can perform. Without good customer relations, customers go elsewhere. Although it takes hard work, patience, and a good disposition to perform good customer service functions, it is well worth the time and effort.

The following are the most important topics that were discussed in this chapter, which should be always kept in mind when dealing with your customers:

Answer the call promptly.

Identify yourself by giving your name and title.

Write down the caller's name and ID number as soon as identification is provided.

Be professional in voice and choice of words.

Listen to what the caller has to say. If (s)he is angry, let her/him get the anger out.

Don't react to a caller's hostility with hostility of your own.

Give out accurate information. If you don't know the answer to a question, take the caller's name and phone number and tell him or her that you will find out and call back.

Stay informed concerning all policies and procedures and know the benefits of the group(s) for whom you are responsible.

Be patient with the caller. He or she might not be familiar with insurance procedures.

Always be supportive of your peers and your company. Acknowledge when a mistake has been made but don't make any derogatory remarks about other personnel or company policies or procedures.

Be empathetic. Many callers are experiencing serious illness, death of a family member, or financial problems.

10

Computer Basics

In this chapter you will learn:

- General knowledge of a basic computer system, its use and purpose.
- To describe the keyboard in its five components: Typewriter Keys, Numeric Keypad, Editing and Cursor Control Keys, Function Keys, Status Lights.
- The three basic types of computer systems that may be utilized in a medical office.
- The pros and cons of computerizing the medical office.

As with most other industries, the majority of providers of service, administrators, and payors are automated. The computer has therefore become an indispensable tool.

Only time and usage will make the medical biller and the health claims examiner accurate and fast on the computer. However, the following information may assist you when entering data.

- Become familiar with the processing program you are using. If you know the fields (spots where specific information is entered), input will significantly increase since less verification and decision-making will be required.
- When learning to use the computer, watch either the video screen or the claim or record. Every effort should be made not to watch your fingers, since it is a difficult habit to break once learned.
- Prepare your claims or medical records so that less shuffling of papers is required (eg, unstaple, arrange by date).
- A comfortable chair that is adjusted to the correct height decreases fatigue.
- Both hands should be free for typing in data. Pens, pencils, and other tools should not be held while entering data.

The computer is actually a combination of three different machines, the computer, the monitor, and the keyboard.

The Computer

The computer is the rectangular box that houses the memory and functional components of the computer. A degree in computer engineering is needed to understand all the inner workings of the computer. However, you should become familiar with a few of these components, such as the power switch, the reset button, the disk drives, and the repairs.

The power switch is the on/off switch for the computer. It can be located anywhere on the computer, but is often found toward the back.

The reset button is often found on the front of the computer. Pressing this button clears the screen and "reboots" or restarts the system. In other words, it achieves the same function as turning the computer off and then on again. Use caution with this button. If you do not save your data prior to pressing this button, it will be lost.

A computer disk drive is simply a place for the storage of information. Usually, a computer contains a "hard drive" within it. The hard drive provides space (memory) for information to be stored within the computer itself.

If there is insufficient memory in the hard drive or if there is a need to make data transportable to another computer or to make a copy of the data, disks are used to record the information on.

In the front of the computer is a slot (or several slots). These are alternate (floppy) disk drives. If the data you are using are stored on a disk, slide the disk into the slot, and "close the door" by turning the small handle near the opening. This handle actually lowers an internal component to allow it to read the information that is stored on the disk. If the door is not closed, the computer will be unable to read the information.

At no time should a medical biller or claims examiner be required to repair the computer. If something is wrong with the system, a computer repair technician should be called for on-site repair or the computer should be returned to a computer service center. Ask your supervisor what procedure to follow. First, however, make sure that all connections are in place at the back of the computer. This is similar to making sure that a television is plugged in before calling a repairman.

There are a number of connections between the computer and its various components, the power source, and peripheral units (eg, modems, fax machines). To ensure that all connections are in place, turn off the computer, then simply look at the back of the computer. If any cords or cables are hanging down, they may be the source of your problem. However, be sure that you know where to plug in the cable before attempting to slide it into any of the slots. Plugging in a cord or cable incorrectly can destroy your machine, your programs, or the machines and programs of others whose computers are attached to yours.

The Monitor

The computer monitor is the screen that is connected to the computer. It is this screen that allows you to see the programs and the data you are working with. There are four items you should be familiar with on the computer monitor: the power switch, the contrast control, the brightness control, and the cursor.

Like the power switch on the computer, this button turns the monitor on and off. When the computer is not in use for an extended period of time, the power switch should be turned off to prevent the image from burning into the phosphor on the screen. Be aware that turning off the monitor does not turn off the computer. Therefore, the data and information you were working on are still there; you simply can't see them.

The contrast control turns the contrast up and down between varying fields. This control is usually used to provide more or less contrast between those sections in a document that have been bolded or highlighted and those that have not.

The brightness control knob changes the brightness of the image on the screen. Adjust this knob so that you can read the screen without difficulty and without glare.

The cursor is the small lighted symbol on the monitor screen, which tells you where you are in the program. Depending on the system, this symbol may look like a bright straight line, a bright blinking line, or a blinking or solid box.

The Keyboard

The keyboard is your primary means of communicating with your computer. The input commands and data are typed in through the keyboard. Its layout roughly resembles that of an ordinary typewriter. To describe the keyboard more clearly, we will divide it into six parts, each with its own function:

1. Keyboard angle adjustment
2. The typewriter keypad
3. The numeric keypad
4. The editing and cursor control keys
5. The function keys
6. The three status lights

Keyboard Angle Adjustment

You can adjust your keyboard to two different positions for your typing comfort. To adjust, push on the adjustable leg handles which are located underneath the keyboard on both sides, and turn them to the desired position.

The Typewriter Keypad

The typewriter area of the keyboard looks and behaves a lot like a standard typewriter keyboard. Like a typewriter, the Shift key produces capital letters. To type the special characters shown above the numbers on the number keys, hold down the Shift key and press the appropriate key. For example, the Shift key with the number 1 produces an exclamation mark (!).

The computer keyboard also includes several special control keys specifically associated with computer operations, including Esc, Ctrl, Alt, and Enter.

Here's a brief explanation of some important typewriter and control keys:

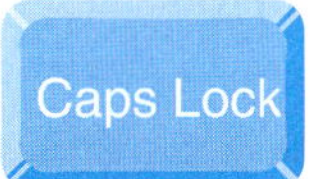

CAPS LOCK—With this key, you can type upper case letters without holding down the Shift key. When Caps Lock is engaged, the indicator light in the upper right-hand corner of the keyboard lights up. The Caps Lock key affects only the 26 letters of the alphabet. To get special symbols, you still need to press the Shift key.

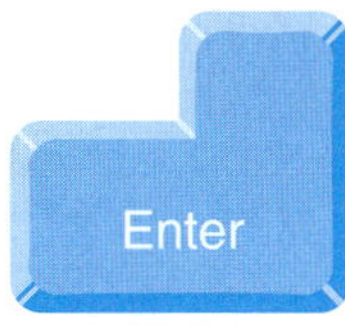

ENTER—This key acts as both the Return key and the Enter key. As a Return key, it ends the line being typed and advances the cursor to the next line. As the Enter key, it is used to execute commands you have typed.

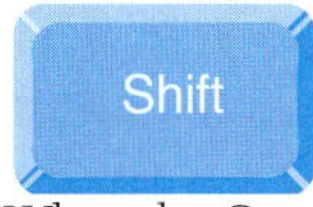

SHIFT—For upper case letters, punctuation, or symbols, either one of the two Shift keys can be pressed. When the Caps Lock key is engaged, the Shift key acts as an "Un-Shift" key, allowing you to type lower case letters.

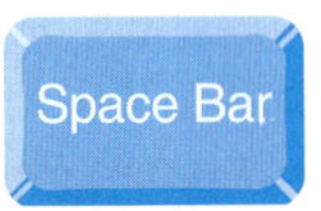

SPACE BAR—Moves the cursor one position to the right. Also erases characters to the right replacing them with blanks.

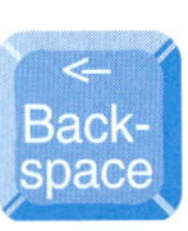

BACKSPACE—Like the Backspace key on a typewriter, this key erases one character to the left of the cursor.

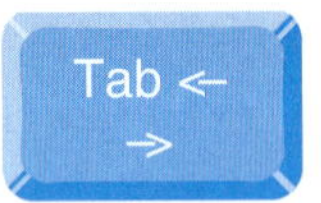

TAB—Like the typewriter Tab key, it moves the cursor to the next tab stop. In some programs the Tab key acts as a margin release to the left if the Shift key is depressed, or moves the cursor one tab spot to the left.

ESC—The Escape key has different functions, depending on the program.

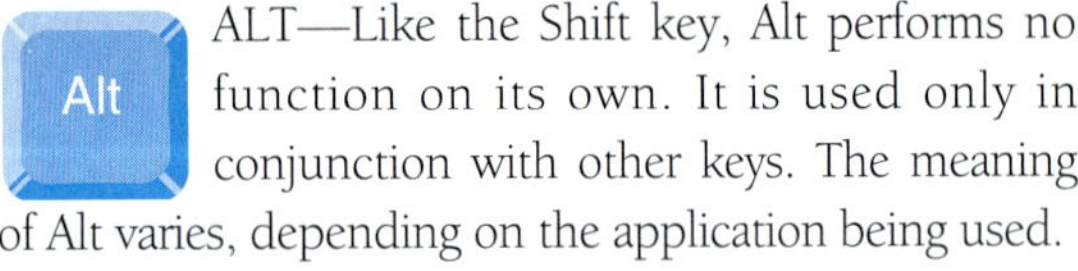

ALT—Like the Shift key, Alt performs no function on its own. It is used only in conjunction with other keys. The meaning of Alt varies, depending on the application being used.

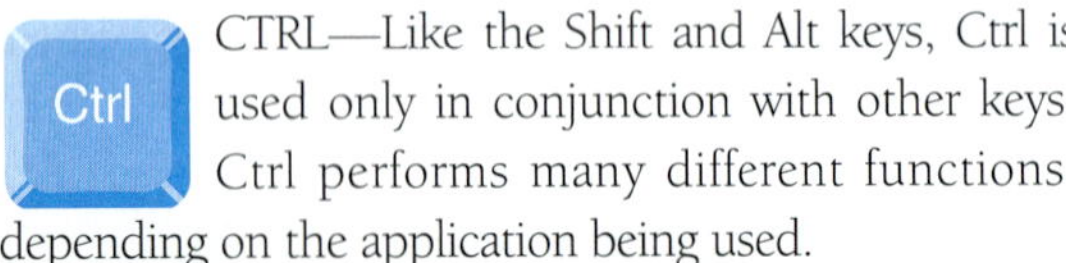

CTRL—Like the Shift and Alt keys, Ctrl is used only in conjunction with other keys. Ctrl performs many different functions, depending on the application being used.

Pressing two or three keys simultaneously can perform a series of unique program control and screen control functions.

To produce the function indicated, press and hold down the first (and second in a series of three) key(s) and press the last key to invoke the corresponding function.

The following list of functions available is by no means comprehensive:

Keys	**Function**	**Description**
Ctrl/Break	Break	Terminates the execution of a program and identifies the line where it stops.
Ctrl/Alt/Del	System Soft Reset	Causes a reload from the diskette or fixed disk.
Shift/Print	Print Screen	Causes all data on the screen to be printed.

The Numeric Keypad

The numeric keypad, located separately from the alphabetic keys, is usually located on the right-hand side of a computer keyboard. The keypad performs a dual function.

With the Num Lock key engaged (indicated by the status light in the upper right-hand corner of some keyboards), the keypad can be used for the rapid data entry of numbers. Without Num Lock, the keypad can be used to move the cursor or to perform special editing features.

A 101-key enhanced keyboard provides a separate keypad for cursor control and editing (located immediately to the left of the numeric keypad). For this reason, most users find it convenient to leave the Num Lock key on, thus allowing for the rapid entry of numbers. If your keyboard is not a 101-key enhanced board, you will probably not want to leave the Num Lock key on.

The following keys operate the same, regardless of whether the Num Lock key is on or off:

ENTER—Works the same as the Enter key on the Typewriter keypad.

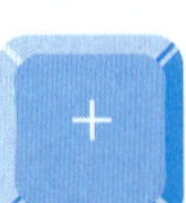

Displays the Plus symbol.

Key		
–	Displays the Minus symbol.	
*	Displays the Asterisk, used for multiplication.	
/	Displays the Slash, used for division.	

The following keys behave differently, depending on the status of the Num Lock key:

Key	Num Lock On	Num Lock Off
1 End	The number 1	END—Moves the cursor to the end of the line.
2 ↓	The number 2	↓—Moves the cursor down.
3 Pg Dn	The number 3	Pg Dn—Moves the cursor down one page, or 25 lines.
4 ←	The number 4	←—Moves the cursor to the left.
5	The number 5	No function.
6 →	The number 6	→—Moves the cursor to the right.
7 Home	The number 7	HOME—Moves the cursor to the screen's upper-left corner.
8 ↑	The number 8	↑—Moves the cursor up.
9 Pg Up	The number 9	PG UP—Moves the cursor up one page, or 25 lines.
0 Ins	The number 0	INS—Insert mode. Characters typed are inserted before text that already exists.
. Del	The Decimal	DEL—(Delete). Erases one character point at the position of the cursor.

Editing and Cursor Control Keys

The 101-key enhanced keyboard contains a separate set of editing keys usually located between the Typewriter and Numeric keypads.

Key	
Home	HOME—Moves the cursor to the first character of the top line of the screen.
↑	CURSOR UP—Moves the cursor up one line for each key stroke.
↓	CURSOR DOWN—Moves the cursor down one line for each key stroke.
→	CURSOR RIGHT—Moves the cursor to the right one character position for each key stroke.

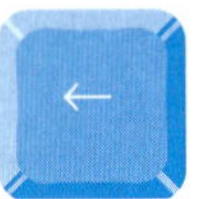

CURSOR LEFT—Moves the cursor to the left one character position for each key stroke.

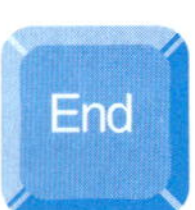

END—Moves the cursor to the right of the last character on the current line.

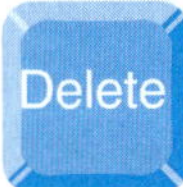

DELETE—Deletes characters at the cursor. All characters to the right will be moved left. If this key is held down, it will erase each character as it reaches the cursor.

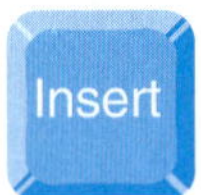

INSERT/TYPEOVER—On Insert, characters typed are inserted before previously typed text, pushing the existing text to the right. On Typeover, existing characters are typed over.

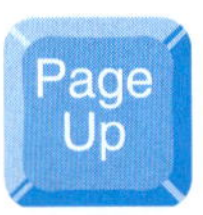

PAGE UP—Moves the cursor up one page, or 25 lines.

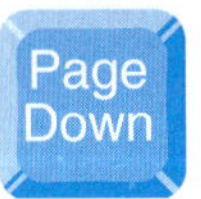

PAGE DN—Moves the cursor down one page, or 25 lines.

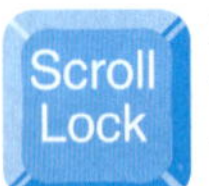

SCROLL LOCK—When pressed, the Scroll Lock light will be illuminated on the keyboard. When the Scroll Lock light is on, it can be turned off by pressing the Scroll Lock key again, which also turns off the Scroll Lock mode of operation. Refer to the computer application program manual for more details on this key.

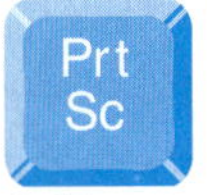

PRINT SCREEN—When pressed, the data displayed on the screen will be printed (if the computer is hooked up to a printer). If the Ctrl key is pressed and held while the Print Screen key is pressed, the printer function will be disabled or enabled.

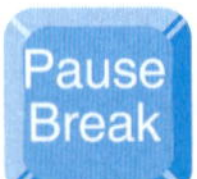

PAUSE BREAK—This key suspends the program execution until another key is pressed. When used with the Ctrl key, the program being run will be terminated.

Function Keys

Along the top of the keyboard or on the left side of some keyboards are 12 function keys that allow complex program commands to be performed with a single keystroke.

Different software programs use function keys for different purposes. Therefore, to properly use these keys, the program-specific user's guide must be referred to. It is highly advisable not to use the function keys without referring to the program instructions, since they may delete data or cancel parts of a program.

The Three Status Lights

The three status lights are usually located in the upper-right corner of the keyboard. They are labeled NUM LOCK, CAPS LOCK and SCROLL LOCK. The Num Lock light, when lit, signifies that the Num Lock function is on, thus causing the keys on the numeric keypad to act as numbers, rather than cursor movement keys.

When the Caps Lock light is on, it signifies that all letters typed on the keyboard will appear as capital letters.

Scroll Lock is a feature that only works with some computer programs. When the Scroll Lock is used in these applications, the cursor is locked onto whatever line it is on when the Scroll Lock button is pushed, and the entire page will move around it. For example, if your cursor is halfway down the page when you hit the Scroll Lock button, your cursor will remain halfway down the page. When you hit the arrow down key, the entire document will move up one line, but the cursor will remain in the center of the screen.

Computer Terminology

With the development of computers, a whole new set of terms had to be created to define items relating to the application and use of these machines. Although "computerese" is a complete language that could take years to understand, the person who uses computers will need to be familiar with a number of terms.

Acoustic Coupler—A device consisting of two rubber muffs enclosed in a box that holds a telephone handset. It permits data to be transmitted by converting digital signals into sound waves. These sound waves travel over the phone lines and into the receiving computer where they are converted back into digital information. The acoustic coupler is a type of modem.

Back-Up—A back-up copy is a duplicate file or set of information contained in a different area of the computer or on magnetic tape or disk. This allows you to recreate information if something should happen to your main file.

Batch—A group of documents, papers, or forms that are related in some way, often by date or batch number.

Bit—Binary digit, the smallest possible unit of memory storage. Eight bits is equal to one byte.

Bug—An error in a computer program.

Byte—A measurement for the storage capacity of computers. A byte is equal to eight bits, or roughly the amount of bits needed to make one character or letter.

Cathode Ray Tube (CRT)—A television-type screen attached to a computer. It is also known as a video display terminal (VDT). CRTs are the forerunners of the modern-day monitor.

Central Processing Unit (CPU)—The brains of the computer. It controls the internal memory and directs the processing and the flow of information.

Command Key—A key or combination of keys that activates a command in a computer program.

Cursor—A small light or bar on the computer screen that indicates the position of the next data entry.

Data Base—A collection of electronically stored data.

Debug—To remove errors from a computer or a software program.

Disk—A device for storing information. There are two main types of disks, a hard disk and a floppy disk.

Disk, Hard—A disk made of hard material, which can be stored inside the computer housing, or outside attached securely by cables and wires.

Disk, Floppy—A plastic diskette that holds data information and is easily transportable. Floppy disks come in two types: $5^1/_4$ inches square and $3^1/_2$ inches square. The $5^1/_4$-inch disks are the forerunners of the $3^1/_2$-inch disks. Storage space on floppy disks is much more limited than on a hard disk. The $3^1/_2$-inch disk is contained in a hard plastic shell. The $3^1/_2$-inch disks are beginning to replace $5^1/_4$-inch disks because they are easier to transport, they are more durable, and they can hold more information. However, their memory storage capacity is still far less than that of a hard disk.

Documentation—An instruction book detailing how to use a computer program or piece of equipment.

DOS (Disk operating system)—A set of programmed instructions that tells the computer how to operate.

Down Time—The time during which a computer is not operating properly.

Format—The way the data are organized or the appearance of the data.

Hard Copy—A printout of information from the computer.

Hardware—The pieces or components of a computer system, which can include the monitor, keyboard, hard disk, computer housing, or modem.

Header—A notation that appears at the top of a page or computer screen.

Input—The act of entering information into a computer, or the information itself.

Interface—The linking of two or more computer systems (ie, computer to computer, computer to printer, computer to modem).

K—A unit of memory storage measurement. A K is equal to 1000 bytes.

Keypad—A device that contains the keys that control mathematical function. This unit is separate from the keyboard.

Memory—The ability of the computer to store data.

Menu—A list of items or computer functions displayed on a computer screen from which the operator can choose.

Modem—A device that can convert outgoing digital data into sound waves to be transmitted across telephone lines and can reconvert incoming sound waves into digital data.

Network—An interconnection of two or more computers.

On-line System—(1) A system in which data that is input is entered directly into the computer and output data is sent directly from the computer to where it is used (printer, modem). (2) A system that works without human intervention between the recording and the processing of material.

Optical Character Recognition (OCR)—A device that can read typed characters and convert them to computer data. Also known as a scanner.

Program—Another word for software.

Prompt—A symbol (often >) that indicates that the computer is ready to receive information.

RAM (Random Access Memory)—A data storage system in which data may be stored randomly and retrieved by specifying its location.

Retrieve—The act of locating a stored file and bringing it up on screen.

ROM (Read-Only Memory)—A data storage system in which information can be read, but not changed. This usually includes permanent programs.

Scrolling—The ability to move from one side of the screen to another, top to bottom, or page by page through a document.

Soft Copy—The information displayed on a computer screen.

Sort—The process by which a computer arranges data in a specified order.

Spooling—A device by which the output from a computer is placed in storage queues to await transmission to a device that moves more slowly than the computer output (ie, the storage of data to a file until data can be read by a printer with a more limited memory capacity).

Terminal—A device or system that can receive information from and send information to a computer system.

Time-sharing—The use of a computer device for more than one purpose at one time (eg, working on one document while another is being sent to the printer) or the use of a system by more than one user at one time.

Voice Activation—The ability of a computer or other device to recognize and respond to verbal commands.

Memorizing these terms and their meanings will help you to communicate in an environment that includes computers.

Manual vs Computer System

One of the first questions that comes to mind when discussing computers is "Why should we use a computer system?" This is immediately followed by "What are the pros and cons of computers?" There are as many answers for these questions as there are places to work and types of work done. The cons usually include the following:

- The cost of the computer equipment (whether purchased or leased).
- The cost of software and computer programs, including taking into account their need to be updated on a regular basis.
- The cost of "transient" computer equipment, including data disks, paper, and printer supplies.
- The cost of hiring and training personnel to run the equipment.
- The cost of hiring and training personnel to maintain the equipment.
- The problems associated with "down time." Also consider what the response time will be for assistance when there is a system failure.
- The possible increased difficulty in retrieving information on short notice.
- An increased possibility of losing the data that you have stored.
- The amount of space lost to the computer system, equipment, and related materials.
- The additional costs associated with installing a computer system. These can include the installation of additional telephone and electrical lines, the cost of the added electricity and telephone usage, any interest on the financing of the computer equipment, consulting costs, and insurance and warranty costs on the system.
- The costs associated with converting your present system to a computerized system.

- Depending on the type of computer system that you use, a possible delay in the time that the information is entered and when the reports or forms are printed.

On the other hand, the following are advantages to using a computer system, especially in the medical office:

- Valuable time is saved because the same data can be transferred from one report to another, eliminating the need for duplicating entries.
- Forms look neater and cleaner since errors can be corrected quickly and easily and a new report generated.
- It is easier to get duplicate copies of a single report or form for those who may need them (ie, medical office, patient, insurer).
- There are fewer errors since the computer can be programmed to do certain functions for you (eg, addition of numbers).
- The overhead may be lower than the cost of maintaining, using, and storing manual files.
- Storage is much easier and less bulky than with paper files.
- There may be better management control, and new updated information may be available more readily.
- The office may run more efficiently.
- Accounts receivable may be maintained more accurately and past due accounts are easier to track and trace, thus increasing collections.
- The option of electronic claims submission becomes available, thus decreasing the time between submission and payment of claims.

In addition, when using an outside computer processing center, the system vendor often maintains more up-to-date files and programs without increased cost to the medical office. There is also the added security of having your files stored in a second location away from the medical office.

Types of Computer Systems

After the decision has been made to go to a computerized system, the medical office needs to determine which type of system best meets their needs. There are three main types of computer systems available to the medical office:

1. The office computer or *in-house system* is self-contained in the office. This means that the system contains all necessary units for the running of the desired programs. This type of system has limited storage capabilities, limited program capabilities, and a limited lifetime. Occasionally, this type of system is referred to as a turnkey system. The term *turnkey* refers to a system that is assembled by the vendor and sold as a package. It implies that the system will do everything it is supposed to do as soon as it is turned over to the purchaser.
2. A *batch system* is used where the medical office collects the data to be entered and sends it to a data processing center. Information may be sent by mail or messenger on a daily or weekly basis. The data processing center then enters the data and prints any reports or other information that the medical office needs. This type of system can accommodate a large number of users, thus sharing the costs of equipment, maintenance, and personnel. Larger computers with increased memory capacity are needed for the batch system. Monthly fees are paid by the medical office to the data processing center. A prime example of this type of system is a medical office that sends their information to be processed by an independent medical biller.
3. The third type of computer system is known by many names, including *interactive, remote terminal, on-line batch,* or *time-share system.* The main idea is that the computer system is held by an outside company, but the medical office rents the use of the computer system for a period of time each day or week. This allows the medical office to enter their own information at their terminal and then transfer the information to the outside company. This type of system allows for quick access to the equipment without the cost outlay associated with purchasing the equipment. Storage and maintenance of the equipment are also handled by the outside company. Such systems

require a computer terminal in the medical office and a transmittal device such as a modem. However, there are some systems in which the information is entered on the medical office computer and transferred to a floppy disk; the floppy disk is then mailed or sent by messenger to the data processing center.

Frustration-Free Computing

According to Murphy's Law, anything that can go wrong, will go wrong. However, a number of techniques will help to eliminate the frustration of losing computer-stored information. These eight techniques should be learned and should become a daily part of your computer life.

1. Save your data often and make back-up copies while working on it. A second copy of the data should be saved to a second file when you are finished. A power surge or brief break in the power supply can erase your entries in less than 1 second.
2. Keep a back-up copy in a different location. A second copy of important data should be stored in a different room or, if possible, a different building. This preserves the data in case of fire, destruction of the building, or water damage.
3. Always date the copies of your files so that you can retrieve the latest disk easily.
4. Use permanent disks or tapes to store copies of financial and confidential records and keep them in a secure, fire-proof spot.
5. Maintain a notebook or log, which shows what you have stored in the computer and the file name it is located under.
6. Set up a system for naming documents so that they will be easily accessible even if you do not have the log.
7. Handle data diskettes properly. This includes the following:

   a. Never touch the magnetic media housed inside the plastic cover. On both the 5¼-inch and 3½-inch floppy disks, there is a hole in the plastic through which the computer reads the information. On the 3½-inch disk, this hole is covered by a piece of sliding metal. On the 5¼-inch disk, it is left open.

   b. Store all disks inside plastic or paper covers to protect them from damage. Insert and remove the disk carefully from the cover to prevent scratching the magnetic media.

   c. Never fold, spindle, or mutilate your disk.

   d. Keep diskettes stored at temperatures between 50° and 125° F. Never leave a data disk exposed to sunlight.

   e. Keep all magnets away from your data disks. Information stored on magnetic medium can be erased when it comes in contact with a magnet. This includes the magnet contained in office supplies such as paper clip holders.

   f. Before touching a data disk, discharge any static electricity you may have picked up by touching a piece of metal or an antistatic mat. Static electricity also demagnetizes and therefore erases the data contained on a disk.

   g. When carrying disks across a carpeted area, place the disk inside its protective sleeve and inside another object such as a disk storage box or between the pages of a book. This will prevent erasure by any static electricity that you may pick up by walking across the carpet.

   h. To prevent any changes to information stored on a data disk, cover the "write protect" notch on the side of the disk. This cut-out notch may be covered with tape or labels. To change the data at a later date, simply remove the tape or label.

   i. Do not write on a disk label with ballpoint pen or pencil; use a felt-tip marker. The pressure applied when writing with pen or pencil may cause indentations on the magnetic media, which the computer cannot read around.
8. If you delete information incorrectly or are unable to retrieve information, immediately remove the disk from the computer if you are working with a floppy disk. Do not save anything on the disk. Many computer files can be reconstructed with

the proper programs, but only if the information hasn't been written over.

Remember that it is far easier to retrieve data that has never been lost than to recreate it from scratch. Taking proper care of your data will ensure that it will be retrievable when you need it.

Summary

Computers have infiltrated all aspects of business life, including insurance and medical offices. Using the computer saves time, produces neater and cleaner reports in as many copies as needed, reduces errors, and allows for electronic submission of data to the insurance carrier.

Learning to use a computer program quickly and accurately, and learning the proper means of storing information will provide the health claims examiner and medical biller with a valuable skill.

Assignments

Complete the Questions for Review.

Questions for Review

Directions: Answer the following questions without looking back into the material just covered. Write your answers in the space provided.

1. The numeric keypad is used for the ______________________ when the Num Lock is on.
2. The space bar performs two functions. What are they?
   a. ______________________
   b. ______________________
3. What two functions does the Enter key perform?
   a. ______________________
   b. ______________________
4. Function keys perform what function? ______________________
   ____
5. The cursor is ______________________

If you were unable to answer any of the questions, refer back to the section and then fill in the answers.

11

Correspondence

In this chapter you will learn:

- To understand the three basic components of effective written communications.
- To understand the role of a fiduciary.
- To understand basic ERISA correspondence requirements.
- To write an effective letter.

Correspondence has become an integral part of the business world today. Without effective written communications, it is virtually impossible for a business to succeed. Written communications have permeated every aspect of the business world, from interoffice memos to correspondence with clients to filed reports. The demand for personnel with effective writing skills has also increased.

Therefore, one of the most important skills that an employee can have is the ability to write clearly and effectively. No one wants to read a dull, boring letter, no matter how short. With effective writing techniques, the dullest subject can be made inviting and exciting.

Remember that the reader will judge you and your company by the types of correspondence that he or she receives. Learn to use effective language, which is clear, concise, and interesting. Of course, your correspondence should also be grammatically correct and properly punctuated.

Before you begin writing the correspondence, think of the audience, whether it is a personal letter to a single customer or a newsletter that will be distributed to many people. It will be easier to tailor your writing when you have a clear picture of the reader.

Effectiveness in writing means being able to evoke the type of response you want your reader to have, whether you want the reader to subscribe to your service or to purchase a product or service. Before beginning to compose a letter, ask yourself the following questions:

- Is this correspondence really necessary? If the answer is no, eliminate it.
- Could this information be easily expressed over the phone? Would it save time to do this? If the answer to these questions is yes, pick up the phone and start saving time.
- Has this information already been expressed in previous correspondence? If the answer is yes, perhaps a photocopy of the previous material or a short note referencing it will suffice.
- Is it vital that this information be written down "for the record?" If the answer is yes, then it must be written.

No one wants to waste time reading through information that is not necessary or that has already been covered. Too many communications of this sort cause your reader to pay less attention when an important piece of correspondence arrives. If the previous questions determine that the information must be written, follow these points:

- Determine what you want to say before you begin to write.
- Determine what action or response you are seeking from the reader.
- After the correspondence has been written, proofread it carefully for clarity, proper spelling, and proper grammar.
- Finally, make sure that the correspondence conveys the message that you intended.

One trick is to read the correspondence aloud. This often illustrates punctuation and grammar errors that might not have otherwise been caught. You are used to speaking, and passages that are awkward to say usually signal that something is wrong in the writing.

There is no prescribed length for a letter. It should be long enough to say what you need to say in clear concise language and short enough that your reader doesn't get lost among too many words. When you have completed your idea and made it clear to the reader, your correspondence is complete. Don't delete information just because you want to keep the correspondence brief. If the subject matter is pertinent and has been presented in an interesting manner, the reader will read it regardless of length.

Let your writing reflect your personality. Correspondence that uses language natural to you is usually most effective. It provides a human link between writer and reader. Be concise, simple, and direct, but be yourself.

Most correspondence is composed of three parts: the opening, the body, and the closing.

The Opening

The first paragraph, and especially the first sentence of your correspondence, is critical. You must gain your reader's attention and interest him or her in reading further, and at the same time make the reader receptive to your ideas. Without the reader's attention, you cannot hope to gain the response you are looking for.

Remember that your reader's first interest is nearly always him- or herself. The reader automatically defines the correspondence according to the personal benefits it will bring. Therefore, you must involve the reader or you run the risk of losing him or her.

The two principal purposes of the opening are to attract attention and to develop interest. Therefore, don't try to say too much in the opening. To be successful, the opening must invite sufficient interest to draw the reader into the body of the correspondence.

The Body

The body of the correspondence is where you present the purpose of the communication. Here, you also let the reader know what you wish to obtain from him or her, if anything. Any additional information that is needed to verify the request or purpose should also be included here if it is succinct enough. If it isn't succinct, a copy of the information should be attached and a reference should be included in the body of the letter (eg, see accompanying account statement).

Make sure to provide enough information for the reader to understand your purpose and desire, but not so much that you overwhelm him or her with information. Here also, keep the information concise and move the correspondence forward.

Clarity and Coherence

Clarity in writing means exactness of language. Clarity in your correspondence results in the reader's understanding what you intended to say. If the meaning is not clear, the entire message has failed, no matter how eloquently it was stated. Remember that your reader cannot respond appropriately if he or she can't figure out what you're asking for.

After writing a piece of correspondence, take a moment to put yourself in the reader's place and read the letter as if you were seeing it for the first time. Ask yourself, "Does this say what I intended it to say?" If not, it needs to be rewritten.

Coherence refers to something "sticking together." In writing, this means that the letter or information follows a logical flow from one idea to the next. Being coherent may require you not to cram too many ideas into a single piece of correspondence. Eliminate any ideas that are not necessary.

If all the information is necessary and the correspondence is still lengthy, consider inserting headings to help the reader know when you are moving from one thought pattern to another.

If your document is not clear and coherent, you will have failed in your attempt to get a message across to your reader. Don't make this mistake. If the letter isn't clear and coherent, it isn't worth sending.

Grammar, Sentence Structure, and Paragraphs

Be sure that your grammar and sentence structure are accurate. The impression your letter creates will be a reflection of you and the company you work for. The last thing you want is your customer thinking they are patronizing a sloppy company.

Paragraphs should be kept short and to the point. A paragraph should end when the thought is complete. The only exception is when you add a transitional thought to the end of the final sentence. A transitional thought is one that leads the reader gently into the idea that will be covered in the following paragraph.

The Closing

The closing is the final chance you have to make your point. It should be a brief summary of the major points contained in the body of the paragraph. Also include a congratulatory or consolatory note if the body of the letter contains good or bad news (eg, I am sorry that these benefits were not covered under your plan and we hope to be of service to you in the future.). Bear in mind, however, that all portions of the correspondence should be kept on a professional level.

Your closing should be fresh, stating what you wish the recipient to do in a new and interesting way so that he or she will feel motivated to carry out your wishes.

Format of the Letter

For your correspondence to be taken seriously, it is important for it to look professional. There are numerous books available that show various styles and formats of letters.

While each company has a preferred format for correspondence, there are several general rules that should be followed. These include:

1. Letters should be neatly typed on 8.5 × 11 paper with 1-inch margins on all sides. Refrain from using decorative typestyles such as script or italics.
2. All information should be single-spaced. However, if you are not indenting the first line of a paragraph, it is appropriate to double space between paragraphs. You should double space between each of the items indicated in numbers three through nine below.
3. Indicate your name, address and, if appropriate, your phone number in the center of the page approximately 1 inch down from the top of the paper. Of course, if you are using paper with an imprinted letterhead, this information is omitted.
4. Indicate the current date.
5. List the name and address of the person to whom the letter is written. Be sure you use the appropriate abbreviations for geographic locations and states.
6. Your salutation or greeting comes next. You can use "Dear Sir," "Dear Madam," "Gentlemen," "Dear Mr. ____," or "Dear Ms. ____."

   The salutation should be placed against the left-hand margin, two spaces below the last line of the recipient's address and two lines above the body of the letter.
7. The body of the letter includes the message to be conveyed to the recipient. Your message should look well balanced and contain the important elements of your request or information. Paragraphs should be single-spaced with either the first line indented, or a double space separating the paragraphs. Lines should be flush against the left margin, however, you may indent the first line of each paragraph five spaces.
8. The complimentary closing is placed two or three lines below the last line of the body. The left side should be even with the top line of your address. Under no circumstances should it extend beyond the right margin. The most common complimentary closings include: "Sincerely," "Cordially," "Yours very truly," and "Yours truly."
9. Your signature should appear directly under the complimentary closing. If you wish, you may follow this with your name typed directly under your signature, with the left margin even with the complimentary closing. If you are including your title, it should be typed on the line following your name, with the left margin even with your name.
10. If your letter is typed by someone other than yourself, your initials should be placed in capital letters flush with the left hand margin. These are immediately followed by a slash (/) and the initials of the person who typed the letter in lower case.
11. If enclosures are included with the letter, the word "Enclosures" should be placed against the left hand margin.

Correspondence Containing Negative Content

When writing letters that contain negative content (eg, letters of denial), say "no" as graciously as possible. Your success in keeping this person as a continued customer depends on your saying "no" nicely. Use positive words and phrases to develop a positive feeling within your reader.

Never give the bad news in the first paragraph because the reader may stop reading without understanding the reason for the decision. In this case, you will have lost the reader without getting the reasons and rationale across in a manner that creates mutual understanding.

Clearly state the reasons for the decision and, if possible, refer the reader to any applicable information to support the company's decision (ie, a copy of the contract provisions or a statement of his or her account). If appeals procedures are applicable, include all the necessary information regarding appeals in your correspondence. This will eliminate unnecessary phone calls at a later date.

Due to time constraints and financial considerations, it may be necessary to respond to your client with a form letter. If the form letter is written in a pleasing tone and uses specific references, you reduce the chances that your recipient will think of it as just another form letter.

If the form letter has been photocopied and is obviously a form letter, consider adding a personal note to the margin that will soften the blow.

ERISA Correspondence Requirements

During the late 1960s and early 1970s, pressures mounted for tighter federal controls over the operation of private employee benefit plans. As a result, the Employee Retirement Income Security Act of 1974 (ERISA) was enacted to cover the areas of participation and vesting, funding, termination insurance, fiduciary responsibility, enforcement, and disclosure of the internal operations of self-funded plans.

ERISA mandates that claims must be processed within a specified period of time from receipt by the plan administrator. In addition, claims that are denied must be fully explained to the participant, also within a specified time period. Claimants must be notified of claims that are being reviewed, the reason for review, and so on. All claims must be acted on by the administrator within 90 days. The maximum extension period is 180 days.

The written notice explaining the disposition of a claim must indicate the following:

- The specific reason or reasons for the denial
- Specific reference to pertinent plan provisions on which the denial is based
- A description of any additional material or information necessary for the claimant to submit and an explanation of why such information or material is necessary
- Appropriate information as to the steps to be taken if the participant or beneficiary wishes to submit his or her claim for review

In summation, ERISA governs every aspect of private pension and welfare plans and requires employers who sponsor plans to operate them in compliance with ERISA standards.

ERISA applies only to noninsured benefit plans. Insured plans are under the regulation of each state's Department of Insurance. For noninsured plans, those that are self-funded, ERISA supersedes any and all state laws insofar as they may now or later relate to any employee benefit plan. ERISA plans are regulated and enforced by the US Department of Labor. Of course, for ERISA to preempt the state's insurance laws in reference to a particular plan, that plan must satisfy ERISA's definition of an eligible plan.

Although this sounds confusing, generally you will be safe in assuming that a plan is governed by ERISA if it is self-funded. In reality, it is much more complicated than that.

The main impact felt by most claims examiners when handling self-funded plans relates to specific benefits. For instance, many states have legislatively mandated that specific types of services, such as infertility testing and treatment or mental health providers and treatment, must be provided for under insured plans. Under an ERISA plan, those mandates may not apply. Since most "civilians" (those not involved in the insurance industry) are not aware of the differences between an insured and a self-funded plan, there can be confusion and Department of Insurance complaints against a plan for noncompliance. In such an instance, the plan basically answers the complaint by informing the commissioner that the subject plan is an ERISA plan and is therefore not subject to regulation by their department.

Other instances in which the examiner must understand ERISA compliance relate to the following:

- The requirement for notification of benefits to plan participants
- Fiduciary responsibility
- The processing of claims

The notification of benefits is provided through a very specific type of document that must be prepared by the plan administrators/trustees. This document must explain to the participants what the benefits are and how they are applied. The document, called a Summary Plan Description, must be filed with the Department of Labor (DOL) within a certain time period from the inception of the plan and every time there are plan changes. Plan members must be notified of any plan changes within a specified period of time.

A fiduciary is a person with legal and moral obligations to care for the affairs of a plan. In essence, a fiduciary is responsible for the well-being of a plan. The fiduciary's conduct is prescribed by tenets of common law and the law of trusts, court interpretations of the law, statutes of the various states, the terms and interpretations of the trust agreement, and certain sections of ERISA. Usually, the fiduciaries of a benefit plan are the trustees.

As you become more involved in the industry, you will become familiar with the differences between ERISA and non-ERISA plans. The latter represents only a summary of the main differences.

Summary

Correspondence is written communication between one person and another. Regardless of the content of the letter or the response you wish to evoke, the main purpose of correspondence is to communicate your thoughts, ideas, and desires to another person. To achieve this, be sure that the correspondence is necessary, formulate your ideas before beginning to write, and determine the action you wish the recipient to take.

Written correspondence should always contain an opening, a body, and a closing. It should also be clear, concise, coherent, and grammatically correct. Combining all these elements will help to achieve effective written communications.

Assignments

Complete the Questions for Review.
Complete Correspondence Exercise 11-1.

Questions for Review

Directions: Answer the following questions without looking back into the material just covered. Write your answers in the space provided.

1. ERISA governs what type of plans? ______________________
2. Effective written communications should have three separate components. What are they?
   a. ______________________
   b. ______________________
   c. ______________________
3. The body of the letter explains the ______________________
4. The Department of Insurance has jurisdiction over ______________________ plans only.
5. A fiduciary is someone who has ______________________ and ______________________ obligations to care for the affairs of a plan.

If you were unable to answer any of the questions, refer back to the section and then fill in the answers.

Exercise 11-1

Directions: Using the stationery contained in the workbook, write a letter to cover each of the following scenarios. In each case, you are the medical biller working for the doctor's office. Addresses and personal information are contained in the patient files that were set up at the end of the Introduction of Medical Claims section.

1. Abby Addison has asked you to write to the insurance company and request a preauthorization and an estimate of the charges that will be paid for her surgery.

2. Bobby Bumble disagrees with the amount that the insurance company has paid on his claim. He requests you to send a letter to his insurance company that asks for an adjustment on the grounds that the Usual, Customary, and Reasonable amount allowed should be higher than that listed.

3. You have not received payment from Cathy Crenshaw for her recent visit to your office. This is the first letter you are sending requesting payment.

4. Daisy Doolittle did not bring in her Medicaid card at her last office visit. A new Medicaid card is issued every month, and you need her to bring in her new card to show that the services will be paid by Medicaid. If she does not bring in the card, she will need to pay for the services.

5. Edward Edmunds had asked you to write Medicare to find out if removal of a birthmark would be covered by Medicare. Medicare has written back to say that the procedure is not covered. You need to inform Mr. Edmunds of this and at the same time let him know that your office would be more than happy to perform the surgery and that he can make payments to cover the charges.

12

Job Search Preparation

In this chapter you will learn:

- To determine your marketing objectives, uniqueness, and audience.
- To prepare a top-notch resume.
- Proper interviewing techniques and appropriate mannerisms and dress.
- To write an effective cover letter requesting a job.
- To present yourself effectively in an interview situation.

Regardless of the career path you have chosen, all the education in the world is worthless if you don't have good job-hunting skills. Without them, you will never gain employment.

Gaining successful employment requires you not just to look for a job, but to market yourself. This works for direct mail advertising companies around the world, and it can work for you, too. It is important to start with a set of written objectives, know what separates you from the competition, and familiarize yourself with your target audience.

Job Search Objectives

First, determine your job search objectives. What responsibilities do you want in the position you are looking for? Is there a title for such responsibilities? What type of work environment do you want? What can you reasonably expect, both in the way of title and salary? Writing down these objectives can help solidify them in your mind and help you formulate a plan of action.

Uniqueness

Most available job openings have numerous people applying for the position. You need to emphasize your uniqueness and the talents that you can bring to the job. What sets you apart from your competitors? Do you have a special talent or area of expertise? Call attention to it. What about a skill you can share with other employees? Highlight it. Let prospective employers know how you can help to train co-workers, saving the company time and money while helping the operation run smoothly. Do you have contacts in a particular industry that might allow your new company to expand its sales in that field? Tell prospective employers these details to set yourself apart from the competition.

Target Audience

Success at finding the right job depends not only on the previous two items, but on looking in the right place. You wouldn't go to a restaurant to find a job as a typist. Likewise, you wouldn't go to a typing pool to find a job as a waiter. Much depends on where you look for a job.

After deciding on the particular organizations offering the best opportunities, find out who are the decision makers. Who would be best for you to contact regarding employment. Get the person's title and name. Find out as much as you can about the person who makes the decisions at the companies you're targeting. What are their professional affiliations (eg, Nebraska Mental Health)? What are their career backgrounds? What are their job-related concerns and corporate responsibilities? The answers to these questions will help you to establish a rapport with the person and help you bring out your commonalities.

Build Your Database

Once you have established your target audience, make an organized collection of information about the company and possible job prospects. Your collection needs to keep track of potential employers, professional contacts, and resources.

Keep detailed and well-organized notes on everyone you speak with who can help you reach your objectives. Always write down the person's name, title, the company or organization name, address, phone and fax numbers, any professional affiliations, the date you spoke or met, how you reached them, what follow-up you should make, and any other relevant information.

Build a file on each company from all the resources available to you. This can include job banks, trade publications, executive search firms, civic groups, alumni associations, social networks, colleagues or co-worker, former employers, and anyone else who can help you. You'll be surprised at how many people you know when you start to write them down.

Resumes and Cover Letters

Now you are ready to develop your resume and cover letter. Think of these items as sales materials for your career. The cover letter should invite and interest your target audience enough that they will read your resume. Your resume is essentially the marketing brochure that gets you in the door. Both need to proclaim the benefits you offer to an employer.

A First-Class Resume

A resume can be your best friend or your worst enemy. A first-class resume is one of the most important items you can have in your job search and can open doors for you. A bad resume will slam them shut. In essence, a resume is your personal representative. It tells the company not only who you are, but the type of person you are. No one would welcome a representative who is sloppy and disorganized. Likewise, your resume should not be full of errors or difficult to read. Your resume is a direct reflection of you. Its goal is to get you an interview and help you to land that great job.

The initial screening of a resume occurs very quickly, sometimes merely scanned for a few seconds. Your format should keep this in mind. The purpose of this quick scan is to weed out the resumes that have obvious typographic errors, are poorly organized, or are substandard in reproduction. If the author of a resume is not careful enough to proofread and correct his or her own resume, why should an employer think the person would be any more conscientious at work? If your resume is hard to read or difficult to file (because of odd-shaped paper), it will undoubtedly end up in file 13, also known as the trash can.

Before you write your resume, do a little research. Find a current book on resume writing. This type of book will give you not only a wealth of information, but good resume samples.

The Basics

Your resume should typically be no longer than one page. It should be printed on white or off-white 8 1/2 by 11" paper. Do not use bright or fancy colors. Professionals in the Human Resources arena prefer one-page resumes. The resumes are easier to read through and yet provide enough information to introduce you and your experience. Don't jeopardize your job opportunities by being long-winded or by listing every minute detail about yourself.

Always be concise and use an active voice in your resume. Action verbs and specific nouns are best when describing your job duties and accomplishments. Don't abbreviate any words; the chance of being misunderstood is not worth saving the space.

The heading of your resume should include your name, address, and telephone number. This should be followed by the body of your resume, which includes the objective or qualifying statement, your professional experience, and your education. Optional information, if there is room at the bottom, would include special skills, personal notes, hobbies, and references.

The following five items should be included on your resume:

1. Name, address, and telephone number: You would be surprised at how many people leave off one or more pieces of this vital information. Make sure that all information is correct. Don't cut corners. Your address should include an apartment number and the zip code, and your phone number should include the area code. The easier it is for an employer to contact you, the better.
2. Objective statement: Some employers and resume writers consider an objective statement to be optional. However, if you have a specific direction, include it. It lets the prospective employer know what your goals are. If you are interested in several different jobs, you might want to replace the objective statement with a qualifying statement. In this way, you won't have to prepare separate objective statements (and resumes) for each job title. Make sure that your resume shows that you have some direction. Your cover letter should also reinforce this.
3. Qualifying statement: A qualifying statement is a way to toot your own horn. It sells you as a potential employee and lists your abilities and experiences. To get ideas for your qualifying statement, read the want ads to see what skills and

characteristics are desired (eg, excellent written and verbal communication skills, ability to handle a variety of tasks, and excellent organizational ability). These are exactly the types of statements that should go into your qualifying section.

4. Work experience: There are a variety of ways to state your experience. The most common approach is to list your employment history in reverse chronologic order, putting your most recent job first. However, if you have had numerous job changes or a gap in employment, you don't necessarily want to emphasize this. Therefore, you might consider using the functional format resume. This lists together all related experiences rather than listing according to date.
5. Education: If you have education or training beyond the high school level, you will want that fact to stand out. Find a way to highlight this so that even when your resume is scanned quickly, additional education can be noticed. The simplest format is to list the degree or certificate, followed by your major or course of study. Follow this with the name and location of the school and year in which you graduated (eg, Certificate of Completion, Health Claims Examiner/Medical Biller, Los Angeles College, Los Angeles, CA, [1994]). Education and training should be listed in reverse chronologic order.

Professional Services

If you need additional help, a number of professional resume services are available. It is essential that your resume look professional. This includes the use of a word processor and a letter-quality printer. If you do not have access to this type of equipment, it may be a good investment to hire someone to type and print it for you.

Edit and Proofread!

You must edit and proofread your resume very carefully. Remember that this single sheet of paper can either help or hurt you in getting a job. It is a direct reflection of you. Before you send it to a potential employer, get a friend to check it for errors and content. Another person often spots things that you have missed.

What to Avoid

The following five items are things to avoid when you are composing your resume. Some of these items may seem obvious, but a surprising number of people make these errors on their resumes.

1. Never send a carbon copy or an inferior quality copy of your resume to an employer.
2. Never use abbreviations; this includes the term "etc." Anything important enough to be stated should be written out. Write it out or leave it out.
3. Do not waste time and space detailing mundane, entry level jobs that have no bearing on your present job search.
4. Do not list a desired salary. Discussions of this sort should be saved for the interview. If you ask for too high of a salary, you may not be granted an interview. If you ask for too little, a prospective employer may wonder what you're worth.
5. Consider the importance of salary, job location, and position desired before you limit yourself. Ask yourself if any of these are more important than a chance for advancement.

The Cover Letter

Your resume provides a potential employer with your qualifications. The cover letter is an introduction to your resume. It invites the potential employer to read further.

The cover letter should be concise and to the point. What you are really trying to say with the cover letter is that you are enclosing your resume and are available for an interview at the prospective employer's convenience. For further information regarding the format and content of a cover letter, refer to Chapter 11.

Letter-Writing Don'ts

The following are items that you should avoid when writing your cover letter:

- Don't include anything in your letter that cannot be substantiated in your interview.

- Don't try to force an interview by using sympathy or any sense of urgency.
- Don't load your cover letter with unnecessary information; just present the important facts. The cover letter should be an addendum to your resume.
- Don't address your letter to a company or a title. Find out the name of the person who holds that title and address it to that person. If not, address it to the department or division that will supervise your work.
- Don't mail a resume without a cover letter.
- Don't forget to include a request for an interview in your cover letter.
- Don't forget to proofread your cover letter, checking for appearance, grammar, and spelling errors.

Marketing Yourself

When marketing your skills, keep in mind the following things:

- Segment your audience.
- Prepare your portfolio.
- Professionally market yourself.

Let's discuss each item individually.

Different people respond differently. Salespeople know this and segment their audience accordingly. You also need to segment your audience to be sure you are presenting the right benefit (talent) to the right market in the right tone. This often means you will have to write several different resumes and cover letters. It's worth it if you want to get the right job. Just be sure your objectives, experience, and message are appropriate to the segment you're trying to sell.

You also might consider creating a portfolio on yourself. This portfolio could include your resume, letters of reference, graphs or charts supporting your accomplishments, samples of previous work, and other informational material. Present the information neatly. A handsome presentation folder conveys a stronger impact than a cover letter and resume alone. Its very size commands more attention. Just don't overload it with too much extraneous information. Present only the best of what you have to offer.

Searching for a job is not enough. Instead, you must professionally market yourself. Take charge of the situation and of your career. Job hunters take what comes along; marketing yourself means more. It means going out and searching for the job you want, then selling yourself until you get it.

Develop a plan that will make things happen. Assemble your resources. Present yourself with purpose, professionalism, and positive energy. Not only is this more effective, but it is better for your morale than just starting another dreaded job search!

The Job Interview

The job interview can be one of the most frightening experiences a potential employee faces. Add to this the knowledge that most working adults make an average of 10 career changes in their lifetime, with each change requiring a number of job interviews. That's a lot of stress to go through. But with knowledge can come the power to take control of the interview and turn fear into success.

Interviewing research indicates that there are four basic components to the interview process:

1. The first 4 seconds
2. The next 5 minutes
3. The main portion
4. The end or closing

It is important to fully understand each of these components so that you can control them and reap the best rewards from the interview process.

The First Four Seconds

First impressions are vitally important. They can put you off to a good start. Or, they can strike a mark against you that will be hard to erase, if an interviewer forms a negative impression.

Eighty percent of a first impression is based on your appearance. For that reason, it is suggested that you dress more formally than you might normally dress on the job. Keep your appearance conservative; flashy styles can be risky.

The handshake is a symbolic gesture of trust. A firm, brief handshake and direct eye contact indicate self-confidence and trustworthiness.

The Next Five Minutes

The next 5 minutes of an interview can often determine whether you get a job offer or not. Studies reveal that interviewers often form an opinion within this 5-minute period. They then seek information that will validate this initial impression. Thus, their opinion influences their decision to either hire or reject the candidate. If the impression was negative, one study reveals, 90% of the time the interviewee was not hired. If the opinion was positive, the candidate received a job offer 75% of the time.

Therefore, your primary goal during this time should be to make sure the initial impression is positive. The following suggestions have been found to be among the most important:

- Make direct eye contact with the interviewer. It gives the impression that you are open and honest and have nothing to hide. Eye contact can actually be equal in power to the sound and tone of the voice.
- Your posture conveys a large message while you're sitting as well as standing. Remaining straight and tall with shoulders back will convey confidence. Leaning forward slightly in your chair will convey interest.
- Never underestimate the power of a smile for opening the lines of communication.

The Main Portion

After the important amenities have been taken care of, the general questioning will begin. Listen carefully to the questions and focus your answers on the job requirements and on highlighting your strengths. Look for any specific problems that the organization may have. Highlight your skills and work history as they relate to their needs. Remember that if they didn't have a need, they wouldn't be interviewing you. Make them believe they need you.

Try to find out as much about the company, the job, and the people as possible. A good interview is a two-way, give-and-take situation. According to numerous studies, interviewers expect you to ask questions. Therefore, strong well-directed questions help to create a positive impression. Be sure to listen carefully to the response, then use the information to strengthen your position.

The personality trait that attracts an interviewer the most is enthusiasm. If you like what you've heard about this company, or what you are hearing in the interview, don't be afraid to let the interviewer know. Be comfortable about revealing your personality and the kind of person you are, but do it with interest, awareness, and energy. Many studies have indicated that individuals are often hired based more on their personality than on their skills.

The middle portion of the interview can present some of your greatest difficulty. Be aware of the hidden agenda behind each question. Is the interviewer trying to find out about your skills, your education, or your background?

If an interviewer continually returns to a specific topic, especially in your past, they are unconsciously telling you that they are questioning the response or that they discern a weakness. Remember to control your responses. Frame your experiences in a positive light and focus on the positive aspects that will most benefit the company.

There is probably at least one situation in your history that you would rather not have come out in the open. This may be a termination, a felony conviction, or a similar problem.

First, determine whether the information will come up during the normal course of the interview or during the background check. Most companies run a preliminary check on their prospective employees. This may include a brief phone call to previous employers and a check of police records.

Research has shown that negative aspects are seen much more negatively when they are revealed bit by bit. The impression is that you may have other things wrong if they ask the right questions to bring them out.

Take control of this situation by disclosing any negative information briefly and forthrightly before you are asked. In this way you can place the best possible light on the situation. Even a termination can be turned from a negative into a positive by sincerely and honestly discussing what you've learned from the experience and what you'll do differently, if you are given the opportunity.

The Closing

Finally, you have reached the closing moments of the interview. Many people begin to lose concentration and relax at this point. Don't! Keep yourself focused. A strong finish may be the difference between you and someone else in a tight race. Show the interviewer that you are still excited about the job, especially now that you know more about it and the company.

Make a strong final note by succinctly summarizing your positive points as they relate to the job. There is nothing wrong with asking when a decision on the candidates will be made. When you have the answer, show your enthusiasm by letting the interviewer know that you will call back the afternoon of the decision.

Interviewing is very much like a game. If you make all the right moves, you will win the job. If you make errors, you won't. In the end, it is all up to you and the way you play.

Getting Paid What You're Worth

The issue of salary will undoubtedly come up, either during the interview or before. Salary is probably the most important issue among workers today; nevertheless, the way in which salary is determined is often one of the least understood. Far too many people see their salary as an extension of themselves and how much they are worth. Often, their point of view is totally unrealistic according to the marketplace.

Let's review four of the most common misconceptions regarding how a salary should be determined:

1. Seeing your monetary compensation as a reflection of your worth as a person. It is not. Your salary is based on your objective value in the marketplace. If your skills are in high demand, you will be paid more than if they were not. This is perhaps the single most common mistake employees make. Their pride tells them that they are too good of a person to work for such meager pay. If you are one of these people, you need to face the fact that the laws of supply and demand determine your market worth, not you. If everyone were able to set their own salary at what they felt they were worth, inflation would increase drastically. You would be making $450 per hour, but a loaf of bread would cost $350.

   Bear in mind that when supply and demand chooses a market value for your work, at least it is an objective value, not a subjective one determined by others. So don't take it personally.
2. Expecting your pay to be determined by your needs. This is the second most common complaint, and we've all heard it. Employees making comments like: "My partner is out of work, and we can't pay our bills on my salary alone." "I'm a single parent with children to feed." "I have to put my children in private school." "This salary barely covers the cost of rent and bills every month. What am I supposed to eat on?"

   The fact is that no employer can afford to pay an employee based on his or her needs. People are funny characters. When they have money, they tend to spend it. In the end, you will probably always need more money than you are presently making. Keep your professional dignity by never basing a request for a raise on these types of appeals.
3. Expecting the length of your employment to determine your market value. No matter how long you've worked at a particular position, if you can offer nothing more than the person who has worked at the job for a year, then both of you will be paid at approximately the same level. Many people expect automatic annual raises. This works fine until a company decides that it is much less expensive to terminate the older employee and hire a new one at the lower salary.

Then the policy doesn't sound so good anymore.

Recognize that your pay reflects the value of the work you do. Granted, more experience usually leads to a higher quality of employee, and often the pay reflects this. However, the lowly box boy in the supermarket, no matter how great a box boy he is, will never earn as much as the supervisor of a department.

4. Expecting your pay to go up as the company's profits go up. This concept ignores a fundamental concept: Employees are not shareholders. They are taking no risks with their money. Those who expect their pay to increase when the company's profits increase almost never suggest that they should take a pay cut when the company has a bad year. Yet one is exactly the same as the other. If an employee wishes to share in a company's profits and if the company is publicly held, the employee should purchase company stock. However, these employees, like the current shareholders, will then run the risk of losing their money if profits fall.

If you, as an employee, recognize these misconceptions about salary, you are less likely to base your request for a raise on flimsy reasons. The next step is to consider what is a valid reason for requesting a raise.

First and fundamentally, you need to make some personal decisions. Ask yourself: "Am I in the right job?" "Do I enjoy what I'm doing?" Regardless of your answer, the next question should be, "Is it more important for me to have money or to be happy?" The truth is that it takes a lot of money to compensate someone for being miserable. And if you are miserable in your job, you are probably not putting forth your best effort. Lack of good effort is definitely not going to get you the raises you would like. So what do you do? First, find the job that is right for you.

The next important principle is that the laws of supply and demand will prevail. If you want to increase your market value, you must increase your worth to the company, usually by increasing your skills and abilities.

The following suggestions can help:

- Adopt an active mentality, not a passive one. No one is going to increase your skills and abilities for you; you have to do it yourself and it takes work.
- Never stop learning. Don't be satisfied with knowing your job inside and out. After you have mastered that, begin learning the other jobs in the company, preferably those of the next step up the ladder. Ask questions, read books, or take classes. Make sure that you become a valuable asset to the company and that you are ready for advancement and promotion when the opportunity comes.
- Make long-range plans rather than waiting for life to just happen to you. Those who sit around never go anywhere.
- Finally, realize that very often a significant change in salary comes from changing jobs, either within your present company or by moving to a different employer. We've all heard comments like "If I were working at the company down the street, I could make more than this!" The obvious response is, "If that's true, then why don't you move?" And if the bosses hear you make such a comment, they may assist your transfer to the company down the street by firing you.

Many employees can't accept the fact that it's either true that their current pay is below market, or it's not. If it's true, why not move on? If it's not, change your market value.

Summary

To find the right job takes more than just a passive look at the classified ads. You must first determine your objectives, your uniqueness, and your target audience. With these topics firmly in mind, write an effective resume and cover letter that will introduce you to a prospective employer.

When you have been granted an interview, keep in mind that the first 4 seconds are the most critical, followed by the next 5 minutes. However, the body of the interview and the closing are also important in determining whether you get a second interview and/or ultimely a job offer.

When it comes to salary, your pay is based on your worth to the marketplace. The higher the demand for your skills, the more value will be placed on them and the higher salary you will be paid. Salary is not determined by your worth as a person, your needs, your length of employment, or the company's profits.

Assignments

Complete the Questions for Review.
Complete the Resume Questionnaire (Appendix 12-1) to assist you in preparing your resume and in interviewing for a job. The more prepared you are, the better your job interview will be.

Complete a resume and a cover letter. Give a copy of your resume to the placement director at the school.

Questions for Review

Directions: Answer the following questions without looking back into the material just covered. Write your answers in the space provided.

1. What three points should your written marketing plan cover?
   a. ______________________________
   b. ______________________________
   c. ______________________________
2. To determine your ______________________, consider the responsibilities you want on your next job, the industry in which you want to work, and what you can reasonably expect in the way of title and salary.
3. Your ______________ should show your target audience that you're worthy of their __________.
4. What is your resume?______________________________
5. Never use an active voice or concise phrasing in your resume. (True or False) ______________
6. A ______________________ is a way to toot your own horn.
7. Don't put anything in your letter that you cannot substantiate in an interview. (True or False) __________
8. You should not job hunt but instead ______________________ yourself.
9. Working adults normally make how many career changes in a lifetime?____________________
10. The only way to achieve a significant increase in pay is to change jobs. (True or False)______________

If you were unable to answer any of the questions, refer back to the section and then fill in the answers.

Appendix 12-1

Resume Questionnaire

First ______________________ M.I. ________________ Last Name ________________

Street ____

City ______________________ State ____________________ Zip ________________

Day Phone ______________ Eve. Phone ______________ Soc. Sec. # ________________

Position Objective:

In the spaces below, enter the Occupational Titles of those positions that you feel you would be best qualified to fill. Opposite each position, enter the total number of years' experience you have. Then indicate your minimum acceptable annual salary. "OPEN" is unacceptable.

Occupational or Professional Title(s)	Years' Experience	Desired Annual Salary
______________________________	__________	$ ____________
______________________________	__________	$ ____________
______________________________	__________	$ ____________
______________________________	__________	$ ____________

Experience Summary:

Please summarize briefly your overall business experience and accomplishments.

____

____

____

Education:

Type of degree, diploma, certificate, or years completed: (ie, HS Diploma, College, # year(s), AA/BA, etc)

Highest Level: Type: ______________________ Major ______________________

Name of School, College or University ______________________________________

Additional Courses/Seminars taken, and/or Awards: ______________________________

____

____

US Citizenship:

Yes ___ No ___ Type of Employment: Full-Time _____ Part-Time _____ Temp _____ Contract _____

Geographic Area: Open to any Area _______ Area Desired ______________________________

Work History:
Under each position title describe your duties, responsibilities, and accomplishments. Be sure to list your "Present or Last Employer" first.

_________Mo/Yr (Present/Last)
Company Name ______________________________
Location (City & State) ______________________________
Position Title ______________________________ Salary $ ______________
Type of Firm or Industry ______________________________
Responsibilities/Accomplishments: ______________________________
____
____

_________Mo/Yr
Company Name ______________________________
Location (City & State) ______________________________
Position Title ______________________________ Salary $ ______________
Type of Firm or Industry ______________________________
Responsibilities/Accomplishments: ______________________________
____
____

_________Mo/Yr
Company Name ______________________________
Location (City & State) ______________________________
Position Title ______________________________ Salary $ ______________
Type of Firm or Industry ______________________________
Responsibilities/Accomplishments: ______________________________
____
____

Other Experience/Accomplishments:
List briefly any additional experience or accomplishments that you would consider significant.

____
____
____
____

Skills/Abilities:

Administrative/Clerical Skills
(Accounting, customer service, legal, personnel, purchasing, training, etc)

Typing speed (_________) WPM
Shorthand (_________) WPM
____ 10-key by touch
____ Data entry
____ Word processing
Computer software (types)
____
____
____
____
____
____
____
____
____
____

Technical/Professional Skills
(Type of design, analysis, computer language(s), operating systems, sales, supervision, planning, organizational, interpersonal, etc.)
____
____
____
____
____
____
____
____
____
____
____
____
____
____
____

Tools & Equipment Operated
PC computer, Mini, Mainframe

Industrial equipment (fork lift, crane, lathes, etc.)

Type(s): ____________________
____
____
____
____
____
____
____
____
____
____
____
____
____
____

Industry Experience:
Please indicate the industries in which you have experience and specify type(s).

___ Agriculture (type)____________________
___ Finance/Insurance (type) ______________
___ Hospitality (type)_____________________
___ Mining (type)_________________________
___ Retail/Wholesale (type) _______________
___ Transportation (type)__________________
___ Construction (type) ___________________
___ Health Care (type) ____________________
___ Manufacturing (type)___________________
___ Public Administration (type) ____________
___ Services (type) _______________________
___ Other_____________________________

Foreign Language(s): ______________________________ Speak ________ Read/Write ________

Security Clearance: ______________________________(For defense-oriented occupations)

I hereby certify that all of the information contained herein is complete and accurate and I agree to report any changes promptly.

Signature:______________________________ Date: ____________________

13

Terminology

In this chapter you will learn:

- To recognize and interpret insurance terms.
- To identify providers by their professional abbreviation to determine appropriateness of services rendered or benefits payable.

It is impossible to bill or handle insurance claims properly without learning and understanding the industry terminology. Without proper terminology, coding of diagnosis and procedures is far less accurate. In addition, there is a higher percentage of error in the filling out and processing of forms. This leads to incorrectly paid benefits and delays in payment.

As with learning anything new, the first step is to memorize the terms of what you are studying. One of the easiest ways to accomplish this is by relating the term, whenever possible, to experiences in your own life. By internalizing the terms, it becomes easier to both remember the meaning and to incorporate the use of the term in your vocabulary. Of course, the more you use the terms during your classroom experiences, the faster and better you will retain the meanings.

Insurance Terminology

The following terms will follow you in your insurance career, regardless of the type of insurance-related employer you work for. Therefore, it is absolutely essential that you learn to use and understand this terminology.

Accumulation Period—Period of time (normally January 1 through December 31) in which to satisfy the deductible, accumulate COB credit reserves, reach maximums, and so on.

Actively-at-Work Requirement—The provision of a group plan that requires an otherwise eligible employee to be actively at work on the day he or she is scheduled to become covered. Furthermore, if the employee is not actively at work on the date that the coverage becomes effective, coverage will be delayed until the date he or she returns to active work. For an eligible dependent who is hospital-confined on the date that coverage was to become effective, the coverage will not become effective until after the dependent's release from the hospital.

Adjustment—A correction of the application of benefits or coding on a claim.

ASO—Administrative Services Only. The provision of services such as actuarial benefit plan design, claim processing, data recovery and analysis, employee benefits communications, financial advice, medical care conversions, preparation of data for reports to governmental units for a self-funded plan, or the like. ASO are provided on a contract basis by an insurer or a Third Party Administrator.

Administrator, Third Party—See Third Party Administrator.

Assignment of Benefits—In health coverage, a method under which a claimant requests that his or her benefits under a claim be paid to a designated person or institution, usually a physician or hospital.

Audit, Claim—Checking the accuracy of claim payments in accordance with the contract provisions of the plan. Eligibility of the claimants and of the providers usually are also verified.

Automatic Annual Reinstatement—A specified amount of money (credit) that may be added to the balance of available lifetime benefits. Usually, this is important only when a member has a catastrophic illness or injury and will be calculated only when lifetime benefits have been exhausted.

Basic Benefits—The portion of a plan of benefits that is not usually subject to a deductible and usually pays from the first dollars submitted by a provider. Generally, a maximum amount is allowed for payment for each basic benefit.

Beneficiary—The person designated or provided for by the policy terms to receive the proceeds from the policy upon the death of the insured.

Benefit—The amount payable by the plan to a claimant, assignee, or beneficiary under each coverage.

COBRA—Consolidated Omnibus Budget Reconciliation Act of 1985. This act provides for continuation of coverage for employees no longer considered eligible by a plan.

Coinsurance—The arrangement by which both the member and the plan share a specific ratio of the covered losses under a policy. For example, the plan may reimburse the provider or member 80% of covered expenses, and the member will be responsible for the remaining 20% of such expenses.

Common Accident Provision—An arrangement that only one deductible will be taken for all members of a family involved in the same accident. Remaining deductibles will be waived on all remaining members for expenses incurred for that accident only.

Concurrent Review—A review performed while a patient is hospitalized to determine whether the stay is medically necessary and for what period of time.

COB—Coordination of Benefits. The process by which claim payors determine who is the primary, secondary, tertiary payor.

CoPay—The amount that the member/insured must pay "out-of-pocket." This would normally be the 20% not paid by the coinsurance. The plan CoPay amount may or may not include the major medical deductible. The policy will state this specific. Also known as the out-of-pocket expense (OOP).

Covered Expenses—The amount of those expenses that are allowable under the plan.

C&R—Customary and Reasonable. See UCR.

Deductible—The amount of covered expenses that must be paid by the insured/member before benefits become payable by the insurer/plan. Usually, this is a calendar year deductible (taken once each calendar year), but not always. The deductible is always taken out of the first eligible expenses submitted each year.

Individual Deductible—The amount of covered expenses that must be paid by the individual family member before benefits become payable by the plan.

Family Deductible—A specified number of family members must satisfy their deductible. The deductible is then considered met for the remaining family members. There are two types of family deductibles: aggregate and nonaggregate or individual.

Aggregate Deductible—All major medical deductibles applied for all family members that are added together to attain the family limit.

Non-Aggregate Deductible—A specified number of individual deductibles must be satisfied before the family limit is met.

DEFRA—Deficit Reduction Act of 1984. Requires that employers with 20 or more employees offer the spouses, age 65+, of active employees, the same coverage offered to younger spouses. See Chapter 3 for details.

DXL—Diagnostic x-ray and laboratory tests.

EIN—Employer Identification Number. A number assigned by the IRS for tax purposes. This number is used by businesses in place of a social security number. (May also be called a taxpayer identification number (TIN).

Eligibility Period—A specified length of time (usually 31 days) following the eligibility date, during which an individual member of a particular group will remain eligible to apply, without evidence of insurability, for coverage under a group life or health plan. A newborn child must be enrolled within 31 days of birth.

ERISA—Employee Retirement Income Security Act of 1974. Governs every aspect of private pension and welfare plans and requires employers who sponsor plans to operate them in compliance with ERISA standards.

Evidence of Insurability—A health questionnaire used to determine a person's physical and mental condition and/or other factual information affecting the acceptance of the applicant's application for health or life coverage. Normally, this is required only when the individual is attempting to obtain coverage after the period of eligibility has lapsed on a group plan. However, this is a common requirement to obtain coverage on an individual policy.

Exclusions—Specified conditions or types of services for which the policy does not provide benefits.

Experience Rating—The process of determining the premium rate for a group risk wholly or partially on the basis of that group's experience (dollars paid out in claims). This also takes into consideration administrative costs, inflation, and probability of the next year's costs.

Explanation of Benefits (EOB)—A statement generated by the claim payor that indicates how the benefits were applied, paid, or denied on a particular claim. It would also show when and to whom the benefits, if any, were paid.

Explanation of Medicare Benefits (EOMB)—Issued by the Medicare claims payor to explain the application of benefits on claims submitted on behalf of Medicare participants.

Extended Benefits—The continued entitlement of a member, under certain circumstances, to receive benefits after the coverage has terminated until either the person is no longer totally disabled or until a specified period of time has elapsed. A doctor's certification of disability is required before benefits can be extended. Usually, such coverage will continue only for expenses incurred for the condition that caused the disability and for a maximum of 12 months following the date of disability or the date that the member is no longer totally disabled, whichever period of time is less.

Full-Time Student—A dependent who is attending a recognized educational facility on a full-time basis. The facility may include vocational schools, colleges, junior colleges, universities, high school, or any other type of institution specified by the plan. The contract must specify the maximum age limit allowed under this provision and the member cannot be the subscriber, employee, or member.

Health Maintenance Organization (HMO)—An alternative from of health care delivery that refers all patients to a set location and provides a full range of health services. All patients must be enrolled in the plan.

Last Quarter Carry-Over—Amounts applied to the deductible in the last 3 months of the calendar year, which are carried over (applied) to the next year's deductible also.

Major Medical Benefits (MM)—The portion of a health plan that pays benefits at a set percentage usually subject to a deductible.

Management Information System—A system that processes data and makes the resulting information available to those who request it.

Maximum(s)—The maximum amount payable by the plan. The maximum may refer to a calendar year or a lifetime max. In addition, it may apply only toward expenses paid under Basic or only toward expenses paid under MM or a combination of all payments, Basic and Major Medical. The policy must specify what type.

Medical While Hospitalized (MWH)—Doctor's visits to a patient while the patient is hospitalized.

Out-of-Pocket Expense (OOP)—Applies to expenses for which the insured is held responsible and must pay "out-of-his-or-her-own pocket," such as the deductible and coinsurance. Also known as CoPay.

OOP Max—The yearly limit on the OOP that the insured is responsible for paying. (Most contracts have this.) When this limit or maximum is reached, the plan pays additional covered expenses at 100% instead of the usual percentage for the remainder of the calendar year.

Pre-Admit Testing (PAT)—Testing performed on an outpatient basis prior to admittance to an inpatient facility.

Peer Review—Independent review by a group of physicians to determine whether the services submitted by another physician are usual, customary, and reasonable for the condition being treated.

Plan Document—The legal document prepared by the fiduciaries of a self-funded/self-insured health and welfare fund. This outlines all the terms and conditions of the plan benefits. The plan document is essentially the same as a policy except that the term "policy" is usually associated with insured plans, whereas a plan document is associated with self-insured plans.

Policy—The legal document issued by the insurance company to the policyholder, which outlines the terms and conditions of the insurance.

Preexisting Exclusion—When specified by the plan, a condition that is treated within a specified time period prior to the effective date of coverage. All charges related to the condition would not be covered at all for a stated period of time, or payment for the condition would be limited to a stated dollar amount.

Preferred Provider Organization (PPO)—A medical group of physicians who negotiate discounted fees and does utilization review and quality assurance in exchange for a referral of a population of patients or monthly per capita payments. The arrangements under this heading vary widely within the industry.

Remittance Advice (R/A)—A bill submitted by a provider.

Subrogation—Contract provision that provides a plan with the authority to recover monies paid on claims that are covered by a third party, such as automobile carriers and lawsuit settlements. See also Third Party Liability Provision.

Summary Plan Description (SPD)—A summary of the plan document that is distributed to the members of a self-funded plan. A copy of the SPD is kept on file at the Department of Labor.

Taxpayer Identification Number (TIN)—A unique nine-digit identification number required by the IRS for a provider or business for tax purposes. See also EIN.

TEFRA—Tax Equity and Financial Responsibility Act of 1982. Requires employers with 20 or more employees to offer active employees age 65 and over and their spouses of the same age the same coverage under any group plan that is offered to younger workers. See Chapter 3 for details.

Terminal Liability—Benefits payable after the termination of a contract.

Third Party Administrator (TPA)—A firm that handles all functions related to the operation of a group insurance/self-funded plan. The kind and number of services provided vary, depending on the contract. As an administrator only, the client uses the money to pay for the health care coverage. The administrator provides the personnel and equipment to perform the services for the client.

Third Party Liability Provision—Provision by a plan that when an injury is covered by a third party (another coverage), reimbursement will be provided to the plan if recovery is made through that coverage. For example, in an automobile coverage, or if a lawsuit is won and damages are recovered, the member would have to pay back the plan the money that the plan paid out for coverage of the injury. See also Subrogation.

Three-Month Carry-Over Provision (C/O)—Eligible charges incurred in the last quarter of the calendar year (October, November, December) and applied toward the member's deductible. These will apply toward satisfaction of the deductible for that member for the subsequent calendar year, also. These monies normally are not applied toward the family limit.

Usual, Customary, and Reasonable (UCR)—Also known as U&C, R&C and C&R. The amount determined to be the maximum allowable by the plan, based on the contract provisions, procedure, date of service, and geographic location of the provider.

Provider Abbreviations

Many types of insurance benefits are based on the type of licensing of the provider and the type of service being provided. Therefore, in order to properly apply these types of benefits, the examiner must understand the various types of licensing available and the types of services that that particular type of provider is allowed to perform. The following is a list of the more common types of licensing that are covered under most contracts and the types of services they usually provide.

CA—Certified Acupuncturist. Usually required for other than an MD or DO. Provider must have this certification to provide acupuncture treatments.

Clinical Psychologist—Licensed to perform psychological testing and therapy. Referral by an MD is not required.

CRNA—Certified Registered Nurse Anesthetist. Certified to administer anesthesia under the direction of an MD.

DC—Doctor of Chiropractic. Performs manual manipulations of the spine and other musculoskeletal areas. Licensed for office visits, x-rays, nutritional supplements, manipulations, ultrasound and physical therapies. All other services should be questioned. Cannot draw blood or perform surgery.

DDS—Doctor of Dental Surgery. Licensed to perform all dental care including dental surgeries and surgeries to the face and jaw.

DMD—Doctor of Medical Dentistry. Licensed to perform dental care including dental surgeries and surgeries to the face and jaw. The only difference between a DDS and a DMD is the school attended; the training and licensing authorizations are the same.

DO—Doctor of Osteopathy. Licensed to perform any service that an MD can. Training is essentially the same as an MD.

DPM—Doctor of Podiatry. Licensed for the care, treatment, and surgery of the feet.

DSC—Doctor of Surgical Chiropody. The same as a podiatrist; deals with foot surgeries. DSC is an old licensing designation that is seldom seen today.

EdD—Doctor of Education. An educational degree, not a licensing. The licensing needs to be obtained. Without appropriate licensing, services by this provider would not usually be covered.

EMT—Emergency Medical Technician. Licensed to administer basic emergency procedures such as CPR. Usually works in an ambulance.

LCSW—Licensed Clinical Social Worker. Licensed to provide psychological counseling. Referral from an MD is required.

LPN—Licensed Practical Nurse. Equivalent to an LVN. LVNs are in California, whereas LPNs are from other states.

LVN—Licensed Vocational Nurse. Lower level (2-year school) nurse, not certified to perform IV-Push (injecting medications directly into a vein) and cannot be a charge nurse on a floor.

MD—Medical Doctor. Licensed to perform any and all medical care/procedures.

MFCC—Marriage, Family, Child Counselor. Licensed to provide psychological counseling and marriage and family counseling. Requires a referral from an MD.

Midwife—Licensed as a registered nurse and certified as a nurse midwife. Usually handles routine maternity cases. Must be associated with an MD or a DO to handle emergency cases.

MSW—Master of Social Work. Licensed to provide family and psychological counseling. Referral from an MD required.

MT—Medical Technologist. Usually works in a laboratory and can draw blood and perform lab testing. An MT also can administer injections and perform EKGs.

Myofunctionist—Licensed to perform myofunctional speech therapy. This is involved with the reeducation of the facial muscles needed to speak and breathe.

NA—Nurse's Aide. Licensed to assist patients not requiring skilled nursing care. Normally employed in skilled nursing facilities, nursing homes. and home health agencies. (Also known as a CNA—Certified Nurse's Aide.)

NP—Nurse Practitioner. Licensed as a registered nurse with additional training to be certified as a nurse practitioner. Must practice under the direction of an MD or DO. Cannot prescribe medicines nor perform surgeries. Normally performs routine examinations and physicals, well baby care, immunizations, and so on.

OD—Doctor of Optometry. An optometrist. Not licensed to perform surgery. Most commonly performs eye refractions, dispenses glasses and contacts.

OT—Occupational Therapist. Licensed to perform occupational therapy. Occupational therapy is the retraining of muscles and nerves, usually in the hands and arms, necessary for the performance of routine daily movements (ie, learning to feed oneself, brush hair, and other activities of daily living.)

PA—Physician's Assistant. A specialized 4-year diploma program that allows the individual to assist an MD with routine care and services. The PA works under the direction of an MD.

Paramedic—Licensed to administer emergency care. Has more extensive training than an EMT. Normally works in an ambulance or for a fire department.

PhD—An educational degree (doctorate) not a licensing. Services by this provider would be covered only when there is also appropriate licensing.

RN—Registered Nurse. Highest-level nursing degree (usually a 3-year program).

RPT—Registered Physical Therapist. Licensed to perform physical (muscle) therapy when services are prescribed by an MD or DO.

Medical Abbreviations and Acronyms

AA	Aortic aneurysm
ABD	Abdomen
ABG	Arterial blood gas
ACTH	Adrenocorticotropic hormone
ADH	Antidiuretic hormone
ADI	American Drug Index
ADL	Activities of daily living
ADR	Adverse drug reaction
AFB	Acid fast bacilli
AFIB	Atrial fibrillation
AFO	Ankle foot orthosis

AG Antigen
AGGLUT Agglutination
AGL Acute granulocytic leukemia
AHS Allied Health Services
AICD Automatic internal cardioverter defibrillator
AIDS Acquired immune deficiency syndrome
AK Above knee
AKA Above knee amputation
AL Aluminum
ALK Alkaline
ALS Amyotrophic lateral sclerosis
AMA Against medical advice
AMI Acute myocardial infarction
AML Acute myelogenous leukemia
ANA Antinuclear antibody
ANS Autonomic nervous system
AODM Adult onset diabetes mellitus
APC Atrial premature contraction
APP Application
AR Accounts Receivable
AROM Active range of motion
ASBD Arteriosclerotic brain disease
ASC Ambulatory surgical center
ASCHD Arteriosclerotic coronary heart disease
ASCVD Arteriosclerotic cardiovascular disease
ASD Atrial septal defect
ASHCVD Hypertensive arteriosclerotic cardiovascular disease
ASHD Arteriosclerotic heart disease
ATN Acute tubular necrosis
AVF Arterio-venous fistula
AVR Aortic valve replacement
AWMI Anterior wall myocardial infarction
AZT Azidothymidine
BBB Bundle branch block
BCG Bacillus calmette guerin
BCP Birth Control Pills
BILI Bilirubin
BK Below knee
BKA Below knee amputation
BLS Basic life support
BMR Basal metabolic rate
BOM Bilateral otitis media
BP Blood pressure
BPH Benign prostatic hypertrophy
BR By Report
BS Blood sugar
BSO Bilateral salpingo oophorectomy
BUN Blood urea nitrogen
BX Biopsy
C&S Culture and sensitivity
CA Cancer
CABG Coronary artery bypass graft
CABP Coronary artery bypass
CAD Coronary artery disease
CAPD Chronic ambulatory peritoneal dialysis
CAVH Continuous arteriovenous hemofiltration
CBC Complete blood count
CBI Continuous bladder irrigation
CBS Chronic brain syndrome
CCF Congestive cardiac failure
CCPD Continuous cycling peritoneal dialysis
CCU Coronary care unit
CEA Carcinoembryonic antigen
CF Cystic fibrosis
CHB Complete heart block
CHD Coronary heart disease
CHDP Child Health and Disability Prevention Program
CHF Congestive heart failure
CKG Cardiokymography
CL Chloride
CML Chronic myelogenous leukemia
CM Centimeter
CNS Central nervous system
COPD Chronic obstructive pulmonary disease
CP Cerebral palsy
CPAP Continuous positive airway pressure
CPK Creatine phosphokinase
CPR Cardiopulmonary resuscitation
CR Creatinine
CRD Chronic renal disease
CRF Chronic renal failure
CRIF Closed reduction internal fixation
CSF Cerebrospinal fluid
CT Computerized axial tomography

CTS	Carpal tunnel syndrome	ESR	Erythrocytic sedimentation rate
CU	Cubic	ESRD	End stage renal disease
CV	Cardiovascular	EST	Electroshock therapy
CVA	Cerebrovascular accident	ESWL	Extracorporeal shock wave lithotripsy
CVD	Cardiovascular disease	EUA	Examination under anesthesia
CXR	Chest x-ray	EUD	Etiology undetermined
D&C	Dilation and curettage	F/U	Follow up
D&E	Dilation and evacuation	FB	Foreign body
D/T	Due to	FBS	Fasting blood sugar
DC	Direct current	FSH	Follicle stimulating hormone
DHS	Department of Health Services	FUO	Fever of undetermined origin
DJD	Degenerative joint disease	FX	Fracture
DM	Diabetes mellitus	GE	Gastroesophageal
DME	Durable medical equipment	GH	Growth hormone
DNR	Do not resuscitate	GI	Gastrointestinal
DOA	Dead on arrival	GTT	Glucose tolerance test
DOS	Date of service	GU	Genitourinary
DPT	Diphtheria pertussis tetanus	GYN	Gynecological
DT	Delirium tremens	H&P	History and physical
DTT	Diphtheria tetanus toxoid	H/O	History of
DUB	Dysfunctional uterine bleeding	HAA	Hepatitis associated antigen
DVA	Department of Veterans Affairs	HBEAB	Hepatitis B antibody
DVT	Deep vein thrombosis	HBEAG	Hepatitis B antigen
DX	Diagnosis	HBP	High blood pressure
EBV	Epstein-Barr virus	HCG	Human chorionic gonadotropin
ECCE	Extracapsular cataract extraction	HCL	Hydrochloride
ECF	Extended care facility	HCT	Hematocrit
ECG	Electrocardiogram	HEENT	Head, eyes, ears, nose, throat
ED	Emergency department	HGH	Human growth hormone
EDC	Expected date of confinement	HIB	Hemophilus influenza B
EDP	End diastolic pressure	HIV	Human immune deficiency virus
EEG	Electroencephalogram	HKAF	Hip knee ankle foot
EGD	Esophogogastroduodenoscopy	HKAFO	Hip knee ankle foot orthosis
EKG	Electrocardiogram	HOSP	Hospital
EMG	Electromyogram	HR	Hour
EMT	Emergency medical technician	HX	History
ENT	Ear nose and throat	HYPERAL	Hyperalimentation
EOB	Explanation of Benefits	I&D	Incision and drainage
EOMB	Explanation of Medicare Benefits	IBC	Iron binding capacity
EPSDT	Early periodic screening, diagnosis and treatment	IBS	Irritable bowel syndrome
		ICF	Intermediate care facility
ER	Emergency room	ICP	Intracranial pressure
ERCP	Endoscopic retrograde cholangiopan-creatography	ICU	Intensive care unit
		IDDM	Insulin dependent diabetes mellitus

IH	Infectious hepatitis
IHD	Ischemic heart disease
IHSS	Idiopathic hypertrophic subaortic stenosis
IM	Intramuscular
INC	Incorporated
INTERMED	Intermediate
INTRACATH	Intracatheter
IP	Inpatient
IPD	Intermittent peritoneal dialysis
IPPB	Intermittent positive pressure breathing
IQ	Intelligence quotient
IUD	Intrauterine device
IUP	Intrauterine pregnancy
IVH	Intravenous hyperalimentation
IVP	Intravenous pyelogram
JODM	Juvenile onset diabetes mellitus
JRA	Juvenile rheumatoid arthritis
KAF	Knee ankle foot
KO	Knee orthosis
KUB	Kidney ureter bladder
L/S	Lumbosacral
LAD	Left anterior descending
LB	Pound
LBBB	Left bundle branch block
LBP	Low blood pressure
LCA	Left coronary artery
LDH	Lactic dehydrogenase
LE	Lower Extremity
LGI	Lower gastrointestinal
LLL	Left lower lobe
LLQ	Left lower quadrant
LMP	Last menstrual period
LOC	Loss of consciousness
LOM	Left otitis media
LP	Lumbar puncture
LPN	Licensed practical nurse
LSK	Liver, spleen, kidney
LSO	Lumbar sacral orthosis
LTC	Long-term care
LUL	Left upper lobe
LUQ	Left upper quadrant
MD	Medical doctor
MEDS	Medications
MG	Milligram
MI	Myocardial infarction
MIA	Medically indigent adults
MINS	Minutes
MM	Millimeter
MMIS	Medicaid Management Information System
MMPI	Minnesota multiphasic personality inventory
MMR	Measles mumps rubella
MONO	Mononucleosis
MRI	Magnetic resonance imaging
MS	Multiple sclerosis
MSL	Midsternal line
MTP	Metatarsal phalanges
MVA	Motor vehicle accident
MVP	Mitral valve prolapse
NA	Sodium
NACL	Sodium chloride
NEC	Not elsewhere classified
NH	Nursing home
NIDDH	Non insulin dependent diabetes mellitus
NKA	No known allergies
NMRI	Nuclear magnetic resonance imaging
NOC	Not otherwise classified
NOS	Not otherwise specified
NP	Nasopharyngeal
NSR	Normal sinus rhythm
NSVD	Normal spontaneous vaginal delivery
O2	Oxygen
OB	Obstetrics
OM	Otitis media
OPD	Obstructive pulmonary disease
OPV	Oral poliovirus
ORIF	Open reduction internal fixation
OU	Both eyes
OV	Office visit
OZ	Ounce
PAP	Papanicolaou
PC	Professional component
PCP	Phencyclidine
PDR	Physicians desk reference
PHP	Prepaid health plan

PID	Pelvic inflammatory disease	S/P	Status post
PIN	Physician identifier number	SBO	Small bowel obstruction
PKG	Package	SED	Sedimentation
PMS	Premenstrual syndrome	SIDS	Sudden infant death syndrome
PO	By mouth	SLR	Straight leg raising
POE	Proof of Eligibility	SNF	Skilled nursing facility
POS	Place of Service	SOB	Shortness of breath
PPD	Purified protein derivative	SOC	Share of cost
PPN	Peripheral parenteral nutrition	SOM	Serous otitis media
PRN	As occasion requires	SQ	Subcutaneous
PRO	Professional Review Organization	SSA	Social Security Administration
PROM	Passive range of motion	SSI/SSP	Supplemental Security Income/State Supplemental Program
PTCA	Percutaneous transluminal coronary angioplasty	SSN	Social Security Number
PTT	Partial thromboplastin time	STD	Sexually Transmitted Disease
PUD	Peptic ulcer disease	SVT	Supraventricular tachycardia
PVC	Premature ventricular contraction	T&A	Tonsillectomy and adenoidectomy
PVD	Peripheral vascular disease	TAB	Therapeutic abortion
QD	Everyday	TAH	Total abdominal hysterectomy
QID	Four times a day	TAR	Treatment Authorization Request
R/O	Rule out	TB	Tuberculosis
RA	Rheumatoid arthritis	TD	Tetanus diphtheria
RAST	Radioallergosorbent test	TIA	Transient ischemic attack
RBBB	Right bundle branch block	TIBC	Total iron binding capacity
RBC	Red blood cell	TKR	Total knee replacement
RDS	Respiratory distress syndrome	TM	Temporomandibular
REM	Rapid eye movements	TMJ	Temporomandibular joint
RF	Rheumatoid factor	TORCH	Toxoplasmosis other rubella virus cytomegalovirus herpes
RHD	Rheumatic heart disease		
RIA	Radioimmunoassay	TOS	Type of service
RLL	Right lower lobe	TPL	Third-party liability
RLQ	Right lower quadrant	TPN	Total peripheral nutrition
RML	Right middle lobe	TSH	Thyroid stimulating hormone
RN	Registered nurse	TSS	Toxic shock syndrome
RO	Rule out	TUR	Transurethral resection
ROM	Right otitis media	TURP	Transurethral resection prostate
RPR	Rapid plasma reagin	UA	Urinalysis
RT	Right	UCG	Urine chorionic gonadotropin
RTC	Return to clinic	UE	Upper extremity
RUL	Right upper lobe	UGI	Upper gastrointestinal
RUQ	Right upper quadrant	UNI	Unilateral
RV	Right ventricular	URI	Upper respiratory infection
RVS	Relative value studies	UTI	Urinary tract infection
RX	Prescription	UV	Ultraviolet

VC	Vital capacity
VD	Venereal disease
VDRL	Venereal disease research laboratory

Medical Symbols

✔, u	Urine
⁒	Urine and defecation
⁄.	Defecation
□,♂	Male
○,♀	Female
↑	Goes up (toe signs)
↓	Goes down (toe signs)
>	Increased, enlarged, more than
<	Decreased, diminished, smaller than, less than
#	Number or pounds
†	Death
*	Birth
c, c̄	With (Latin: cum)
s̄	Without
+	Plus; excess; acid reactions; positive
−	Minus; deficiency; alkaline reaction; negative
±	Plus or minus; either positive or negative; indefinite
≅	Approximately, equals
≮	Not less than
≯	Not greater than
≤	Equal to or less than
≥	Equal to or greater than
≠	Not equal to
°	Degree
%	Percent

Summary

Understanding proper medical and insurance terminology is essential to both the health claims examiner and the medical biller. Without this knowledge, there will be a higher percentage of errors in both the filling out of forms and the payment of benefits.

Assignments

Complete the Questions for Review.
Complete Terminology Assignments 13-1 through 13-5.

Questions for Review

Directions: Answer the following questions without looking back into the material just covered. Write your answers in the space provided.

1. Define adjustment. ______________________________
2. The amount payable by the plan to a claimant, assignee, or beneficiary under each coverage is called a ______________________________
3. What does TIN stand for? ______________________________
4. An ______________________________ is licensed to perform any and all medical care or procedures.
5. What does LUQ stand for? ______________________________

If you were unable to answer any of the questions, refer back to the section and then fill in the answers.

Exercise 13-1

Directions: Define the following terms.

1. Eligibility Period ______________________________
2. Family Deductible ______________________________
3. Last Quarter Carry-Over ______________________________
4. Plan Document ______________________________
5. Common Accident Provision ______________________________
6. Exclusions ______________________________
7. Coinsurance ______________________________
8. Assignment of Benefits ______________________________
9. Basic Benefits ______________________________
10. Adjustment ______________________________
11. Beneficiary ______________________________
12. Benefit ______________________________
13. Maximum(s) ______________________________
14. Preexisting Exclusion ______________________________
15. Subrogation ______________________________

Exercise 13-2

Directions: Write the correct title for the following licensing abbreviations in the space provided.

1. DDS ______
2. EMT ______
3. LPN ______
4. MFCC ______
5. OT ______
6. PA ______
7. MD ______
8. DPM ______
9. CA ______
10. DC ______
11. OD ______
12. EdD ______
13. MSW ______
14. MT ______
15. RPT ______

Exercise 13-3

Directions: Write the correct definition for the following abbreviations in the space provided.

1. BP ______
2. CAPD ______
3. DOA ______
4. D&C ______
5. F/U ______
6. ER ______
7. HR ______
8. FB ______
9. LLQ ______
10. LE ______
11. AK ______
12. BK ______
13. RUQ ______
14. OB ______
15. NH ______

Exercise 13-4

Directions: Match the following abbreviations with their meanings. Write your answer in the space to the left of the abbreviation.

Column 1

_______ 1. ASO

_______ 2. COBRA

_______ 3. MWH

_______ 4. EIN

_______ 5. HMO

_______ 6. EOB

_______ 7. DEFRA

_______ 8. OOP

_______ 9. SPD

_______10. ERISA

_______11. TEFRA

_______12. PPO

_______13. UCR

_______14. MM

_______15. PAT

Column 2

a. The 1984 act that requires employers with 20 or more employees to offer the spouses, age 65+, of active employees the same coverage offered to younger spouses.

b. A summary of the plan document that is distributed to members of a self-funded plan.

c. A group of physicians who have negotiated discounted fees and do utilization review and quality assurance in exchange for a referral of a population of patients or monthly per capita payments.

d. The providing of services such as actuarial benefit plan design, claim processing, data recovery and analysis, and other administrative services for a self-funded plan.

e. The government act that requires employers with 20 or more employees to offer active employees age 65 or over and their spouses of the same age the same coverage under any group plan that is offered to younger workers.

f. Testing performed on an outpatient basis prior to admittance to an inpatient facility.

g. The amount determined to be the maximum allowable by the plan, based on the contract provisions, procedure, date of service, and geographical location of the provider.

h. Doctor's visits to a patient while the patient is hospitalized.

i. The government act that governs every aspect of private pension and welfare plans and requires employers who sponsor plans to operate them in compliance with these standards.

j. The portion of a health plan that pays benefits at a set percentage usually subject to a deductible.

k. A statement generated by the claim payor that indicates how the benefits were applied, paid, or denied on a particular claim.

l. An alternative form of health care delivery that refers all patients to a set location and provides a full range of health services.

m. The government act that provided for continuation of coverage for employees no longer considered eligible for a plan.

n. Applies to expenses such as the deductible and coinsurance that the insured is expected to pay for.

o. A number assigned by the IRS for tax purposes. This number is used by businesses in place of the social security number.

Exercise 13-5

Directions: Write the correct definition for the following symbols in the space provided.

1. ∵ ______________________
2. ∴ ______________________
3. ↓ ______________________
4. > ______________________
5. * ______________________
6. ≠ ______________________
7. c, $\bar{c}$ ______________________
8. ○, ♀ ______________________
9. ± ______________________
10. = ______________________
11. # ______________________
12. † ______________________
13. ≮ ______________________
14. $\bar{s}$ ______________________
15. □, ♂ ______________________

14

Reference Books

In this chapter you will learn:

- To recognize the *Merck Manual, PDR,* Medical Dictionary, *CPT,* and *ICD-9* and explain their use.

A reference book is a source of information to which a reader or consulter is referred. In health claims billing, coding, and examining, there are a number of books that are utilized as reference books. These include the *International Classification of Diseases–9th Revision Clinical Modification (ICD-9)*, *Physician's Current Procedural Terminology (CPT)*, *Relative Value Study (RVS)*, *Physicians' Desk Reference (PDR)*, the medical dictionary, and the *Merck Manual*. We will discuss each of them briefly in this chapter. The *ICD-9* and *CPT* each have their own chapter to discuss their use in further detail. Use of the *PDR* is covered in Chapter 16.

ICD-9

The *International Classification of Diseases–9th Revision Clinical Modification* is an indexing of conditions that serves a dual purpose for health benefits personnel. Mainly, it enables the medical biller and the claims examiner to convert English-language descriptions of an illness, injury, or other condition into a numerical code. Secondly, it allows for the classification of diseases for statistical purposes.

Symptoms, diseases, injuries, and routine services are identified with either a three-, four- or five-digit code, which may be entirely numerical or a combination of alphanumeric.

The *ICD-9* consists of three volumes:

Volume I–A tabular listing of diseases.

Volume II–An alphabetical listing of diseases by English-language description.

Volume III–A numerical and alphabetical listing of surgical or nonsurgical procedures that may be performed by a physician.

The order of use and the degree of use of each of these volumes varies. However, Volume III is not widely used by medical billers unless they work in a hospital setting. Many hospitals use the *ICD-9* procedural codes for billing rather than the *CPT* procedural codes.

CPT/RVS

The *Physician's Current Procedural Terminology (CPT)* is a systematic listing for coding the procedures or services performed by a physician. Within this text the word "physician" is used generically to apply to any provider of services other than a hospital or other facility. Each procedure is identified with a five-digit numerical code. The purpose of the *CPT* book is to provide a uniform method of accurately describing medical, surgical, and diagnostic services, which facilitates an effective means of communication among physicians, patients, and claim administrators.

The *Relative Value Study (RVS)* is another reference book used for coding physician services. The *RVS* preceded the *CPT* and was, in fact, the basis on which the *CPT* was designed. Consequently, the purpose of the *RVS* is the same as that of the *CPT*. These two manuals are referred to interchangeably even though the rules guiding their usage differ somewhat. Therefore, it is important for the examiner to know which standard is specified by the plan being processed so that the appropriate rules can be used.

The *CPT* and *RVS* each have six major sections:

1. Evaluation and Management–99201-99499
2. Medicine–90001-99199
3. Surgery–10000-69999
4. Anesthesia: CPT–0010-0199; RVS–99100-99140
5. Radiology/Nuclear Medicine–70000-79999
6. Pathology & Laboratory Tests–80000-89999

Physicians' Desk Reference

The *Physicians' Desk Reference* or *PDR* enables a lay or claims person to determine whether a pharmaceutical product is a prescription or nonprescription drug and lists some of the properties (eg, manufacturer, chemical make-up, side effects, appearance) of a specific drug. This is a very important distinction since most health plans do not cover nonprescription drugs.

The *PDR* is divided into six sections:

1. Manufacturers' Index
2. Product Name Index
3. Product Category Index
4. Product Identification Section
5. Product Information Section
6. Diagnostic Product Information

The first five sections are used by billing and examining personnel. Each of these sections will be covered in greater detail in Chapter 16.

Medical Dictionary

Medical dictionaries list medical terms and their definitions, synonyms, illustrations, and supplemental information. Numerous medical dictionaries are on the market. These dictionaries can be very helpful in assisting the biller and examiner to identify diagnoses, their symptoms, prognosis, and common treatment protocols. The use of a dictionary can assist the medical biller and the claims examiner in both coding the claim and determining whether or not the diagnosis or service is allowable under a plan. As a rule, this manual should be used mainly for verifying a diagnosis or affected body area or checking definitions and the spelling of terms. For greater detail on symptomatology and treatment protocols, the *Merck Manual* is more definitive. As with most dictionaries, entries are arranged alphabetically.

When using the medical dictionary, it is important that you first read through the foreword and any instructions or general guidelines contained in the front of the book. Since each publisher uses different symbols and information, you must read these instructions to understand the symbols and terms and their meanings.

In addition to basic definitions, many medical dictionaries include other information regarding the word or term. These can include the following 14 pieces of information:

1. The etymology of the word (ie, the original language and meaning).
2. The pronunciation of the word.
3. Biographical information on diseases, symptoms, conditions, procedures, or cures that have been given an eponym (named after a person, such as Addison's disease).
4. Synonyms. Often diseases or conditions are known by more than one name. In these instances they are listed as synonyms in the dictionary (eg, Addison's disease: adrenocortical hypofunction).
5. Abbreviations. If a word or term has a standard abbreviation in the medical community, this abbreviation is often listed in the medical dictionary.
6. Etiology. The causes of the disease.
7. Treatment. Common medical treatments are stated for some diagnoses or conditions. It is understood that this may not be the only effective medical treatment and that specifics of the treatment are not given.
8. Cross-reference. Cross-references for treatments may be included, allowing the user to locate possible drugs or treatments that may prove to be effective.
9. Prognosis. A generalized prognosis for the disease is given. At times it will include a prognosis for patients who are not treated and for those that are.
10. Nursing implications. The implications of care of the patient are listed. This may include the need for monitoring of certain conditions or vital signs.
11. Nursing diagnosis cross-reference. Some dictionaries list an appendix of nursing diagnoses and implications. Certain diseases or conditions will be cross-referenced to this section.
12. Subentries. Subentries contain more specific information regarding a term or condition and list some of the different types of conditions that can occur. For example, the subentries under the

term "acid" can include acetic a., boric a., citric a., fatty a., and sulfuric a., as well as many others. It is understood that a small letter followed by a period refers to a repetition of the original term or condition. In the example above, the "a." would stand for the word "acid."

13. Illustration cross-reference. An illustration occurs in the dictionary–placed either near the word or under another heading–which illustrates either the term or a portion of the definition. The user is directed to the correct page or term under which the illustration can be found.
14. Cautions or warnings. Certain terms or conditions have a warning placed within the definition. This is most often used with drugs and treatments. This warning can include any side effects or adverse reactions or conditions that can occur from use of the drug or treatment. Often this caution or warning is in boldface or marked off within a section to help call attention to it.

When using the medical dictionary, it is imperative that the medical biller and the health claims examiner read through the entire entry. If terms are used in the definition that the medical biller or health claims examiner does not understand, the unknown word should also be looked up, either in the medical dictionary (if it is a medical term) or in a standard dictionary (if it is not).

There are numerous diseases, conditions, or terms that are very similar to each other in spelling or pronunciation, but vastly different in meaning. It is important to use the proper term and its proper spelling when billing, coding, and examining a claim.

Merck Manual

Even the most experienced examiner occasionally has questions regarding the appropriateness of services for a reported diagnosis. The *Merck Manual* is relied on within the medical profession to assist in identifying the symptomatology, prognosis, treatment protocols, etiology, and other miscellaneous information regarding diagnoses.

When an examiner receives a claim with unusual services based on the diagnosis, using the *Merck Manual* may assist in identifying whether or not the treatment is appropriate for the reported diagnosis or symptoms.

The *Merck Manual* has two main sections: a listing of diseases and an index. The index is arranged alphabetically by disease. To look something up, simply turn to the index to find out what page the disease information is on.

The information provided includes the diagnosis, symptoms, prognosis, and treatment. If the treatment provided is not consistent with the diagnosis, it may be forwarded to a medical review board or a consultant, causing delays in the processing of the claim.

Summary

The *ICD-9*, the *CPT*, the *PDR*, the medical dictionary, and the *Merck Manual* are the reference books most commonly used by medical billing and health claims examining personnel.

The *ICD-9* is used to code diagnoses and conditions. The *CPT* is used to code procedures and services rendered by providers. Use of the *PDR* assists in determining whether a drug is prescription or nonprescription and lists some of the properties (ie, manufacturer, chemical make-up, side effects, appearance) of a specific drug. Medical dictionaries list medical terms and their meanings, and the *Merck Manual* can assist in determining whether a service or procedure is appropriate for a given diagnosis or condition.

Medical billers and health claims examiners should familiarize themselves with the use of each of the reference books just discussed. Without their proper utilization, delays and denials can result in claims submitted to payors.

Assignments

Complete the Questions for Review.

Questions for Review

Directions: Answer the following questions without looking back into the material just covered. Write your answers in the space provided.

1. Which manual is used for coding diagnoses? ______________________________

   ____
2. Name the two manuals that serve the same purpose and may be referred to interchangeably.

   a. ______________________________

   b. ______________________________
3. The full name of the *PDR* is ______________________________.
4. If you needed to verify a diagnosis, affected body area, or spelling of terms and definitions, you would probably refer to the ______________________________.
5. ______________________________ is useful in determining the appropriateness of services for a reported diagnosis.

If you were unable to answer any of the questions, refer back to the section and then fill in the answers.

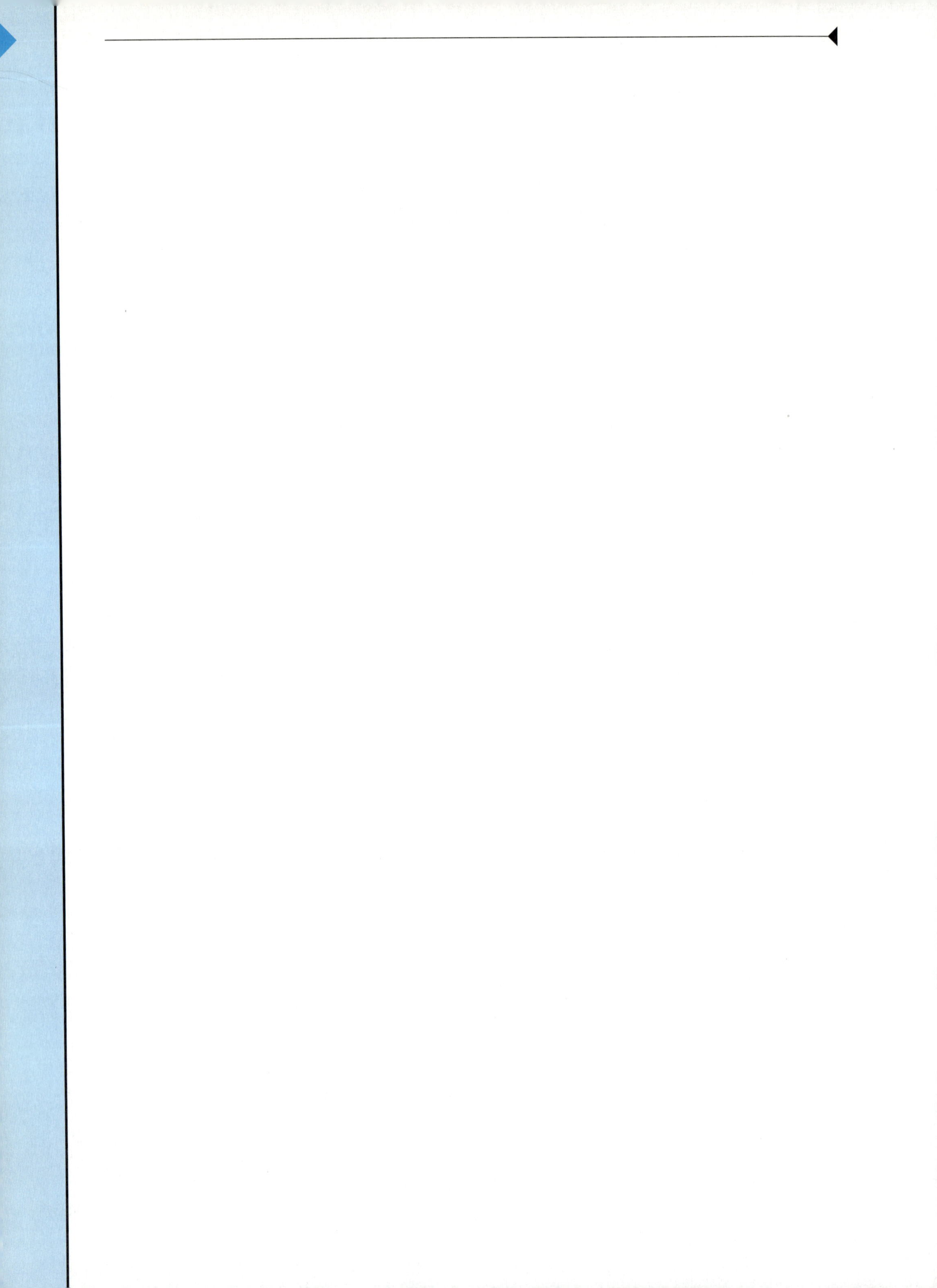

15

ICD-9

In this chapter you will learn:

- How to convert the English-language description of an illness or injury into a numeric ICD-9 diagnostic code.
- How to translate an ICD-9 code into an English-language description of the condition.

The *International Classification of Diseases, 9th Revision, Clinical Modification (ICD-9)* is a coding system devised to provide standardization of coding of diseases, impairments, and symptoms by the medical and insurance industry.

As our world becomes more and more computerized, new ways have been sought to classify and categorize all types of information. The health care industry is no exception.

History of the ICD-9

The *ICD-9* is a statistical coding of medical diagnoses and procedures that has been around (under different titles) since the early 1900s. It is based on the World Health Organization's (WHO) International Classification of Diseases (ICD).

The WHO originally came up with the ICD as a means of compiling data on morbidity and allowing hospitals and clinics to restore and retrieve diagnostic data.

In 1950, The Veterans Administration and the U.S. Public Health Service each began tests on the use of the ICD for hospital indexing. In 1951, New York City's Columbia Presbyterian Medical Center adopted the ICD-6th Revision (with modifications) for use in its medical records department. A few years later the Commission on Professional and Hospital Activities adopted the ICD with similar modifications for the use of hospitals participating in the Professional Activity Study.

Finally, the U.S. National Committee on Vital and Health Statistics (through its subcommittee on hospital statistics) reviewed the ICD and the various modifications and proposed uniform changes.

In 1956, the American Hospital Association and the American Association of Medical Record Librarians (later known as the American Medical Record Association) undertook a study of the efficacies of coding systems for diagnostic indexing. Their study concluded that the ICD provided a good framework for hospital indexing.

In 1977, the National Center for Health Statistics convened a steering committee to provide advice and council on revisions that should be made to the *ICD-9*. This created the ICD-9CM, which is a clinical modification of the WHO's *ICD-9*.

Upon release by the U.S. Department of Health and Human Services, numerous publishing companies print their version of the information contained in the *ICD-9*. These versions all contain the same basic information. However, various options are added in an effort to make their book more preferred. These options can include color coding, tabs, numerous symbols, and various instructions and aids.

The choice of which publisher's version of the *ICD-9* to use is simply a matter of individual or company choice.

Contents of the ICD-9

The ICD-9CM comprises three volumes:

- Volume I–the tabular or numerical listings, books 1 and 2
- Volume II–the alphabetic listings, books 1 and 2
- Volume III–a numeric listing of surgical procedure codes

Correct ICD-9 coding is important because this coding is often used as the statistical basis for clients to review the plan benefits in order to provide the most effective coverage for their members while controlling health care costs.

Many computerized claims processing systems use these codes to determine the benefits to pay on a claim. Incorrect coding can lead to incorrect benefit payments.

Let's look at each of the volumes in greater detail.

Volume I

Volume I is structured numerically according to body system. It is used when:

An ICD-9 code is provided, but there is no language description of the diagnosis.

A language diagnosis is included, but an ICD-9 is

not indicated and the terms used by the provider cannot be found in Volume II. If you can identify the body system, you may be able to locate an appropriate ICD-9 code.

Table 15-1 shows the organization of Volume I.

Table 15-1: Organization of ICD-9 Volume I

Number	Body System/Classification
00–13	Infective and Parasitic Diseases
14–23	Neoplasms
24–27	Endocrine, Nutritional, Metabolic Diseases
28	Diseases of the Blood and Blood-Forming Organs
29–31	Mental/Nervous Disorders
32–38	Diseases of the Nervous System and Sense Organs
39–45	Diseases of the Circulatory System
46–51	Diseases of the Respiratory System
52–57	Diseases of the Digestive System
58–62	Diseases of the Genito-Urinary System
63–67	Complications of Pregnancy, Child-birth and the Puerperium
68–70	Diseases of the Skin and Subcuta-neous Tissue
71–73	Diseases of the Musculoskeletal System and Connective Tissue
74–75	Congenital Anomalies
76–77	Certain Causes of Perinatal Morbidity and Mortality
78–79	Symptoms, Senility and Ill-Defined Conditions
80–86	Fractures, Dislocations, Sprains and Internal Injuries
87–90	Lacerations
91–99	Other Accidents, Poisoning and Violence (nature of the injury)
V0–Y24	Miscellaneous Informative Codings (a particular diagnosis is not indicated)
E800–E99 9	Supplementary Classification of External Causes of Injury and Poisoning

Volume II

Volume II is the alphabetical listing of diagnoses. This section is most commonly used first. It is divided into four sections:

1. an alphabetical index of diseases and injuries
2. a table of drugs and chemicals
3. an alphabetical index of external causes of injuries and poisonings (accidents) (E codes)
4. a listing of factors affecting the health status of an individual (V codes).

Volume III

Volume III of the *ICD-9* is used for coding diagnoses and procedures performed in a hospital. Volume III contains both a tabular listing and index. The tabular listing has procedures arranged according to body sections. The 16 body sections are arranged as follows:

1. Operations on the Nervous System
2. Operations on the Endocrine System
3. Operations on the Eye
4. Operations on the Ear
5. Operations on the Nose, Mouth and Pharynx
6. Operations on the Respiratory System
7. Operations on the Cardiovascular System
8. Operations on the Hemic and Lymphatic System
9. Operations on the Digestive System
10. Operations on the Urinary System
11. Operations on the Male Genital Organs
12. Operations on the Female Genital Organs
13. Obstetrical Procedures
14. Operations on the Musculoskeletal System
15. Operations on the Integumentary System
16. Miscellaneous Diagnostic/Therapeutic Procedures

The index has procedures listed in alphabetical order. Thus, it is the easiest way to look up a procedure. Medical billers should confirm their choice of code by looking in the tabular listing and checking all referrals, exclusions and notes included.

How to Use the ICD-9

The *ICD-9* is structured to move from a general diagnosis to a more specific diagnosis by adding on digits. It uses three-, four- or five-digit codes. Three-digit codes are the most general. By adding additional digits, a more precise diagnosis is identified.

The requirements of various processing systems or clients vary. Some may require very precise coding, and the use of five digits would be required.Others may not require such precision, so only three or four digits would be used.

When doing ICD-9 coding, the medical biller should always code to the last possible digit. This includes four- and five-digit subclassifications wherever they occur.

General Guidelines

Some basic guidelines should be kept in mind when coding and using the *ICD-9*. Many of these guidelines were first established by the Health Care Financing Administration (HCFA), which oversees the Medicare Program for the United States. After a recommendation or guideline has been adopted by the HCFA or Medicare, private payors and carriers usually adopt the same guidelines shortly thereafter.

Following are 16 general guidelines to keep in mind when trying to locate the proper ICD-9 code:

1. Read through the introduction of the *ICD-9* to be sure that you understand any color coding, symbols, abbreviations, and terms that the book uses.
2. Always use both the Index listing (Volume II) and the Numeric Listing (Volume I). Volume II alone will not give you any exclusions, referrals, or instructions for the codes, including the need for four- or five-digit subclassification.
3. Always code the principal diagnosis. The principal diagnosis is the condition that is established as being chiefly responsible for requiring the patient to seek medical care.
   a. Do not code symptoms nor the suspected condition if a final diagnosis is indicated. Symptoms and suspected conditions are usually accompanied by the following terms: "probable," "suspected," "questionable," or "Rule out (R/O)."
   b. It is understood that some conditions will not be fully diagnosed until test results have provided further understanding of the condition. In such cases, code conditions to the highest degree of certainty for the encounter. For example, many codes contain a fourth or fifth digit, which are for "unspecified" conditions or types. Often this will be indicated by the abbreviation NOS for "Not Otherwise Specified." These codes are acceptable if this is the highest level of certainty documented by the physician at this encounter.
   c. The term "Rule-Out" (R/O) is routinely submitted by some providers. This is not a diagnosis and is often not allowable under a plan. Whenever possible, the final diagnosis or the symptoms that prompted the testing should be used for coding.
4. Code only the diagnosis determined by the physician and any complications. Do not list any codes for previous conditions that were previously treated and that no longer exist.
5. Code diagnosis to the highest number of digits possible. For example, do not use only three digits to describe a condition when four- and five-digit subclassifications exist for that category. Many payors will return such claims requesting additional information. Be sure that you follow a category all the way up to the three-digit classification. Often the coding of four and five digits is listed under the main category heading, not under each separate diagnosis or condition.
6. The main diagnosis, condition, or reason for the encounter should be listed first. All other conditions that coexist at the time of treatment and that affect the treatment are to be coded following the main reason. If several conditions equally resulted in the encounter, the doctor or medical biller is free to list whichever he or she chooses first.
7. When a patient is seen for ancillary diagnostic services only, the appropriate V code should be listed first, and the diagnosis or condition that is

the underlying reason for the tests should be listed second. If a second code is not listed, delays in claim processing or denial of benefits may result. For example, if a chest x-ray is taken (coded V72.5) and no second code is listed, the claim may be denied if there are no benefits for routine chest x-rays. Without the second code the health claims examiner will often assume that the x-ray is for routine screening, not for a specific condition.

8. When a patient is seen for ancillary therapeutic services only, the appropriate V code should be listed first, and the diagnosis or condition that is the underlying reason for the services should be listed second. If a second code is not listed, delays in claim processing or denial of benefits may result.For example, if a child receives physical therapy services (code V57.1) due to cerebral palsy (code 343) and no second code is listed, the claim may be denied if there are no benefits for routine physical therapy. Without the second code the health claims examiner will often delay or deny benefits until they receive further information.
9. Diagnosis codes for chronic diseases or conditions may be coded as often as needed when the patient has repeated encounters for the chronic disease or condition.
10. Diagnoses that relate to earlier episodes of care or are chronic and have no bearing on the current treatment are to be excluded.
11. When billing for surgical procedures, use the correct code to indicate the diagnosis or reason for the surgery. If a postoperative diagnosis is different from the preoperative diagnosis, and the postoperative diagnosis is known at the time the claim is submitted, you should code the postoperative diagnosis.
12. Adjectives (acute, chronic, and the like) may appear as subterms. For example, the diagnosis of Acute Pelvic Inflammatory Disease may be located in the following manner:
    a. Look up the condition—disease
    b. Under disease, refer to the subheading (site) of pelvis, pelvic
    c. Locate the specific condition—inflammatory (female) (PID)
    d. Finally, locate manifestation—acute—614.3
13. Cross-reference to synonyms, closely related terms and code categories beginning with "See" and "See also." For example: Pelvic-peritonitis (See also peritonitis, pelvic, female).
14. Carefully read any and all notes under the main term. These can include exclusions, referrals, and examples of diagnoses or conditions.
15. Carefully note any modifiers associated with the main term. Compare these with any qualifying terms used in the diagnosis statement.
16. Watch for subterms listed under a main term. Subterms become more specific the farther down they go.

These guidelines should be memorized and used whenever you are looking up an ICD-9 code. They will ensure a higher degree of accuracy and a higher rate of correct benefit payment on claims.

Main Terms

The Alphabetic Index is arranged by condition, disease, or syndrome. These identifying names are called the Main Terms and are the keys by which this volume is structured. The Main Terms usually identify disease conditions rather than locations. The Main Terms may be listed as proper medical terms or as outmoded, ill-defined terms or as eponyms. Eponyms are illnesses or conditions named after a person (eg, Gerhardt's disease). Certain conditions may be listed under more than one term.

For example, in the following examples, the Main Terms are italicized.

Streptococcal *tonsillitis*–This can be located in two ways:

- under tonsillitis (subheading streptococcal)
- under infection (subheading streptococcal, site—sore throat)

Streptococcal is not a condition; it is the type of organism involved in an infection.

Some other examples include the following:

dislocated shoulder

pulmonary *edema*
pelvic *abscess*
prolapsed uterus
fractured radius
sick sinus *syndrome*
chronic *hepatitis*
external *hemorrhoids*

Once you have identified the code in the indexed listing (Volume II), cross-reference your selection with the Tabular listing in Volume I. This will ensure that you have selected the proper code. It will also allow you to code to the highest degree of specificity.

Be sure to research any exclusions, referrals ("see also"), and examples to ensure that your code is correct. Also be sure to refer to the three- and four-digit classification headings. These headings often have further information or list the fourth and fifth digits that apply to all following codes in that classification.

For example, let's use the dislocated shoulder mentioned previously. The index lists the three-digit classification for a dislocated shoulder as 831. However, a four-digit classification will tell whether the injury is open or closed, and a five-digit classification will pinpoint the diagnosis as to the more precise location of the injury. Also, note that a chronic or recurrent shoulder dislocation has an entirely different three-digit classification of 718.

Now turn to classification 831 in the tabular listing. You will see that the five-digit subclassifications are listed directly below the three-digit classification heading. This is followed by the three-digit classifications and the four-digit classifications.

The reason for this order can be better understood when you look at the codes 800–804. Each of these codes is for a fracture of the skull. The five-digit codes that immediately follow the classification heading can be used with any of the three- or four-digit classifications that begin with the numbers 800, 801, 803, or 804. The classifications for 804 appear several pages following this one. This is why it is important to always look back to the four- and three-digit classification headings when coding.

Exceptions

In some instances, the *ICD-9* is organized differently so that the Main Terms do not identify disease conditions. These exceptions include:

- Obstetric conditions, which are found under "Delivery," "Pregnancy," or "Puerperal." (*Puerperal* refers to the period immediately following delivery.)
- Complications of medical and surgical conditions, which are located under "Complications." However, they can also be found under the condition. For example, "evisceration" of an operative wound can be found under evisceration and complication. It is recommended that you look under the condition.
- Late effects of diseases and injuries, which are under the Main Term "late effects."
- In some situations, a claim or bill may provide a "diagnosis" that is not an illness or injury per se. For example, exposure to, history of, problem with, or vaccination are not diagnoses but may be considered appropriate Main Terms.

Appropriate sites and/or modifiers are listed in alphabetical sequence under the Main Terms with further subterm listings as required. For example, the diagnosis of Open Tibia/Fibula Fracture may be located as follows:

See Fracture heading
Locate tibia as a subheading
Site—with fibula
Description—open = 823.92

Neoplasms

A neoplasm is a growth (tumor) that results from abnormal cell activity. Selecting an ICD-9 code for a neoplasm involves identifying the following factors:

- the pathologic status of the growth—benign or malignant
- the site of the growth (eg, breast, lung, bladder)
- the cell type (eg, oat cell)

This information is not always provided on medical

reports, claims, or bills. Therefore, as with any other diagnosis, the code selected will be based on the available information. The more information provided, the more specific the code.

For coding growths, you need to become familiar with the ICD-9 Neoplasm Table (NT) located in Volume II. This table is organized alphabetically by site (location). Since the site is not always known, there is an entry for "unknown site or unspecified."

On the right side of the NT are six columns from which to select an ICD-9 code based on the given diagnosis. The terms used in these columns are defined as follows:

Malignant primary—Primary means that the site of the tumor is the point of origin of the neoplasm. Malignant means that the cancer or growth is growing. Malignant growths will spread throughout the body until they kill the patient.

Malignant secondary—Secondary means that the site of the tumor in question is not where the disease originated. It has spread to this location from the primary site.

Malignant CA in situ—In situ means that the malignant growth is still localized in one area and has not spread.

Benign—Localized growth that does not spread (metastasize) and is not usually terminal.

Uncertain Behavior—Usually a particular type of growth is either always malignant or always benign. There are, however, some growths that may be either. In cases in which the information does not establish which type of manifestation is present and the growth could be either, this coding may be used. As a rule, this column should be used only when the neoplasm's behavior is stated to be uncertain by a pathologist or physician or is listed as such in the Alphabetic Index.

Unspecified—A growth is unspecified when it is not identified as benign or malignant and the type of growth is always one or the other.

The first step in coding growths is to determine whether the growth is benign or malignant. If the status is indicated, go directly to the Table under either the malignant or benign column, according to the site of the growth. Choose the malignant column based on the specifics of the diagnosis—primary, secondary, or in situ.

For example:

DX: Benign Breast Tumor
ACTION:
1. Find "breast" alphabetically.
2. Look at the benign column.
3. The code is 217.

DX: CA In Situ–Uterus
ACTION:
1. Find "uterus" alphabetically.
2. Look under Malignant-CA in situ.
3. The code is 233.2.

DX: Brain Tumor
ACTION:
1. Find "brain" alphabetically.
2. Look under Unspecified.
3. The code is 239.6

If a growth is identified as malignant, but is not further identified as primary, secondary, or CA in situ, assume that it is primary.

The terms CA, cancer, carcinoma, and sarcoma always indicate a malignancy. Other terms, like fibroma and adenoma, require you to check the alphabetical listing (not the NT) of Volume II to determine whether the condition is benign or malignant. Subsequently, the proper column in the NT can be referenced.

For example:

If the diagnosis on the bill is:	Look under the Main Term:
Pelvic Fibroma	Fibroma
Adenoma	Adenoma
Adenosarcoma	Adenosarcoma
Papilloma, eyelid	Papilloma
Osteosarcoma	Osteosarcoma

In most cases, looking under the appropriate Main Term will direct you to the correct column in the NT. In some circumstances, however, you will be given a valid ICD-9 code by the provider and you will not need to reference the NT at all.

Lesions

Although lesions are similar to neoplasms, they are treated differently by the *ICD-9*. Lesions should be handled as indicated in the following statements:

If the diagnosis simply states "lesion," look under the Main Term "lesion" alphabetically in Volume II.

If the diagnosis is "benign lesion," look under the Main Term "lesion."

If the diagnosis is "malignant lesion," look under one of the malignant columns in the NT in Volume II.

Sprains/Strains

Sprains and strains are coded according to the site of injury. Strains of the musculoskeletal system are included under the Main Term, Sprain. There is a separate Main Term reference for strains that are not related to the musculoskeletal system (such as eyestrain). If the location of the musculoskeletal strain or sprain is unknown, use code 848.9 (musculoskeletal system). Normally, 848.9 is used as a temporary code while additional information is requested from the member or provider. However, this procedure varies from company to company.

Dislocations

As with strains and sprains, dislocations are coded according to the site of injury. Code 839.8 should be used if the exact injury site is unknown. (See previous paragraph.)

A closed dislocation includes simple, complete, partial, uncomplicated, and unspecified (type). Open includes infected, compound, and dislocation with a foreign body.

"Chronic," "habitual," "old," or "recurrent" dislocations may be coded as "dislocation, recurrent, and pathologic."

Fractures

As with strains, sprains, and dislocations, fractures are coded according to the site of injury.

Closed fractures include the following descriptions, with or without delayed healing:

comminuted	linear
depressed	march
elevated	simple
fissured	slipped epiphysis
greenstick	spiral
impacted	unspecified

Open fractures include the following, with or without delayed healing:

compound	infected
missile	puncture with or without a foreign body

Assume that the fracture is closed unless there is wording that indicates otherwise.

When multiple fractures are involved, it is easier to look under the names of the bones involved than to look under "Fracture, multiple."

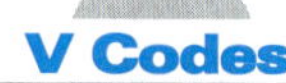

V Codes

The V code listing is a supplementary listing of factors that affect the health status of the patient. Often there are reasons for an encounter that relate to a disease or condition, but do not constitute a diagnosis. There are three main types of occurrences:

1. When a person who is not ill has an encounter with a health care provider for a specific purpose that is not in and of itself a disease or condition. These encounters can include a visit from a person who is getting a vaccination or a check-up, who is acting as an organ or tissue donor to another person, or who wants to discuss a problem that is not considered a disease or condition (ie, fertility problems, genetic counseling).
2. When a patient with a chronic or recurring condition visits a health care provider for service associated with treatment of that condition. This can include a cast change, dialysis for renal disease, monitoring of pacemaker, and other similar situations.
3. When a situation arises that influences the person's health, but is not a disease or condition.

Such situations include exposure to potential health hazards (eg, tuberculosis, polio), animal bites that require rabies vaccination, and the fact that a person's physiology or family history suggests a factor that should be borne in mind when treatment is received (ie, carrier of suspected infectious diseases, history of cancer or other diseases, allergies to medicines).

When doing diagnosis coding in circumstances 2 and 3 above, the V code should be used as a supplementary code (not the primary diagnosis code). The diagnosis or condition that underlies the reason for the treatment (circumstance 2) or that caused the patient to seek medical attention (circumstance 3) should be coded as the primary diagnosis.

V codes are arranged according to the following headings:

V01–V09 Persons with potential health hazards related to communicable diseases
V10–V19 Persons with potential health hazards related to personal and family history
V20–V29 Persons encountering health services in circumstances related to reproduction and development
V30–V39 Liveborn infants according to type of birth
V40–V49 Persons with a condition influencing their health status
V50–V59 Persons encountering health services for specific procedures and aftercare
V60–V68 Persons encountering health services in other circumstances
V70–V82 Persons without reported diagnosis encountered during examination and investigation of individuals and populations

As a medical biller you should examine the V codes and familiarize yourself with the situations they define.

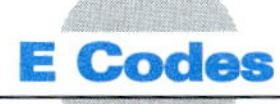

E Codes

The E code listing is a supplementary classification of external causes of injury and poisoning. E codes are used to indicate a cause of the injury, not the injury itself. Therefore, an E code should always be a supplementary code, not a primary diagnosis code.

For example, let's code a patient who was struck by a car as a pedestrian and suffered a fractured femur. The diagnosis would be fractured femur (code 821.00), and the cause would be pedestrian struck by automobile (E814.7).

To correctly code E codes, consult the index located in section 3 of Volume II (behind the table of drugs and chemicals). This index is used the same way the index to diseases and conditions is used. First, locate the cause in the index, then turn to the tabular listing to confirm your choice and to ensure correct four- and five-digit subclassifications.

The beginning of the E code section contains definitions of the terms involved in describing causes. The medical biller should familiarize himself or herself with these definitions because they are vital to proper coding.

When coding transport accidents, the following headings are used:

Aircraft and spacecraft (E840–E845)
Watercraft (E830–E838)
Motor Vehicle (E810–E825)
Railway (E800–E807)
Other road vehicles (E826–E829)

If you are coding an accident that involves more than one type of vehicle, the order listed above should be followed.

For example, let's code an accident between a car and a streetcar. Since a streetcar is considered a railway vehicle, the car would take precedence. Therefore, you would look under the motor vehicle section to find motor vehicle accident involving collision with train (E810). The four-digit subclassification would then be added to this number to describe the activity of the patient at the time of the accident (see motor vehicle accident section heading).

If you are coding machinery accidents (nontransport vehicles), you should use category E919.x. This allows for a broad description of the type of machinery and activity that made up the cause of the injury. If you wish to provide a more detailed description, the Internal Labor Office has created a Classification of

Industrial Accidents According to Agency. However, this classification should be used in addition to the appropriate E code, not in place of it. Some versions of the ICD-9 reproduce this classification listing.

Billing Tips

The medical biller should be aware of a number of factors when entering ICD-9 codes on the claims that they submit for payment. These factors can cause delays in benefit payments and sometimes even denial of benefits.

However, always remember that to file a false claim is considered fraud, and there are severe penalties for fraud. When taking the above factors into consideration, the medical biller should also remember that the claim should be filled out according to the actual diagnosis or conditions that exist and the actual procedures performed. To alter a medical record or a claim just to meet the criteria listed below is to perform a criminal act.

Five important factors to be aware of in billing are:

1. The diagnosis coded must support the services rendered. On the HCFA-1500, the diagnosis that relates to each procedure performed is placed next to the procedure code. Therefore, each procedure performed should have a diagnosis that substantiates the need for that procedure. If the procedures performed are not supported by the diagnosis (eg, an x-ray of the foot is taken when the diagnosis is a concussion), benefits for the procedure will be denied. Likewise, claims submitted on a UB-92 may be denied if the diagnosis does not support the need for the goods or services listed in the itemized billing statement.
2. The medical biller is limited to the available number of spaces on the billing form. Only four codes may be entered on the HCFA-1500 claim form and 10 on the UB-92. If more conditions exist than there are spaces on the form, there are three options:
   a. List only the main conditions up to the number of spaces provided.
   b. On the HCFA-1500, if more than six procedures were performed, you may submit on more than one claim form. For example, the doctor may treat a patient who was a pedestrian struck by a car. If the patient had multiple injuries, those procedures that were related to the head and upper body injuries could be billed on one claim form and those procedures relating to the lower body injuries could be billed on a second claim form. Both claim forms should contain the correct E code (E814.7) and the date of the accident.
   c. If you strongly believe that additional diagnostic information is needed to process the claim or substantiate the services provided, you may attach a medical report or other supporting documentation to your claim. However, it should be noted that this information may be ignored by the health claims examiner, or it may result in a delay to allow time to review the information.
3. The location of service must be substantiated by the diagnosis and the procedures rendered. There are two factors related to this condition:
   a. If the location of service is clearly inappropriate for the services rendered, there will be problems in the payment of the claim. For example, if the diagnosis indicates heart disease and the service provided is a heart transplant, then the location of services cannot be a doctor's office.
   b. Many people will go to a place that is convenient rather than to the place where it is appropriate that they should go. The greatest abuse of this situation is people using the hospital emergency room for situations that are not true emergencies. If the diagnosis listed indicates that the condition was not an emergency, many payors will pay the claim based on the appropriate place of treatment. Since emergency room services cost much more than those same services performed in a doctor's office, this can result in a large discrepan-

cy between the amount billed and the amount received from the payor.

4. The diagnosis must match the level of services provided. When coding procedures, the complexity of the medical condition and the level of service rendered (ie, minimal, limited, brief, expanded, comprehensive) should be substantiated by the diagnosis listed. If the diagnosis and the complexity of services do not match, often the level of services will be downgraded (see following section on Downgrading of Codes/Benefits) to match the diagnosis.
5. The diagnosis must substantiate service frequency. Often patients need repeated services to alleviate chronic conditions. However, if there is no alleviation of the symptoms or no benefits are received from the continued treatment, payors may deny some or all of the treatments.

Concurrent Care

Often reimbursement problems arrive when two doctors are seeing a patient at the same time for two unrelated medical conditions. This is known as concurrent care. Claims were frequently denied as duplication of services when the patient was seen by two physicians on the same day, when no duplication actually occurred.

Prior to 1992, there was a CPT modifier (-75) that notated concurrent care. This modifier has since been dropped. Now there are two ways to ensure the greatest possibility of payment from the payor:

1. Submit two separate claim forms, one for each physician, which list two completely separate diagnoses and the related services that were provided.
2. If the separate providers were members of the same medical group and payment is to be made to the medical group, then all services should be submitted on the same claim form. However, two separate diagnoses should be listed, and the procedures performed for each should be substantiated by the referencing of the separate diagnosis next to the procedure.

Downgrading of Codes/Benefits

Diagnoses that do not fit the previously mentioned criteria may cause the health claims examiner to downgrade the codes or the benefits paid. Downgrading is a process of reducing a code of a higher value to one of a lower value so that the procedures, locations, and frequency of service are appropriate to the diagnosis given. This can result in the loss of millions of dollars for the health care provider and his or her patients.

For example, if the diagnosis does not support the level of services provided, a lower level will be assigned. If the diagnosis given does not substantiate the procedures, payment on the procedures will be denied as medically unnecessary. If the location is inappropriate for the service provided, the claim will either be delayed or denied, or the benefits will be paid as if the services were rendered at the appropriate place (as in emergency services being paid at office services rates when no true emergency occurred).

If claims are submitted to Medicare with any of the above-mentioned discrepancies in place, the claim will automatically be returned to the provider without payment of any benefits. The provider must then resubmit a properly completed claim.

If the provider refuses to submit the correct ICD-9 codes, fines may be levied or the provider may be barred from participating in the Medicare program.

Summary

The *ICD-9* is the primary book used when coding diagnoses on health claims. It is made up of three volumes. Volume I is the tabular listing of diagnoses and conditions. Volume II is the indexed or alphabetic listing of diagnoses and conditions. Volume III is the tabular and alphabetic listing of procedures.

To accurately look up a diagnosis, the medical biller should locate the Main Term for the condition under the indexed listing in Volume II. The numeric code gained should then be checked against the information provided in Volume I, and all referrals, exclusions, and additional digit subclassifications should be consulted to ensure that the right code has been chosen.

The same process is used when coding procedures

in Volume III. First, consult the index, then cross-reference the code with the information provided in the tabular listing.

It is vital for the medical biller to understand each of the three volumes of the *ICD-9* and how to use them.

It is also important for the medical biller to understand the importance of how diagnoses or ICD-9 codes relate to the other information on a claim form. Diagnoses that do not substantiate services rendered, match the proper location of services, or otherwise conflict with additional information on the claim form will result in delays and denials of benefit payments.

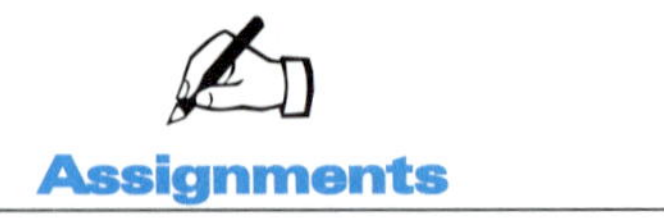

Assignments

Complete the Questions for Review.

Complete ICD-9 exercises 15-1 through 15-3. Correct the exercises upon completion. If you are billing correctly less than 90% of the time, more practice is needed.

Questions for Review

Directions: Answer the following questions without looking back into the material just covered. Write your answers in the space provided.

1. Volume __________ is the tabular listing of diagnoses.
2. If only a language description of the condition is provided, Volume __________ should be used to locate the numerical listing.
3. Main Terms are used to identify the ______________________________.
4. Benign lesions are listed in the Neoplasm Table. (True or False) ______________________________
5. Always assume fractures are "open," unless otherwise indicated. (True or False) ______________________
6. The more digits in the code, the more general the diagnosis. (True or False) ______________________
7. Obstetric-related conditions are handled differently than other Main Terms. (True or False) ____________
8. "Rule Out" is a definitive diagnosis. (True or False) ______________________________
9. Volume II is used in some instances to determine whether a neoplasm is ____________________ or ____________________.
10. One important use of ICD-9 codes by clients is ______________________________.

If you were unable to answer any of the questions, refer back to the section and then fill in the answers.

Exercise 15-1

Directions: Look up the following ICD-9 codes in Volume I and write the corresponding English-language description in the space provided.

	Code	Description
1.	091.69	1. ______
2.	142.8	2. ______
3.	203.8	3. ______
4.	239.5	4. ______
5.	282.4	5. ______
6.	282.61	6. ______
7.	322.0	7. ______
8.	391.0	8. ______
9.	464.3	9. ______
10.	711.37	10. ______

Exercise 15-2

Directions: Look up the following ICD-9 codes in Volume I and write the corresponding English-language description in the space provided.

Code	Description
1. 780.1	1. ______________________
2. 250.71	2. ______________________
3. 711.15	3. ______________________
4. 727.43	4. ______________________
5. 730.22	5. ______________________
6. 741.93	6. ______________________
7. 802.22	7. ______________________
8. 902.41	8. ______________________
9. V04.5	9. ______________________
10. E912	10. ______________________

Exercise 15-3

Directions: Based on the condition, look up the appropriate ICD-9 code and write it and the Main Term in the space provided.

Condition	Code(s)	Main Term
1. Tuberculous pleurisy	________	________
2. Nontoxic nodular goiter	________	________
3. Pernicious anemia	________	________
4. Bacterial meningitis	________	________
5. Tricuspid valve disease	________	________
6. Upper respiratory infection	________	________
7. Bronchitis	________	________
8. Acute bronchitis	________	________
9. Gangrene secondary to diabetes	________	________
10. Normal delivery	________	________
11. Metacarpus osteoarthrosis	________	________
12. Apnea	________	________
13. Exposure to hepatitis	________	________
14. Gallbladder disease	________	________
15. Acne	________	________

Exercise 15-4

Directions: Based on the condition, look up the appropriate ICD-9 code and write it in the space provided.

Condition	Code
1. Mexican typhus	1.______________
2. Endometrium squamous metaplasia	2.______________
3. Orbital melanoma	3.______________
4. Corii degenerative melanosis	4.______________
5. Cerebrum medullomyoblastoma	5.______________
6. Lipoidica necrobiosis	6.______________
7. Rosacea acne	7.______________
8. Artificial insemination	8.______________
9. DPT inoculation	9.______________
10. Unexplained night sweats	10.______________
11. Swimmer's ear	11.______________
12. Heart palpitations	12.______________
13. Paramacular lesion of the retina	13.______________
14. Rectal leukoplakia	14.______________
15. Plasma cell leukemia not in remission	15.______________

Exercise 15-5

Directions: Based on the condition, look up the appropriate ICD-9 code and write it in the space provided.

Condition	Code
1. Proximal fibular open dislocation	1.______________
2. Gangrene of the tunica vaginalis	2.______________
3. Obstructed gangrenous hernia	3.______________
4. Hypercholesterolemia	4.______________
5. Dysfunctional amenorrhea	5.______________
6. SIDS	6.______________
7. Glomerulohyalinosis diabetic syndrome	7.______________
8. Gonococcal salpingo-oophoritis	8.______________
9. Bladder neck stricture	9.______________
10. Popliteal thrombophlebitis	10.______________
11. Cooper's disease	11.______________
12. Superior mesenteric artery syndrome	12.______________
13. Renal artery thrombosis	13.______________
14. Recurrent urethritis	14.______________
15. Enuresis	15.______________

Exercise 15-6

Directions: Based on the condition, look up the appropriate ICD-9 code and write it in the space provided.

Condition	Code
1. Giant cell carcinoma	1.__________
2. Dermatofibroma protuberans	2.__________
3. Leydig cell tumor	3.__________
4. Glomangioma	4.__________
5. Intramuscular lipoma	5.__________
6. Sebaceous cyst	6.__________
7. Leukemia	7.__________
8. Oat cell lung carcinoma	8.__________
9. Papillary hydradenoma	9.__________
10. Mucoid adenoma of the auricle	10.__________
11. Juxtaglomerular tumor	11.__________
12. Malignant insulinoma	12.__________
13. Basophil adenoma of the nose	13.__________
14. Malignant renal intraductal papilloma	14.__________
15. Abdominal fibromatosis	15.__________

Exercise 15-7

Directions: Based on the condition, look up the appropriate ICD-9 code and write it in the space provided.

Condition	Code
1. Diabetes mellitus	1. ______________
2. Endogenous obesity	2. ______________
3. Essential hypertension	3. ______________
4. Inguinal hernia	4. ______________
5. Tendon sheath ganglion	5. ______________
6. Borderline glaucoma	6. ______________
7. Glioblastoma of the forearm	7. ______________
8. Ulcerative gastroenteritis	8. ______________
9. Hallux valgus	9. ______________
10. Heart disease	10. ______________
11. Heat prostration	11. ______________
12. Epidural hematoma of the brain	12. ______________
13. Internal hemorrhoids	13. ______________
14. Familial hypercholesterolemia	14. ______________
15. Endocrine imbalance	15. ______________

Exercise 15-8

Directions: Based on the condition, look up the appropriate ICD-9 code and write it in the space provided.

Condition	Code
1. Hypothyroidism	1.________________
2. Fetal alcohol intoxication	2.________________
3. Diabetic Iritis	3.________________
4. Loss of appetite	4.________________
5. Embryonal liposarcoma	5.________________
6. Degenerative macula	6.________________
7. Necrosis of the liver	7.________________
8. Ameloblastic sarcoma	8.________________
9. Septicemic salmonella	9.________________
10. Squamous cell carcinoma of the skin, in situ	10.________________
11. Cuboid infected fracture	11.________________
12. Recurrent elbow dislocation	12.________________
13. Weight gain failure	13.________________
14. End-stage renal disease	14.________________
15. Thyroid disease	15.________________

Exercise 15-9

Directions: Based on the condition, look up the appropriate ICD-9 code and write it in the space provided.

Condition	Code
1. Degenerative nephritis	1. ____________
2. Neurofibromatosis	2. ____________
3. Cardiovascular observation	3. ____________
4. Tibial osteosarcoma	4. ____________
5. Stirrup otosclerosis	5. ____________
6. Ruptured spleen	6. ____________
7. Skin sepsis	7. ____________
8. Anaphylactic shock	8. ____________
9. Sesamoiditis	9. ____________
10. Carotid artery stenosis	10. ____________
11. Post status asthmaticus	11. ____________
12. Capsulitis of the knee	12. ____________
13. Glue ear syndrome	13. ____________
14. Tattoo removal	14. ____________
15. Trichinosis	15. ____________

Exercise 15-10

Directions: Based on the condition, look up the appropriate ICD-9 code and write it in the space provided.

Condition	Code
1. Costochondral pain	1. ________
2. Food poisoning	2. ________
3. Spurious polycythemia	3. ________
4. Prolapsed cecum	4. ________
5. Psoriasis	5. ________
6. Manic-depressive	6. ________
7. Hydrocephalic fetus	7. ________
8. Exhaustion	8. ________
9. Fibromyositis	9. ________
10. Mammary fibrosis	10. ________
11. Psychological strain	11. ________
12. Bronchial carcinoma	12. ________
13. Plasma cell sarcoma	13. ________
14. Corneal scarring	14. ________
15. Metacarpal villous adenoma	15. ________

Exercise 15-11

Directions: Based on the condition, look up the appropriate ICD-9 code and write it in the space provided.

Condition	Code
1. Biphasic mesothelioma of the bladder	1.________
2. Uterine fibroids	2.________
3. Microglioma of the brain	3.________
4. Melancholia	4.________
5. Menopausal syndrome	5.________
6. Hereditary methemoglobinemia	6.________
7. Complications of gallbladder surgery	7.________
8. Thrombotic thrombocytopenic purpura	8.________
9. Apoplexy of the brain	9.________
10. Ruptured thoracic aneurysm	10.________
11. Pseudoleukemia infantum	11.________
12. Overdose of anesthesia	12.________
13. Normocytic myelophthisic anemia	13.________
14. Corpus cavernosum contusion	14.________
15. Subdural brain bruising	15.________

Exercise 15-12

Directions: Based on the condition, look up the appropriate ICD-9 code and write it in the space provided.

Condition	Code
1. Nervous twitch	1.__________
2. Hurthle cell	2.__________
3. Pregnant with twins	3.__________
4. Twisted umbilical cord (during delivery)	4.__________
5. Metastasis to the pancreas	5.__________
6. Semilunar cartilage cyst	6.__________
7. Endometrioid cystadenocarcinoma of middle lobe of lung	7.__________
8. Premature heart contractions	8.__________
9. Severe sunburn of the back	9.__________
10. Chemical burn of gums	10.__________
11. Struck by a falling object	11.__________
12. Deaf mute	12.__________
13. Cruveilhier's disease	13.__________
14. Cholecystic chlamydial disease	14.__________
15. Alzheimer's disease	15.__________

Exercise 15-13

Directions: Based on the condition, look up the appropriate ICD-9 code and write it in the space provided.

Condition	Code
1. Fractured mandible, open	1. ________
2. Fractured larynx	2. ________
3. Fractured femur, subtrochanteric	3. ________
4. Fractured tibia and fibula	4. ________
5. Compound Fx, trochanter	5. ________
6. Fx skull with concussion	6. ________
7. Fx ribs (six), open	7. ________
8. Sprained ankle	8. ________
9. Strain, knee	9. ________
10. Sprain, elbow	10. ________
11. Sprained foot	11. ________
12. Eye strain	12. ________
13. Dislocated joint (infected)	13. ________
14. Dislocated jaw, recurrent	14. ________
15. Dislocated collar bone, open	15. ________

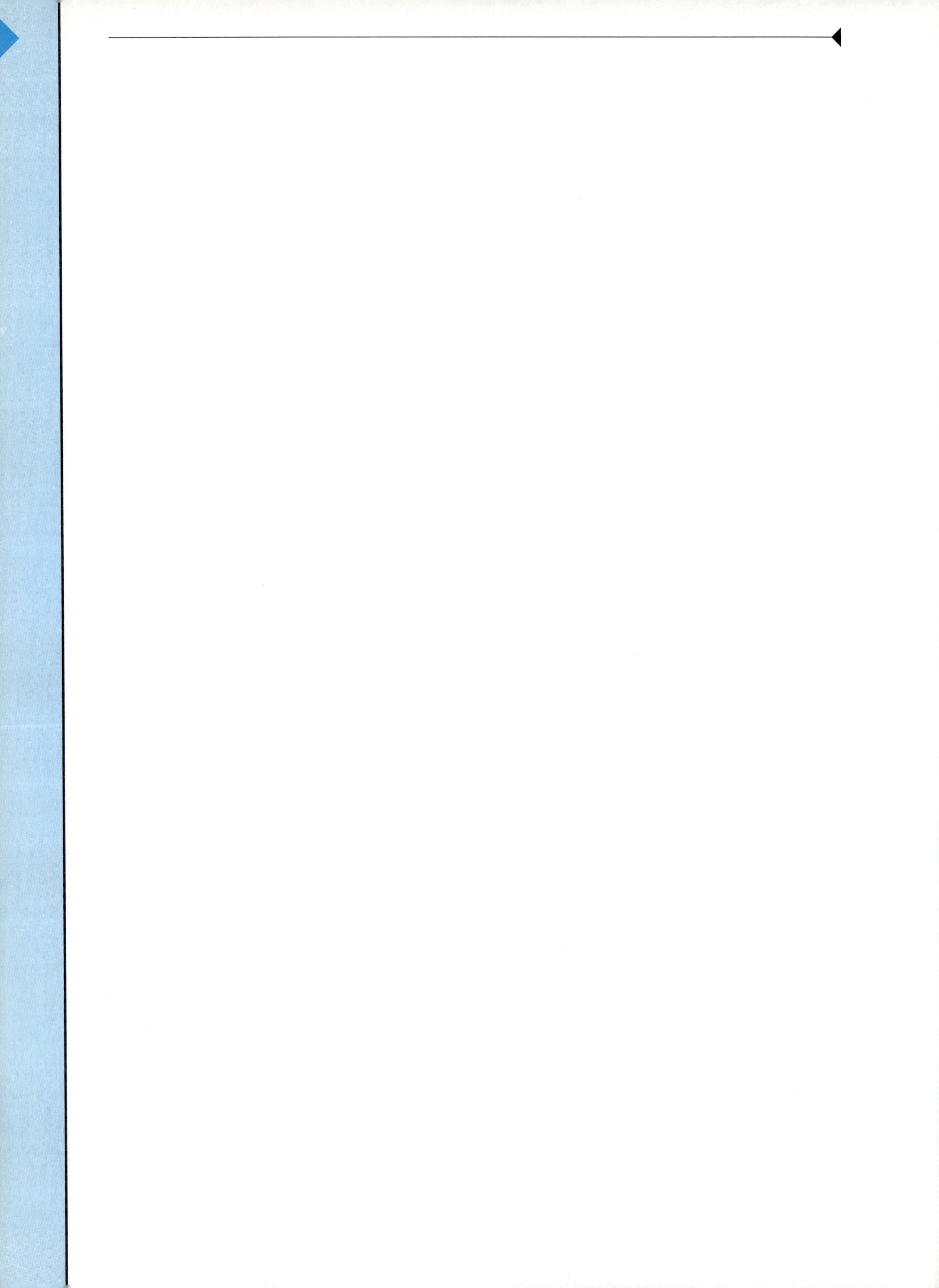

16

Medications and the Physicians' Desk Reference

In this chapter you will learn:

- To determine if a drug is a prescription or a non-prescription drug.
- To understand the sections of the *Physicians' Desk Reference* and the information each section contains.
- To properly use the *Physicians' Desk Reference*.

Medications are drugs used to treat diseases, symptoms, or discomforts (eg, pain medications). Prescription medications are usually covered under benefit plans in one of two ways: (1) under a separate, free-standing plan for outpatient, prescription medicines only or (2) under Major Medical as any other eligible expense, subject to all applicable deductibles, co-payments, limitations, and exclusions.

Service Plans

Separate prescription service plans are usually handled by third-party administrative (TPA) organizations, which establish networks of participating pharmacies and then assume responsibility for the claims processing. Such plans usually include some if not all of the following five components:

1. The claimant is not required to pay for his or her prescription with a large cash outlay. Instead, a small specified co-payment amount, chosen by the group, is paid by the claimant for each prescription (these co-payments usually range from $2.00 to $15.00).
2. The pharmacy accepts an identification card as evidence that payment will be made by the plan; it then bills the plan for the unpaid balance.
3. A claim form is not required from the cardholder. The pharmacy bills the TPA directly.
4. The member is required to go to a participating pharmacy to fill prescriptions. Otherwise, the claimant will be responsible for the full payment of the medication, or a reduced percentage may be paid by the TPA. In this case, the claimant would have to submit the prescription to the TPA for payment consideration.
5. Each prescription filling will provide a supply for a specified number of days—usually a 30-day maximum.

Typically, service plans exclude the following six types of expenses:

1. Devices or medical/surgical supplies of any type such as bandages, gauze, and the like. Hypodermic needles and syringes may be covered for diabetics.
2. Contraceptive drugs, even though the medication may have been prescribed for other than contraceptive purposes.
3. Drugs dispensed while the member is confined in a facility, including those given on the day of discharge.
4. Immunization agents, biological sera, blood, plasma, or other blood agents.
5. Investigational or experimental drugs.
6. Health foods, food supplements, vitamins, and appetite suppressants.

As with most other plan provisions, the covered and excluded charges vary from plan to plan. Therefore, the provisions must be verified.

Major Medical Plans

Most Major Medical plans include as covered expenses drugs requiring a written prescription from a licensed physician. Such drugs must be necessary for the treatment of an illness or injury.

Major Medical plans process drug claims on the following basis:

- The claimant must pay the full cost of the prescription and then submit it to the plan administrator for reimbursement (a copy of the prescription receipt is required, indicating the date purchased, the name of the medication, the number of pills and dosage prescribed, and the name of the ordering physician).
- Medications are subject to all of the regular plan provisions including the deductible and coinsurance.
- The claimant can go to the pharmacy of his choice. The charge is usually not subject to UCR (usual, customary, and reasonable) determinations.
- Any amount of the medication can be purchased at one time (based on the number of dosages pre-

scribed by the physician).

Similar to the separate drug plan, Major Medical plans characteristically exclude the following types of expenses:

- Devices or medical/surgical supplies of any type such as hypodermic needles, syringes, bandages. (Although not covered as a prescription, these types of expenses may be covered under Major Medical as supplies.)
- Contraceptive drugs. Some plans cover contraceptive medications if not prescribed for contraceptive purposes.
- Drugs dispensed while the member is confined in a facility (may be covered as a hospital expense) and drugs dispensed on the day of discharge (take-home medication).
- Investigational or experimental drugs.
- Health foods, food supplements, vitamins, and appetite suppressants. Vitamins may be covered if the diagnosis from the physician is for a specific vitamin deficiency and it can be supported with a laboratory test.

Miscellaneous Guidelines

The following three guidelines usually apply regarding drugs:

1. Drugs dispensed by a dentist for dental-related conditions may be covered if necessitated due to pain, infection, or other condition. In these instances, the dental-related condition is considered an illness.
2. Drugs dispensed in an MD or DO's office, requiring a prescription, usually qualify for payment under Major Medical. Over-the-counter (OTC: non-prescription) drugs are not covered at all.
3. Drugs dispensed by persons other than MDs or DOs, usually represented by chiropractors, naturopaths, optometrists, and psychologists are usually not covered because, by law, these license designations are not allowed to prescribe or dispense drugs or medications that require a prescription.

To determine whether the drug is a prescription medication, the claims examiner may be required to refer to the *Physicians' Desk Reference (PDR)* manual.

Physicians' Desk Reference

The *PDR* is published annually with supplements published as necessary during the year. The manual comprises the following sections:

Manufacturer's Index (white)—arranged alphabetically by manufacturer, then by drug name. The name and address of the manufacturer are included. This section includes prescription and non-prescription drugs. The related information has been provided by the manufacturer.

Product Name Index (pink)—arranged alphabetically by brand name or generic name (if provided). Prescription and non-prescription drugs are included.

Product Category Index (blue)—arranged alphabetically by drug action category, that is, according to the most common use of the drug. If the drug is an antidepressant, it is listed under the antidepressant category; if it is an antacid, it is listed under the antacid category, and so on.

Product Identification Section (gray)—arranged alphabetically by manufacturer, then by brand name. This section contains the actual size and full-color reproductions. Only the reproductions submitted by the manufacturer are included.

Product Information Section (white)—arranged alphabetically by manufacturer, then by brand name. Most pharmaceuticals are described by indications and usage, dosage, administration, description, clinical pharmacology, supply warnings, contraindications, adverse reactions, overdosage precautions and other miscellaneous information.

Diagnostic Product Information (green)—arranged alphabetically by manufacturer, then by product. This section provides a description of diagnostic products only.

Medical billers and claims examiners use the Product Information Section (white) the most. However, since generic drugs are cheaper than brand name medications, many plans encourage their members to purchase generically and offer increased payment incentives. Therefore, use of the Product Name Index (which includes both brand name and generic names) is increasing. For instance, instead of paying generic drugs at the plan's regular coinsurance rate of 80%, 100% may be payable. As with all benefits, this varies widely by plan.

Definitions

Controlled Drugs—Drugs that are more tightly controlled by federal mandates due to their addictive, experimental, toxic, or other highly volatile properties. In this group, four classifications range from the least controlled to the most controlled. Even the least controlled of the Controlled Drugs is more highly regulated than regular prescription medications.

Legend Drug—A drug requiring a prescription. The "legend" always appears on the label.

Legend, Prescription—The pharmaceutical manufacturer's warning on the label: "Caution: Federal (United States) law prohibits dispensing without a prescription."

Non-legend Drug—A drug not requiring a prescription.

Over-the-Counter Drug (OTC)—A drug that may be purchased without a prescription. Also known as a non-legend drug.

Proprietary Drug—A drug that is patented or controlled by a manufacturer. The manufacturer copyrights the trade or brand name. This is not the same as the generic name, which identifies the drug's chemical composition.

Symbols

The following symbols appear in the various sections of the PDR, usually to the right side of the drug name. If nothing appears to the right, the drug is not a legend medication.

OTC—Over-the-Counter drug. A prescription is not required and it is usually not covered under benefit plans.

Rx—Prescription required for purchase.

CI-CIV—Controlled substance. Prescription always required.

O—Identi-Code symbol. It is a manufacturer's identification code. This symbol does not indicate whether or not a prescription is required. It is placed directly on the medicine (if in pill form).

TM—Registered Trademark.

Summary

Medications are drugs used to treat diseases, symptoms, or discomforts. The two ways in which coverage is provided for the payment of drugs is under a service plan and under a Major Medical plan. However, drugs that do not require a prescription (over-the-counter drugs) are generally not covered by either plan.

The *Physicians' Desk Reference (PDR)* can be used to determine whether or not a drug is a prescription drug. In addition, the *PDR* lists drug manufacturers, product names, product categories, product identification (pictures), specific product information, and diagnostic product information.

Assignments

Complete the Questions for Review.
Complete PDR Exercises 16-1 through 16-3.

Questions for Review

Directions: Answer the following questions without looking back into the material just covered. Write your answers in the space provided.

1. What are medications? ____________________
2. Explain the difference between a legend and a non-legend drug. ____________________

   ____
3. Name the six sections of the *PDR*.
   a. ____________________
   b. ____________________
   c. ____________________
   d. ____________________
   e. ____________________
   f. ____________________
4. Controlled drugs can be purchased over the counter. (True or False) ____________________
5. Usually, with a Service Plan, the member is required to go to what kind of pharmacy? ____________________

If you were unable to answer any of the questions, refer back to the section and then fill in the answers.

Exercise 16-1

Directions: Look up the following medications in the *PDR.* In the space provided, indicate whether or not the drug is prescription by writing in the status symbol. Also, write the trade name if the generic name is given, and write the generic name if the trade name is given. The manufacturer's name is indicated in parentheses.

	Name	Symbol
1. Fluorouracil (Roche)	__________	__________
2. Proventil	NA	__________
3. Spectazole	__________	__________
4. Fenfluramine Hydrochloride (Robins)	__________	__________
5. Valium Injectable	__________	__________
6. Purinethol	__________	__________
7. Psyllium Hydrophilic Mucilloid	__________	__________
8. Metaproterenol Sulfate	__________	__________
9. Pentazocine Hydrochloride (Winthrop)	__________	__________
10. Basaljel Capsules (Wyeth)	__________	__________
11. Dilantin Injection (parenteral)	__________	__________
12. Sotradecol Injection (Elkins-Sinn)	__________	__________
13. Aldomet Tablets (Merck)	__________	__________
14. Mandol (Lilly)	__________	__________
15. Ferancee Chewable Tablets (Stuart)	__________	__________

Exercise 16-2

Directions: Write at least one diagnosis for which the indicated medication is normally used.

1. Atromid ______
2. Inderal LA ______
3. Theophylline ______
4. Ortho-Novum ______
5. Boric Acid 5% ______
6. Sus-Phrine Injection ______
7. Tofranil ______
8. Lanoxin ______
9. Diethylstilbestrol ______
10. Parafon Forte ______

Exercise 16-3

Directions: List the manufacturers of the following medications as listed in the 1994 PDR.

Medication	Manufacturer
1. Xylocaine 2% Jelly	__________
2. Decadron Tablets	__________
3. Visine Extra Eyedrops	__________
4. Flagyl Tablets	__________
5. Capoten	__________
6. Similac Natural Care	__________
7. K-Lor Powder Packets	__________
8. Bactrim Suspension	__________
9. Wytensin Tablets	__________
10. Hytrin Tablets	__________
11. Jevity	__________
12. Tenex Tablets	__________
13. Lidocaine 5% Ointment	__________
14. Sudafed 12 Hour Capsules	__________
15. Zantac 150 and 300 Tablets	__________

17

CPT Coding

In this chapter you will learn:

- To name the six sections of the *CPT* and *RVS* reference books.
- To use the *CPT* to code procedures.
- Proper use of CPT vs. HCPCS codes.
- To properly code services.

The *Current Procedural Terminology (CPT)* is the most commonly used coding reference manual by medical billing and claims examining personnel in the health care industry. The CPT provides a listing of descriptive terms and identifying codes for reporting medical services and procedures performed by physicians. It uses a 5-digit code to identify procedures and services, which not only simplifies reporting, but allows for compilation of data by computer. (The term physician is used generically to refer to any provider of service other than hospitals or other facilities.) The purpose of the CPT is to provide a uniform language that will accurately describe medical, surgical, and diagnostic services.

The CPT was originally created by the American Medical Association in 1966. Since that time it has undergone extensive revisions. Revisions are made every year with other updates created as needed. Due to the extensive changes that sometimes appear, it is important to use the correct version of the CPT. Using an outdated CPT may result in using codes that have been changed or deleted, thus causing delays or denials in claim payments.

Inclusion in the CPT does not constitute endorsement by the American Medical Association or anyone else as to the efficacy of the procedure for a given diagnosis or condition. It also does not imply any insurance coverage or payor provisions of a procedure by its inclusion or exclusion.

The Relative Value Study (RVS) is a listing of procedures and their appropriate codes, along with a unit value that has been assigned to the procedure. (For further information regarding the use of the RVS, please see the UCR Chapter in Volume II.) Often the CPT and the RVS are mentioned interchangeably. However, the CPT, not the RVS, should be used when coding procedures. When coding or processing claims, it is important for the biller or examiner to understand the difference between the two books and to use the appropriate book when billing or processing claims.

The CPT and RVS reference books have six major sections:

Section		Codes
1. Evaluation and Management		99201–99499
2. Surgery		10000–69999
3. Anesthesia:	CPT	00100–01999
	RVS	10000–69999
4. Radiology/Nuclear Medicine		70000–79999
5. Pathology and Laboratory Tests		80000–89999
6. Medicine		90701–99199

Modifiers

Modifiers are 2-digit codes that can be added to CPT codes to denote unusual circumstances. These modifiers more fully describe the procedure that was performed. In addition, modifiers alter the valuation of the procedure by increasing or decreasing the allowed amount. For example:

Modifier -80 denotes the work of an assistant surgeon. Since the assistant surgeon is merely assisting and is not responsible for the primary care of the patient, he or she is paid substantially less. Most plans allow assistant surgeons to be paid at 20% of the normal surgeon's fee.

Modifier -20 denotes microsurgery. Since microsurgery is more difficult than standard surgery, most plans allow an additional 25% for this type of surgery.

Some adjustments to allowed amounts are listed in the CPT Coding book. However, these adjustments are set by the insurance carrier or the plan document. (For example, see the assistant surgery section in the XYZ Corporation contract.) Before processing claims with modifiers, claims examiners should check the contract and company policy regarding modifiers.

Most modifiers are for use with surgical codes. Modifiers -22, -23, -32, -47, and -51 are also appropriate to use with anesthesia coding.

The list in Table 17-1 is intended to acquaint you with modifiers. For a more complete listing, please consult the surgery and anesthesia sections of the CPT book.

Table 17-1: Sampling of Modifiers and Their Meanings

Modifier	Meaning and Use
- 20	Microsurgery
- 22	Unusual services
- 23	Unusual anesthesia
- 26	Professional component
- 32	Mandated services
- 47	Anesthesia by surgeon
- 50	A bilateral procedure
- 51	Multiple procedures, but not bilateral
- 52	Reduced services
- 54	Surgical care only
- 55	Postoperative management only
- 56	Preoperative care only
- 58	When an asterisk (*) procedure is carried out at the time of the initial office visit and this procedure constitutes the major service provided at that visit
- 64	Co-surgeons
- 66	Surgical team
- 80	Assistant surgeon
- 90	Reference (outside) laboratory

Unlisted Codes

Listed at the end of each CPT section and subsection are "unlisted codes" (sometimes called junk codes). These are the codes that end in "99." Procedures that are unusual or new and, therefore, do not have a designated code to describe them are coded by the appropriate unlisted code (based on body section or type of service). These codes are to be used only when no other appropriate code is available.

The following coding sections deal specifically with using the CPT manual. Since this is the main reference manual used by medical billing and claims examining personnel, it is vitally important that its usage be thoroughly understood. You should also go through the general guidelines listed in the CPT to assist in coding each section.

Evaluation and Management

Evaluation and management codes designate procedures used to evaluate the patient's condition and to assist the patient in managing that condition.

The key components in determining the proper code are history, examination, and medical decision making.

Additional components that are considered include counseling, coordination of care, nature of presenting problem, and time.

For further instructions regarding proper coding, please see the general guidelines contained in the CPT Coding book.

The appropriate CPT section involved is 99200–99999. (The previous code range indicated in parentheses lists the code range prior to 1992 when an extensive revision of the CPT was last done.)

Office Visits 99201–99215

(Previously 90000–90090)

An office visit is face-to-face treatment between a physician and a patient in the physician's office, clinic, or outpatient department of a hospital. Any type of licensed professional provider can bill for an office visit. An office visit code does not specify the type of service performed other than that the patient is seen by a physician.

Specialized care such as chiropractic, physical therapy, psychiatric counseling are in their own coding sections. Specialized care is coded based on the type of treatment provided, not the place (location) of service. For instance, a chiropractic adjustment is coded 97260 and indicates that a manipulation of the spine was performed. The place of the treatment could be anywhere although it is usually in an office.

If care is provided outside of the normal office hours, codes 99050 through 99054 are used in addition to the regular office visit code. This allows for the provider to obtain extra compensation for the inconvenience of care provided outside the usual business hours.

If the physician does not give a complete language description of the type of visit and does not use a CPT code, most payors use a designated default code, which is usually either 99211 or 99212. (This is a payor-designated procedure, so it varies by company.)

Acute Care 99221–99238

(Previously 90200–90282)

Inpatient hospital care or acute care is also known as Medical While Hospitalized (MWH). The patient is admitted into a facility and the physician visits the patient in the hospital. Multiple types of MWH benefits are available. However, regardless of the type of benefit, all are based on the same coding foundations. The payment of this and all other benefits is covered in detail in the Benefit Structures section of Volume II.

As with office visits, the coding for these services are based on whether the patient is a new or established patient with the physician, the time, and the complexity of the case.

Normally, the claim form indicates the place of service as a facility and usually, either through a language description or through coding, indicates whether the services were inpatient or outpatient. In order for an MWH benefit to be payable, the admission type must be inpatient. The standard claim form, HCFA-1500, has some important blocks that can help in the identification of hospitalizations:

Block #16—Dates of total disability

Block #18—Hospitalization dates, date admitted, and date discharged

Block #32—Name and address of the facility where the services were provided

Although it is not uncommon for these blocks to be left uncompleted, always check them since they can provide verification as to whether the care provided was inpatient. Start now to learn to use all the clues provided when coding claims.

Consultations 99241–99263

(Previously 90600–90643)

Usually, a consultation is provided by a specialist who has been requested to provide an opinion only. The specialist examines the patient at the request of another physician. The specialist may request diagnostic services and may make therapeutic recommendations to the referring physician. However, the specialist does not usually take over the day-to-day treatment or management of the patient. In fact, for the service to qualify as a consultation, the physician cannot be responsible for the regular management of the patient.

If the physician subsequently assumes responsibility for the routine care of the patient, the services should be coded as visits and not consultations, even if billed as consultations. (The initial consultation would be allowed as such.) If the consultant is seeing the patient, in addition to the regular attending physician, 99231–99233 should be used.

Second Surgical Opinion Consultations (SSO) 99271–99275

(Previously 90650–90654)

A second opinion is designed as a benefit to the patient by confirming the need for surgeries that have a reputation for being done needlessly.

Many plans provide a special benefit called an SSO benefit, which provides 100% payment on services provided by a second, independent specialist whom the patient consults prior to the scheduling of an elective, nonemergency surgery.

Normally, for an SSO benefit to be payable, the following requirements must be satisfied:

1. The second- or third-opinion physician must be totally uninvolved with the original recommending physician. Therefore, he or she cannot be part of the same medical group and will often be picked by the administrator, medical management firm, or payor.
2. The consultation must be completed prior to the scheduling of the surgery.
3. The second-opinion physician cannot perform the recommended surgery.

Depending on the plan, failure to obtain an SSO

may result in:

1. Complete denial of all charges for the surgery and related services.
2. Application of a special, reduced coinsurance. For instance, instead of paying 80% of the expenses, 50% would be paid. Noncompliance penalties vary substantially.
3. No change of benefits. In this case, the SSO is considered to be a benefit for the member and is not utilized to penalize for noncompliance.

Emergency Department Services 99281–99288

(Previously 90500–90590)

When a patient goes to the outpatient or emergency department of a hospital, there is usually a physician in attendance who has a contract to provide professional care at the facility. The contracting physician's charges may appear on the hospital bill or may be billed separately.

Many hospitals have two types of outpatient departments: the emergency room (ER), and outpatient medical clinics.

If the patient wants to have his or her regular physician in attendance and the physician is called in from outside the hospital to provide services, code 99056 should be used.

If the patient visits thc outpatient clinic of a facility, regular office visit coding should be used since a clinic is conceptually the same as an office; that is, the same doctors see the same patients, visits are scheduled the same as in an office, the treatment provided is the same as what would be provided in an office, and so on. In essence, the physician is using the facility as his or her office.

Skilled Nursing Care (SNF) 99301–99313

(Previously 90300–90370)

A skilled nursing facility is a specially qualified facility that has the staff and equipment to provide skilled nursing care or rehabilitation services and other related health services.

Often, an individual is admitted to a Skilled Nursing Facility (commonly referred to as an SNF) from an acute care facility. This occurs because the acuteness of the patient's condition has been stabilized and only time and continued noncritical treatment are required.

Custodial Care 99321–99333

(Previously 90400–90470)

Custodial care is primarily for the purpose of meeting the personal, daily needs of the patient and could be provided by personnel without medical care skills or training. For example, custodial care includes assistance with walking, bathing, dressing, eating, and other activities. Skilled nursing personnel are not required for this nonmedical type of care, which is commonly referred to as "meeting the daily living needs" of the patient. Most plans do not provide coverage for these types of services, and, if they do, payment is very limited. If there is a question whether care is custodial or not, copies of the provider's nursing notes or the Admit and/or Discharge Summary reports should be requested.

Home Services 99341–99353

(Previously 90100–90170)

As the name implies, home services are visits provided by a physician in the patient's home. Today, home visits are extremely rare. The coding of these services is based on the same factors as office visits. In the absence of a proper description, use code 99351.

Preventive Medicine 99381–99429

(Previously 90750–90778)

Preventive medicine is, as the name implies, routine, well-care provided when there is not an active illness or disease. If there is any credible diagnosis indicated, do not code as preventive. (Some of the services may still be considered preventive and not covered, such as immunizations.) In such a case, the visit may be covered as not preventive whereas the immunizations and some tests would be preventive. Each case must be decided on its individual circumstances.

Nervous/Mental Care and Treatment 99401–99492

(Previously 90801–90899)

Nervous/mental care and treatment includes psychotic and neurotic disorders, organic brain dysfunction, alcoholism, and chemical dependency.

The language description on the claim form generally indicates "psychotherapy" or "individual therapy" or "group therapy." The ICD-9 coding is usually in the range of 290.00 to 319.00. The providers of service are usually an MD (usually a psychiatrist) or a clinical psychologist.

Most benefit plans require a referral by an MD if one of the following providers is indicated: MFCC (Marriage, Family, and Child Counselor), LCSW (Licensed Clinical Social Worker), or MSW (Master of Social Work).

These CPT codes are used only when psychiatric counseling or therapy is provided. If such therapy is not provided, even if the service is performed by one of the above licensed providers, a different code range should be used.

Most plans pay a reduced benefit for this type of treatment. There may be a limit on the number of visits per year or per lifetime, along with a dollar limit per visit, per calendar year, or per lifetime. Also, many plans cover only certain provider licensing. Therefore, it is very important to read the plan document prior to processing any psychiatric care claims.

Surgery

The surgical section of the CPT book is arranged according to the body system, (eg, integumentary, musculoskeletal). Within each body system, the surgeries are arranged according to their anatomic position from the head down.

Table 17-2 shows the organization of surgical codes.

The RVS lists unit values for surgical procedures, which include the surgery, local anesthesia and the normal, uncomplicated follow-up care associated with the procedure for the time period indicated in the column titled "Follow-up Days."

Block Procedures

Block procedures are multiple surgical procedures performed during the same operative session, in the same operative area, usually in the integumentary system. The objective of these codes is to handle multiple repe-

Table 17-2: Organization of Surgical CPT Codes

CPT Codes	System
10000–17999	The integumentary system—the skin, hair, and nails
19000–19499	Breast—Due to the commonality of procedures in this area, a separate section has been set aside for it.
20000–23929	Musculoskeletal system, the trunk sections (head and body)—Fracture and dislocation codes are at the end of each musculoskeletal section.
23930–26989	Musculoskeletal system, upper limbs—This section is arranged so that the first codes are for the upper arm and elbow, then a section on the forearm and wrist, and finally a section for the hands and fingers.
26990–28899	Musculoskeletal system, lower limbs—These codes are for the pelvis and hip, then the tibia, fibula and ankle, foot and toes.
29000–29799	Musculoskeletal system, casting, and strapping only (all areas)
29815–29883	Musculoskeletal system, arthroscopy (all areas)
30000–32999	Respiratory system
33010–37799	Cardiovascular system
38100–38999	Hemic and lymphatic system
39000–39599	Diaphragm
40490–49999	Digestive system
50010–53899	Urinary system
54000–55899	Male genital system
56000–58999	Female genital system
59000–59899	Maternity care, delivery, abortion
60000–60699	Endocrine system
61000–64999	Nervous system
65091–68899	Eye (ocular) system
69000–69979	Auditory system–Divided into the outer ear, middle ear and inner ear
93501–93553	Cardiac catheterizations

titions of the same service. A block procedure consists of a primary code and subsequent modifying codes.

For example:

10000 is for incision and drainage of one sebaceous cyst.

10001 is for incision and drainage of the second sebaceous cyst.

10002 is for each additional sebaceous cyst.

Other block procedures include 11050–11052, 11100–11101, 11200–11201, 95005–95006 and 95019–95021.

Asterisk Procedures

Asterisk procedures are those surgical procedures denoted by an asterisk (*) to the left of the CPT code and that require special handling. If an asterisk follows a CPT code, the following six rules apply:

1. The listed value is for the surgical procedure only.
2. Pre- and postoperative care is to be added on a fee-for-service basis. That is, billing should be allowed for pre- and postoperative care.
3. If an asterisk procedure is done during an initial visit of a new patient, and it is the major service at that visit (it has the highest RVS unit value), the code 99025 is given for the initial visit and payment is allowed.
4. If an asterisk procedure is done during a visit which includes other significant identifiable services, it should be coded according to the appropriate visit code as well as the initial procedure an applicable follow-up care.
5. If an asterisk procedure during the normal follow-up care of a different procedure, the asterisk procedure may be coded. However, the visit is not coded and allowed since it falls under the normal follow-up of the previous procedure.
6. If an asterisk procedure requires hospitalization, hospital visits are allowed in addition to the procedure.

By Report Procedures

Some procedures are so unusual or variable that it is impossible to determine a standard UCR or unit value allowance. These procedures are called By Report (BR) procedures. The RVS may refer to these procedures as Relative Value Not Established (RNE). BR and RNE procedures have to be referred to a professional review unit, a supervisor, or consultant for review to determine the allowance. To be properly reviewed, a copy of the operative report is required. The anesthesia record may also be needed. If the operative report is not submitted with the claim, the claim should be pended and a copy requested prior to referral.

Multiple or Bilateral Procedures

Multiple procedures are more than one surgical procedure performed during one operative session. Bilateral procedures are surgeries that involve a pair of similar body parts (eg, breasts, eyes).

There are two main types of multiple or bilateral procedures:

Same Time, Different Operative Field, Incision, or Orifice

When more than one surgery is performed during the same operative session but through a different orifice (opening) or incision or in a different operative field, 100% of the actual charge or UCR (or scheduled amount) is allowed for the major procedure and 50% of UCR (or actual charge, whichever is less) is allowed for each additional procedure.

Bilateral procedures follow the same rules as multiple procedures performed through different incisions. Multiply the UCR allowance for the single procedure by 150% or 1.5. If, however, there is an established bilateral procedure code, that code would be allowed at 100% only because the units have already been assigned at 1.5% of the single procedure.

Same Time, Same Operative Field, Incision or Orifice

Usually, when multiple procedures are performed during the same operative session through the same incision, orifice, or operative field, the additional procedures are considered to be incidental.

An incidental procedure is one that does not add significant time or complexity to the operative session. In such a case, the allowable amount will be that of the major procedure only. No additional amount will be allowed for the extra procedures. However, if the additional procedures are not incidental, then the rules for handling multiple procedures explained above would be applied. That is, the major procedure would be considered at 100% of UCR and the lesser at 50%.

For example, let's say that the following bill is received from the provider:

	Billed Amt	UCR
Tonsillectomy (42821)	$600.00	$600.00
Eustachian Tube Inflation (69400)	300.00	200.00

Following the rules previously indicated, we would allow 100% of the major procedure plus 50% of the lesser procedure. Therefore, in this example, the allowable amount would be 100% of $600 + 50% of $200 for a Total Allowance of $700.

It is important to understand which procedure is the primary procedure and which is the secondary procedure since we don't want to penalize the patient for an incorrect billing.

For example, let's look at the same procedures as those just mentioned in the following way:

	Billed Amt	UCR
Tonsillectomy (42821)	$300.00	$600.00
Eustachian Tube Inflation (69400)	600.00	$100.00
Total	$900.00	$700.00

By referring to the RVS, we can tell that the major procedure is the tonsillectomy, which allows 16.39 units, whereas 69400 allows only 1.39 units. Therefore, using the multiple surgery rules but following the doctor's billing the allowed amount would be:

100% of $600.00 up to the actual charge of	$300.00
50% of $200.00 or the actual charge, whichever is less	+100.00
Total Allowance would be	$400.00

As you can see, incorrect billing could substantially reduce the amount of the claim payment if the insurance company chooses not to use global UCR (comparing the total bill to the total UCR).

Assistant Surgery

As mentioned briefly in the modifiers section, some surgical procedures require an assistant surgeon. When billing or examining for assistant surgeon services, the modifier -80 should be added to the appropriate CPT code.

For further information, see the Surgery Chapter in Volume II.

Anesthesia

The CPT code range for anesthesia is 00100–01999. The RVS code range for anesthesia is 10000–69999 (same as surgery). When coding anesthesia claims, it is preferable to include both the ASA (RVS) and CPT codes.

For example:

Anesthesia for total ankle replacement 01486/27702

Anesthesia unit values are listed in the RVS for procedures that require anesthesia administered by an anesthesiologist. Remember that local anesthesia is never allowed separately. Therefore, anesthesia benefits are those that are allowed on procedures that require more than a local anesthesia. These units (for all schedules) are used under the following conditions:

- The anesthesia is personally administered by a licensed physician.
- The physician remains in constant attendance during the procedure for the sole purpose of rendering the anesthesia service.

Basic/Base Units

The basic or base anesthesia units are designed to allow for the usual pre- and postoperative care, the administration of the anesthetic, and the administration of fluids and blood incident to the anesthesia or surgery. Remember that the surgical unit values include surgery, local infiltration, digital block, or topical anesthesia.

Time Units

The length of time that a patient is under anesthesia determines the amount of money that will be considered allowable for the procedure. Anesthesia time begins when the anesthesiologist starts to physically prepare the patient for the induction of anesthesia in the operating room area (or its equivalent). The time ends when the anesthesiologist is no longer in constant attendance, usually when the patient is ready for postoperative supervision. This time should always be indicated on the claim form when billing for anesthesia services.

Modifiers

All anesthesia services are billed by use of the anesthesia 5-digit procedure code plus the addition of a physical status modifier. The use of other optional modifiers may be appropriate.

Physical status modifiers are represented by the initial P followed by a single digit from 1 through 6.

P1—A normal healthy patient

P2—A patient with mild systemic disease

P3—A patient with severe systemic disease

P4—A patient with severe systemic disease that is a constant threat to life

P5—A moribund patient who is not expected to survive without the operation

P6—A declared brain-dead patient whose organs are being removed for donor purposes

Optional modifiers denote special conditions. The following are the valid anesthesia 2-digit modifier codes:

- 22 Unusual services
- 23 Unusual anesthesia
- 32 Indicates mandated services
- 47 Anesthesia by surgeon
- 51 Multiple procedures, but not bilateral

Qualifying Circumstances

Many anesthesia services are provided under particularly difficult circumstances because of factors such as extraordinary condition of the patient, notable operative conditions, or unusual risk factors. This section includes a list of important qualifying circumstances that significantly impact on the character of the anesthetic service provided. These procedures would not be reported alone, but would be reported as additional procedure numbers qualifying an anesthesia procedure or service. More than one may be selected.

99100—Anesthesia for patient of extreme age, under 1 year or over 70 years

99116—Anesthesia complicated by utilization of total body hypothermia

99135—Anesthesia complicated by utilization of controlled hypotension

99140—Anesthesia complicated by emergency conditions

Emergency conditions need to be specified. An emergency is defined as existing when delay in treatment of the patient would lead to a significant increase in the threat to life or body part.

Radiology

The radiology section of the CPT is arranged according to the anatomic position, that is, by body part, starting at the head and moving downward toward the feet. Knowledge of anatomy will make it much easier to localize which area of this section to refer to. This section is divided into four subsections. They are listed below with their CPT codes:

1. Diagnostic radiology—70010–76499
2. Diagnostic ultrasound—76506–76999
3. Therapeutic radiology—77299–77799
4. Nuclear medicine—78000–79999

Diagnostic x-rays are flat or two-dimensional pictures of a particular body part or organ. X-rays are created by sending low-level radiation through the body onto a sheet of film. The image on the exposed piece of film looks like a negative from a roll of camera film. X-rays are most useful for looking at bones and dense tissue since softer tissue is not clearly defined.

Ultrasonography provides a more definitive type of picture than x-rays. Instead of using radiation, sound waves are bounced off the desired structure. The pattern and amount of sound returned constitute what forms a picture of the organ. This type of viewing is less potentially damaging than x-rays. This is why ultrasound scanning can be used during pregnancy, whereas x-rays should not.

Radiation oncology services is the use of radiation to treat a condition. This treatment is used in conjunction with chemotherapy to treat malignant cancers. Normally, radiation therapy is composed of multiple treatments and does not include a "picture" of the body part. It is done for treatment purposes only, not for diagnostic reasons.

Nuclear medicine combines use of radioactive elements and x-rays to image an organ or body part. Certain radioactive elements collect in different organs. Therefore, to see whether an organ is working effectively or to see whether it is enlarged, for example, a radioactive element is injected into the patient, then pictures are taken of the organ at specified intervals to see how, where, and how much of the element collects in a specific organ.

CT scans (computed tomography) are 360-degree pictures of specified body areas. This scan provides a three-dimensional picture of the area and is used to help identify tumors and cancers located in the interior of the organ. CT scans are much more definitive than x-rays.

Pathology

Laboratory examinations are the analysis of body substances to determine their chemical or tissue type make-up. Body fluids or tissues are collected and then either run through analyzing machines or looked at under a microscope to identify any abnormal substances or tissues.

CPT codes 80002–80092 refer to various types of panel tests. Panel tests are composed of multiple tests that are combined and run from one specimen. The number of tests determines which code to use. It is not uncommon today for providers to do what is known as "unbundling" when billing. Unbundling occurs when a provider bills separately for each test performed even though all the tests came from the same specimen and were done simultaneously. In this instance, the provider gets significantly more money for doing nothing additional. When a bill is received unbundled, the examiner needs to rebundle it (see Laboratory Profile Index). An example of unbundling is shown in the following bill:

Bill from Doctor	CPT Code	Charges	Coding by Examiner	Charge
Albumin	82040	$15.00		
Calcium	82310	20.00		
Chlorides	82435	25.00		
Cholesterol	82465	25.00		
Creatinine	82565	15.00		
Glucose	82947	10.00		
Potassium	84132	15.00		
Sodium	84295	15.00		
BUN	84520	30.00		
Uric Acid	84550	25.00	80110	$195.00
Total		$195.00		

In this example, all the billed charges should be combined together and coded under one panel code. Benefits would then be determined based on the one code.

Lab Coding Specifics

There are many laboratory tests that are commonly ordered by most doctors. The following is a list of some of those services with general coding and billing guidelines.

1. Urinalysis—If unspecified, use code 81000.
2. Glucose—If unspecified, use 82947.
3. Pregnancy testing—If unspecified, use 84702.
4. TB Tine Test (86585)—Often, this test is covered only if the diagnosis is for a respiratory condition (eg, URI, rhinitis). If no diagnosis is indicated or if the condition is not a respiratory illness, deny the charge as routine.
5. Culture and sensitivity—If billed for a "culture and sensitivity" lab, use codes 87181–87192. A culture lab does not usually include a sensitivity study. However, a sensitivity study must include the culture. If the billing is for a culture with no indication of a sensitivity study, use codes 87040–87163.
6. Pap smears—Usually a covered expense if the patient is being treated for a valid gynecologic condition, eg, vaginitis, pelvic pain, dysmenorrhea. If 88155 is billed and the diagnosis is menopause-related, the test should not be considered routine since this code includes a hormonal evaluation. Routine Pap smears are not covered unless specified in the plan benefit schedule as a covered expense.

   Routine Pap smears are billed in various ways, such as

a. Pap to rule out (R/O) malignant neoplasm
b. Screening for abnormal pathology
c. Screening for malignant neoplasm
d. Pap smear class II, III, or IV are ok to pay as they reflect an abnormal tissue sample. Class I is routine or normal.

7. Handling/collection charges—Normally coded 99000–99002. This charge usually appears on the physician's bill when the specimen is obtained in the office but sent out to an outside laboratory for analysis.
8. EKG and other cardiac procedures, codes 93000–93350—Considered laboratory expenses.

For laboratory coverage, it is important to establish whether the tests are being done as part of a routine check-up or because the patient has symptoms that are being diagnosed. Also, the testing must be appropriate for the reported symptoms. In other words, some tests would be routine for some diagnoses but not for others. This type of discrimination is learned through experience and time.

The remaining subsections of this section are based on the type of analysis being performed. The subsections are the following:

81000–81099	Urinalysis
82000–84999	Chemistry and Toxicology
85000–85999	Hematology
86000–86999	Immunology
87001–87999	Microbiology
88000–88299	Anatomic Pathology
88300–88399	Surgical Pathology
89050–89399	Miscellaneous

Component Charges

Whenever a lab or x-ray test is performed, there are two distinct services that are actually performed.

The first service is the taking of the specimen or x-ray. This charge should include the expense for the personnel performing the test and the cost of the necessary equipment. This is called the Technical Component and is denoted by adding modifier -27 to the CPT code.

The second service is for the interpretation or the reading of the results of the test. This is called the Professional Component and is denoted by adding modifier -26 to the CPT code.

An independent pathologist or radiologist often bills separately for the interpretation report. This interpretation-only charge is called a professional component (PC) charge.

The use of modifier -26 applies in the following situations: (1) the provider of service is an independent radiologist or pathologist, and (2) the place of service may be inpatient or outpatient hospital, or it may be billed as an office expense but it is noted that the actual test was done by someone other than the physician.

PC charges used to be limited to instances in which hospital charges were involved. However, it is becoming more common to see this occurring on doctor's claims since it increases revenues for the medical community and since independent laboratories and radiologists are becoming more common.

Medicine

This is nonsurgical or medical care services. Nonsurgical services include optometry care, chiropractic care, acupuncture treatment, physical therapy and hospital care. The appropriate CPT section involved is 90701–99199.

Immunizations 90701–90749

Immunizations are considered to be preventive treatment. Therefore, an active illness or disease is usually not present.

Therapeutic Injections 90782–90799

These codes are used for therapeutic injections (those required in the treatment of an illness or disease). They are not routine, preventive injections.

The types of therapeutic injections include the following:

Subcutaneous—just below the outermost level of skin

Intradermal—just below the second level of skin, the dermis

Intramuscular—into a muscle

Intra-arterial—into an artery

Intravenous—into a vein

Allergy injections should be coded 95115–95117, unless otherwise directed. Most antibiotics are injected intramuscularly.

Biofeedback 90900–90915

Biofeedback is training a person to consciously control automatic, internal body functions. For instance, through conscious control, some body rhythms that control the constriction of blood vessels, beating of the heart, and so on, can be increased or decreased. This type of treatment can be used for a variety of illnesses or symptoms. A common use is for the control of intractable pain.

Biofeedback is controversial because its effectiveness is very hard to prove or disprove. In addition, it does not cure anything. Instead, it is used as a tool in dealing with the symptoms of a condition, not in its treatment. Generally, most plans do not cover biofeedback, or if it is covered, it is very limited and only covered for certain diagnoses.

Dialysis 90935–90999

Dialysis is a maintenance procedure used for End-Stage Renal Disease when the kidneys cease functioning. Note that this is not really a treatment because it is only handling the functions normally performed by the body. (However, it is still referred to generically as "treatment.") For a patient with this disease to survive, the blood-cleansing function must be performed artificially by one of three processes currently available: hemodialysis, CAPD—continuous ambulatory peritoneal dialysis, or transplantation of a new kidney.

Most hemodialysis is performed at private dialysis centers. A small percentage of the patients have a machine in their own home. The fees for dialysis are usually billed on a monthly basis. When coding, either the actual dates of service should be indicated or a monthly from/through date is used. Normally, the insurance carrier provides coverage only for the first 18 months of treatment. After that time, Medicare becomes the primary payor (refer to the Medicare section for additional information). If the dialysis is performed in an acute facility, you may be billed separately for the facility fees and the physician fees. Remember, the CPT codes are only to be used on physician services. Dialysis treatment runs about $5,000 per month.

CAPD is performed by the patient at home. The peritoneum of the stomach is used to cleanse the blood. Surgery is required for the implantation of catheters and the construction of the internal bag (made of the peritoneum) to hold the dialysate fluids. Monthly supplies must be purchased, and there will be monthly examination charges by the attending physician. This type of treatment runs approximately $2,000 per month.

Transplants are coded in accordance with the surgery section of the CPT.

Ophthalmology 92002–92499

Ophthalmology care is provided by either an optometrist or an ophthalmologist (MD). Most health plans do not cover routine vision care services related to the refraction and subsequent prescription of glasses or contact lenses. If they are covered, however, the benefits are usually very limited in both the dollar allowance and the time restraints and are often provided under a separate vision care plan or benefit. Therefore, always be sure to verify plan benefits prior to processing a vision claim. However, also be aware that not all vision care is routine. Some vision care is essential for the proper care and treatment of eye diseases. Most payors have a listing of payable diagnoses, but even then the important point will be what type of services are being provided. Prescriptive services for glasses or contact lenses will still be considered routine. (Except, possibly, if the lens of the eye has been removed, as in cataract surgery.)

Orthoptics is a retraining of the muscles that control vision. Some plans allow for this therapy for certain conditions such as strabismus and binocular vision. If the plan does allow the therapy, it is usually very limited and may require a second opinion from an ophthalmologist.

Otorhinolaryngologic Services 92502–92599

(Ear, Nose, and Throat)

Otorhinolaryngologic services are for the care and treatment of the nerves of the hearing organs. Some of the services entail regular hearing tests. Other services are very complex diagnostic tests performed when it has been determined that there is a hearing loss but the cause of the loss has not been established. As with vision services, this care is often restricted under many health plans.

Cardiovascular 92950–93979

The cardiovascular section is very large, and it is heavily used by the medical biller and the claims examiner. The following codes are some of the more commonly billed services:

93000—EKG
93010—EKG Interpretation and Report Only
93015—Cardiovascular Stress Test
93224—24-Hour EKG Monitoring

As a rule, the codes from 93000 through 93350 and 93600 through 93979 are considered to be DXL (Diagnostic X-ray and Laboratory) expenses. Codes 93501 through 93553 are considered surgical procedures.

It is important to carefully review the description of the procedure prior to coding, since many examiners are not familiar with the differences between procedures. However, with careful consideration, the proper code can be determined. It is usually easier to start with the code supplied by the provider and then verify it for accuracy.

Physical Therapy 97010–97799

Physical therapy is the science of physical or corrective rehabilitation or treatment of abnormal conditions of the musculoskeletal system through the use of heat, light, water, electricity, sound, massage, and active, passive or restrictive exercise.

This therapy often follows surgery or an injury to a joint or muscle. When either of these events occurs, the muscles attaching to the affected joint become weak or atrophied. Consequently, to restore full movement, concentrated therapy to the affected area is required. Physical therapy treatments may include functional activities, mobility training, manipulation, physical modalities, assessment, instruction, and specialized testing or therapeutic exercises.

Although physical therapy is usually performed by a Registered Physical Therapist (RPT), it is not uncommon for chiropractors (DC), podiatrists (DPM) and osteopaths (DO) to also bill for these services.

Occupational therapy is a type of physical therapy. The objective of this treatment is to either restore normal movement, or, in the case of paralysis, to teach the patient alternative ways of dealing with his or her handicap to meet the demands of everyday living. Occupational therapy is normally billed by an Occupational Therapist (OT), a hospital or a rehabilitative facility.

Speech therapy is for the purpose of improving speech and verbal communication skills. It is usually performed by a speech therapist.

Physical Medicine 97010–97145, 97260, 97261

Physical medicine is the manipulation and physical therapy associated with the nonsurgical care and treatment of the patient. The most common form of physical medicine is chiropractic manipulation of the spine. Theoretically, any joint can be involved; the most common is the spinal area.

The chiropractor's scope of practice is limited in most states. For instance, in California, chiropractors are not allowed to draw blood or prescribe prescription medicines. The limitations vary by state.

Due to overutilization of chiropractic services, there has evolved an intense monitoring and restricting of payment for chiropractic services. Such restrictions may limit the number of visits per year, per month or per condition, along with specifying daily money maximums or limiting the number of modalities that may be performed in a single visit. As a result, it is important to check the coverage and the administrative policies, which vary from payor to payor.

Many chiropractors use an accident diagnosis, 84x.xx series, for billing purposes. Unless an accident or injury has actually occurred with a date, place, and circumstance indicated, the coding should be changed to reflect a noninjury skeletal condition, 72x.xx. (This varies by administration.)

Miscellaneous Services

The remaining part of this section of the CPT is composed of miscellaneous services. These services are usually billed only by specialists within a given field. It is important to take time to look through this section to become aware of what services are listed. A brief explanation of the remaining sections is provided below.

Gastroenterology (91000–91299)—Services related to the digestive system, esophagus, stomach, intestines.

Pulmonary (94010–94799)—Treatment and testing of the respiratory system, in relation to lung function.

Allergy and Immunology (95000–95199)—Allergy testing and desensitization (allergy shots).

Neurology (95805–95999—Nerve and muscle testing. May be considered lab or medical.

Chemotherapy (96400–96549)—Administration of chemotherapy agents, usually for treatment of cancer. These codes do *not* include the cost of the chemical.

Special Dermatology Procedures (96900–96999) —Skin treatment.

Case Management Services (99361–99373)—Initiation and coordination of a health care treatment team. Only required in very complex cases involving multiple body systems.

Special Services and Reports (99000–99199)—Miscellaneous services not covered elsewhere. Includes critical care services that are usually considered to be hospital or emergency care.

The following medicine codes are often considered to be diagnostic testing (DXL) or surgical (this varies from payor to payor):

DXL	Surgery
91010–91052	91000, 91055
91060, 91065, 91122	91100
92100–92140	92880
92512–92599	
93000–93255	92975–92984
93280–93350	93501–93553
93561–93640	93650
93720–93790	
93850–93960	
94010–94620	
94680–94770	
95000–95082	
95819–95958	99170

Billing Tips

The following are billing tips on using the CPT:

- As long as you document the time you spent and the reason why, you can bill for the higher level E&M codes (and get the higher reimbursement).
- Make sure the diagnosis code you submit is consistent with the level of the visit you are billing for.
- Assign a person to recheck all codes, prior to the claims leaving the office.
- If the code you are submitting is a high-level code or is unusual, include documentation to support the services when the claim is submitted.

Summary

The CPT is used for coding procedures and services rendered by a provider. It provides a uniform means of reporting and allows for computer compilation of data.

The CPT reference book has six major sections. The correct code is located according to the section that pertains to the service or procedure performed.

Modifiers are 2-digit codes that can be added to CPT codes to denote unusual circumstances. These modifiers more fully describe the procedure that was carried out.

CPT coding is one of the most vital functions that a medical biller performs. Without proper CPT coding, claims will be denied, delayed, or simply returned for correction.

Assignments

Complete the Questions for Review.

Complete CPT Coding exercises 17-1 through 17-25. If you are getting less than 90% accuracy in your coding, the need for more practice is indicated.

Questions for Review

Directions: Answer the following questions without looking back into the material just covered. Write your answers in the space provided.

1. What are Evaluation and Management codes? ____________________
2. What is physical medicine? ____________________
3. In what order is the CPT surgical section arranged? ____________________
4. When is modifier -80 used? ____________________
5. Modifier -50 is used when billing for preoperative care only. (True or False) ____________________

If you were unable to answer any of the questions, refer back to the section and then fill in the answers.

Exercise 17-1

Directions: Look up the following Physician Service CPT Codes and write the corresponding English-language description in the space provided.

	Code	Description
1.	99201	
2.	99341	
3.	99221	
4.	99301	
5.	99321	
6.	99281	
7.	99241	
8.	90701	
9.	99273	
10.	90945	

Exercise 17-2

Directions: Look up the following Physician Service CPT Codes and write the corresponding English-language description in the space provided.

	Code	Description
1.	96900	
2.	96400	
3.	90844	
4.	93041	
5.	94150	
6.	90900	
7.	92557	
8.	95857	
9.	95819	
10.	94620	

Exercise 17-3

Directions: Look up the following Physician Service CPT Codes and write the corresponding English-language description in the space provided.

	Code	Description
1.	91000	
2.	92002	
3.	92504	
4.	93000	
5.	97010	
6.	99238	
7.	99221	
8.	99204	
9.	95822	
10.	97261	

Exercise 17-4

Directions: Based on the description of the Physician Service, look up the appropriate CPT code and write it in the space provided.

Description	Code
1. Office visit, evaluation of established patient, medical decision low complexity, expanded problem history.	1. ________
2. Rest home visit, evaluation of new patient, medical decision making moderate complexity, expanded problem history and exam.	2. ________
3. Admission to hospital, initial hospital care, straightforward medical decision, detailed history and exam.	3. ________
4. Subsequent hospital care, medical decision of moderate complexity, expanded problem.	4. ________
5. Admission to SNF, established patient, medical decision of low complexity, detailed history, comprehensive exam.	5. ________
6. Limited follow-up care in a convalescent facility, straightforward medical decision, problem-focused history and exam.	6. ________
7. Emergency department care, minimal care, straightforward medical decision, problem-focused.	7. ________
8. Initial inpatient consultation, new patient, medical decision of moderate complexity, comprehensive history and exam.	8. ________
9. Complex initial consultation, office, medical decision of high complexity.	9. ________
10. Follow-up minimal consultation, office, straightforward medical decision making, problem-focused history and exam.	10. ________

Exercise 17-5

Directions: Based on the description of the Physician Service, look up the appropriate CPT code and write it in the space provided.

Description	Code
1. Diathermy with paraffin bath	1. ____________
	____________
2. Tar and ultraviolet bath, dermatology	2. ____________
3. Manipulation for physical therapy by physician, one area	3. ____________
4. Electrocardiogram, complete	4. ____________
5. Provocative testing, for allergies	5. ____________
6. Heart electroconversion	6. ____________
7. Gonioscopy	7. ____________
8. Psychoanalysis	8. ____________
9. Biofeedback for high blood pressure	9. ____________
10. IV therapy for anaphylactic shock, 1 hour	10. ____________

Exercise 17-6

Directions: Based on the Physician Service description, look up the appropriate CPT code and write it in the space provided.

	Description	ICD-9 Code	CPT Code
1.	Glaucoma provocative test	______	______
2.	Diabetic minimal check-up, established	______	______
3.	Hearing loss comprehensive testing	______	______
4.	Allergen immunotherapy injection for grass	______	______
5.	Physical therapy for skeletal pain, 45 minutes	______	______
			______
6.	F/up newborn care, in the hospital	______	______
7.	Problem-focused f/up visit to Shady Oaks Rest Home, advanced senility	______	______
8.	Emergency high complexity admit to Hoag Memorial Hospital, pulmonary edema	______	______
9.	Manipulation with hot packs and traction and ultrasound, physical therapy for low back pain	______	______
		______	______
			______
			______
			______
10.	Therapeutic phlebotomy for URI	______	______

Exercise 17-7

Directions: Based on the Physician Service description, look up the appropriate CPT code and write it in the space provided.

Description	Code
1. Informational book of diabetes care	1. ______
2. Specimen handling fee	2. ______
3. Newborn resuscitation	3. ______
4. Subsequent detailed hospital visit	4. ______
5. Group psychotherapy by a physician	5. ______
6. Emergency department care at hospital, problem-focused, tetanus-toxoid injection	6. ______ ______
7. Supplies, office	7. ______
8. 25-minute conference with interdisciplinary health team re case management	8. ______
9. Rapid desensitization, 45-minute allergy immunotherapy	9. ______
10. Cardiopulmonary resuscitation	10. ______

Exercise 17-8

Directions: Based on the Physician Service description, look up the appropriate CPT code and write it in the space provided.

	Description		Code
1.	IPPB treatment, initial	1.	________
2.	45-minute individual psychotherapy	2.	________
3.	Color vision exam	3.	________
4.	Extended f/up visit, critical care, 1 hour	4.	________
5.	Prosthetic training, 35 minutes	5.	________
			________
6.	Peritoneal dialysis for May, age 35	6.	________
7.	Psychological testing, 5 hours	7.	________
8.	Infusion of calcium, 1.5 hours	8.	________
			________
9.	SSO, extensive, high complexity	9.	________
10.	Tetanus injection for cut due to rusty can	10.	________

Exercise 17-9

Directions: Based on the Physician Service description, look up the appropriate CPT code and write it in the space provided.

Description	Code
1. Intermediate ophthalmologic exam and evaluation for continued care	1. ______
2. Pediatric pneumogram	2. ______
3. Typhoid vaccination	3. ______
4. Initial comprehensive consultation, office, moderate complexity	4. ______
5. ER problem-focused exam for suture removal	5. ______
6. Initial hospital visit, normal newborn	6. ______
7. Allergy injection	7. ______
8. Allergen serum, 1 vial, single antigen	8. ______
9. Hearing aid exam	9. ______
10. Initial problem-focused consultation, office	10. ______

Exercise 17-10

Directions: Based on the Physician Service description, look up the appropriate CPT code and write it in the space provided.

Description	Code
1. F/up consultation for complications of diabetes/inpatient, expanded problem moderate complexity	1. ________
2. Injection of penicillin	2. ________
3. Problem-focused initial ER exam for severe congestion	3. ________
4. Comprehensive exam for new patient with severe arthritis, office, moderate complexity	4. ________
5. Contact lens prescription	5. ________
6. Pulmonary stress, testing	6. ________
7. Emergency department f/up for suture removal, problem-focused	7. ________
8. Discharge from hospital	8. ________
9. Detailed office visit; subsequent initial hospital comprehensive admission and history, low complexity	9. ________ ________
10. Minimal office visit, established patient	10. ________

Exercise 17-11

Directions: Based on the DXL Service description, look up the appropriate CPT code and write it in the space provided.

Description	Code
1. Urinalysis	1. __________
2. Complete chest x-ray	2. __________
3. EKG, complete	3. __________
4. CBC	4. __________
5. MRI of left hip joint	5. __________
6. Lipid panel	6. __________
7. Erythropoietin bioassay	7. __________
8. CT scan of the abdomen with contrast	8. __________
9. Cardiovascular stress test with exercise, interp. only	9. __________
10. Cholecystography with contrast	10. __________
11. Streptokinase, antibody	11. __________
12. HIV antigen	12. __________
13. Ultrasound for gestational age, limited	13. __________
14. Doppler EKG, complete	14. __________
15. Facial nerve function study	15. __________

Exercise 17-12

Directions: Based on the DXL Service description, look up the appropriate CPT code and write it in the space provided.

Description	Code
1. Ova and parasites, concentration and identification	1. ________
2. Blood potassium	2. ________
3. Estradiol, RIA (placental)	3. ________
4. General toxicology screen	4. ________
5. Cyanocobalamin bioassay (vitamin B_{12})	5. ________
6. Lithium levels, interpretation and report only	6. ________
7. Serum albumin	7. ________
8. Needle biopsy ultrasonic guidance, complete	8. ________
9. Unilateral renal venography, complete	9. ________
10. MRI w/contrast, brain	10. ________
11. Entire spine, myelography, super. & inter.	11. ________
12. Cervicocerebral angiography, with catheter including vessel origin	12. ________
13. Basic dosimetry, radiation therapy	13. ________
14. Laryngography w/contrast super. & inter.	14. ________
15. Protozoa antibody tube, guide	15. ________

Exercise 17-13

Directions: Based on the DXL Service description, look up the appropriate CPT code and write it in the space provided.

Description	Code
1. Wet mount for ova and parasites	1. ________
2. Huhner test and semen analysis	2. ________
3. Platelet survival study	3. ________
4. Intermediate radiology therapeutic treatment planning	4. ________
5. CT, lumbar spine w/o contrast	5. ________
6. A/P abdominal x-ray, single view	6. ________
7. Intravenous KUB, pyelography	7. ________
8. B-scan retroperitoneal echography, limited	8. ________
9. Infusion of radioelement solution	9. ________
10. Salivary gland function study	10. ________
11. SMA-18, panel	11. ________
12. Serum cholesterol, total	12. ________
13. Blood ethchlorvynol	13. ________
14. X-ray knee, A/P and lateral	14. ________
15. Feces screening for lipids, qualitative	15. ________

Exercise 17-14

Directions: Based on the DXL Service description, look up the appropriate CPT code and write it in the space provided.

Description	Code
1. Ascorbic acid (vitamin C), blood	1. ________
2. Desipramine, assay	2. ________
3. Digoxin, RIA (reduced services)	3. ________
4. Histamine test	4. ________
5. Galactose test (reference laboratory)	5. ________
6. Cephalogram, orthodontic (professional component)	6. ________
7. X-ray hand; minimum of three views	7. ________
8. Duodenography, hypotonic	8. ________
9. Pelvimetry, with or without placental localization	9. ________
10. X-ray forearm, A/P and lateral (professional component)	10. ________
11. Gases, blood Po_2 by manometry	11. ________
12. Heparin assay	12. ________
13. Hepatitis Be antigen (HBeAg)	13. ________
14. Necropsy (autopsy); forensic examination	14. ________
15. Russell viper venom time, diluted	15. ________

Exercise 17-15

Directions: Based on the DXL Service description, look up the appropriate CPT code and write it in the space provided.

Description	Code
1. Radiologic exam, hand, two views	1. ____________
2. Bone age studies	2. ____________
3. Xeroradiography	3. ____________
4. Mammography, unilateral	4. ____________
5. Echography, spinal canal and contents	5. ____________
6. Tuberculosis, intradermal	6. ____________
7. Theophylline, assay	7. ____________
8. Urinalysis, chemical, qualitative	8. ____________
9. Obstetric profile	9. ____________
10. Iron binding capacity, serum, chemical	10. ____________
11. Radiologic examination, abdomen single view	11. ____________
12. Radiologic exam, hip, unilateral	12. ____________
13. Glucose tolerance test, 3 specimens	13. ____________
14. FSH	14. ____________
15. Hepatitis panel	15. ____________

Exercise 17-16

Directions: Based on the Surgical Service description, look up the appropriate CPT code and write it in the space provided.

Description	Code
1. Excision of mediastinal cyst	1. ________
2. Pyelotomy, with exploration	2. ________
3. Repair, laceration of palate; up to 2 cm	3. ________
4. Resection of external cardiac tumor	4. ________
5. Wedging of clubfoot cast	5. ________
6. Puncture aspiration of cyst of breast	6. ________
7. Removal of foreign body, intraocular, anterior chamber	7. ________
8. Mastoidectomy, complete	8. ________
9. Open treatment of ankle dislocation	9. ________
10. Nipple/areola reconstruction	10. ________
11. Hysterotomy, abdominal	11. ________
12. Cholecystectomy	12. ________
13. Amniocentesis, any method	13. ________
14. Spinal puncture, lumbar, diagnostic	14. ________
15. Acne surgery, removal of comedones	15. ________

Exercise 17-17

Directions: Look up the following Surgical Service CPT Codes and write the corresponding English-language description in the space provided.

	Code	Description
1.	29804	
2.	56441	
3.	69300	
4.	43842	
5.	38200	
6.	40650	
7.	27030	
8.	32405	
9.	23000	
10.	16035	
11.	32604	
12.	32800-80	
13.	56620	
14.	69400	
15.	54100	

Exercise 17-18

Directions: Based on the Surgical Service description, look up the appropriate CPT code and write it in the space provided.

Description	Code
1. Routine obstetric care w/antepartum care, vaginal	1. ________
2. Excision of tonsil tags	2. ________
3. Direct repair of aneurysm, carotid—assistant	3. ________
4. Arthroscopy, ankle surgical removal of FB	4. ________
5. Excision of lesion of pancreas—assistant	5. ________
6. Ureterectomy, with bladder cuff (separate procedure)	6. ________
7. Radical abdominal hysterectomy—assistant	7. ________
8. Tenotomy, subcutaneous, toe, single	8. ________
9. Synovectomy, intertarsal	9. ________
10. Pericardiocentesis, initial	10. ________
11. Biopsy of liver, percutaneous needle	11. ________
12. Catheterization, urethra, simple	12. ________
13. Treatment of incomplete abortion	13. ________
14. Incidental appendectomy—assistant	14. ________
15. Urethroplasty, first stage—assistant	15. ________

Exercise 17-19

Directions: Look up the following Surgical Service CPT Codes and write the corresponding English-language description in the space provided.

	Code	Description
1.	45000	
2.	54125-80	
3.	59515	
4.	62268	
5.	19364-80	
6.	24900-80	
7.	30400	
8.	34401	
9.	56405	
10.	61860	
11.	65820	
12.	50240-80	
13.	44155	
14.	33120-80	
15.	28001	

Exercise 17-20

Directions: Based on the Surgical Service description, look up the appropriate CPT code and write it in the space provided.

	Description		Code
1.	Excision or curettage of bone cyst or benign tumor, talus or calcaneus	1.	________
2.	Removal of permanent pacemaker	2.	________
3.	Renal biopsy, percutaneous by trocar	3.	________
4.	Partial hymenectomy or revision of hymenal ring	4.	________
5.	Myringotomy	5.	________
6.	Thoracoplasty	6.	________
7.	Repair blood vessel, direct, neck	7.	________
8.	Colostomy or skin-level cecostomy	8.	________
9.	Circumcision, using clamp, newborn	9.	________
10.	Salpingo-oophorectomy, complete	10.	________
11.	Bronchoplasty, graft repair—assistant	11.	________
12.	Tracheoplasty, cervical	12.	________
13.	Closed treatment of metacarpal fracture, single w/o manipulation	13.	________
14.	Cryotherapy	14.	________
15.	Open treatment of distal tibial fracture of fibula only	15.	________

Exercise 17-21

Directions: Based on the Anesthesia Service description, look up the appropriate CPT code and write it in the space provided.

Description	Code
1. Vaginal hysterectomy	1. ________
2. Total ankle replacement	2. ________
3. Tympanotomy	3. ________
4. Angioplasty	4. ________
5. Lithotripsy, extracorporeal shock wave with water bath	5. ________
6. Radial orchiectomy, inguinal	6. ________
7. Repair of cleft palate	7. ________
8. Vulvectomy	8. ________
9. Venous thrombectomy, direct or catheter	9. ________
10. Complete amputation of penis	10. ________
11. Percutaneous liver biopsy	11. ________
12. Amniocentesis	12. ________
13. Repair of ruptured achilles tendon, with or w/o graft	13. ________
14. Pneumocentesis	14. ________
15. Corneal transplant	15. ________

Exercise 17-22

Directions: Based on the Anesthesia Service description, look up the appropriate CPT code and write it in the space provided.

Description	Code
1. Excision of mediastinal cyst	1. ________
2. Pyelotomy, with exploration	2. ________
3. Repair, laceration of palate, up to 2 cm	3. ________
4. Resection of external cardiac tumor	4. ________
5. Wedging of clubfoot cast	5. ________
6. Puncture aspiration of cyst of breast	6. ________
7. Removal of foreign body, intraocular	7. ________
8. Mastoidectomy, complete	8. ________
9. Open treatment of ankle dislocation	9. ________
10. Nipple/areola reconstruction	10. ________
11. Hysterotomy, abdominal	11. ________
12. Cholecystectomy	12. ________
13. Amniocentesis, any method	13. ________
14. Spinal puncture, lumbar, diagnostic	14. ________
15. Acne surgery	15. ________

Exercise 17-23

Directions: Based on the Anesthesia Service description, look up the appropriate CPT code and write it in the space provided.

Description	Code
1. Routine obstetric care w/antepartum care, vaginal	1. ________
2. Excision of tonsil tags	2. ________
3. Anoscopy	3. ________
4. Arthroscopy, ankle surgical removal of FB	4. ________
5. Laryngoscopy	5. ________
6. Proctoscopy	6. ________
7. Bronchoscopy	7. ________
8. Ophthalmoscopy	8. ________
9. Femoral artery ligation	9. ________
10. Orchiopexy, unilateral or bilateral	10. ________
11. Biopsy of liver	11. ________
12. Catheterization, urethra, simple	12. ________
13. Treatment of spontaneous abortion	13. ________
14. Adrenalectomy	14. ________
15. Urethroplasty, first stage	15. ________

Exercise 17-24

Directions: Based on the Anesthesia Service description, look up the appropriate CPT code and write it in the space provided.

Description	Code
1. Laminectomy	1. ________
2. Sigmoidoscopy	2. ________
3. Renal biopsy, percutaneous	3. ________
4. Liver transplant (recipient)	4. ________
5. Myringotomy	5. ________
6. Thoracoplasty	6. ________
7. Repair blood vessel, direct, neck	7. ________
8. Pneumocentesis	8. ________
9. Circumcision, using clamp, newborn	9. ________
10. Salpingo-oophorectomy, complete	10. ________
11. Bronchoplasty, graft repair	11. ________
12. Tracheoplasty, cervical	12. ________
13. Treatment of closed metacarpal fracture, single	13. ________
14. Cryotherapy	14. ________
15. Treatment of closed distal tibial fracture	15. ________

Exercise 17-25

Directions: Look up the following Anesthesia Service CPT Codes and write the corresponding English-language description in the space provided.

	Code	Description
1.	01392	______
2.	00630	______
3.	01130	______
4.	00830	______
5.	00104	______
6.	01402	______
7.	01772	______
8.	00540	______
9.	01380	______
10.	01999	______
11.	01732	______
12.	00212	______
13.	00102	______
14.	01272	______
15.	01460	______

18

HCFA-1500 Billing Form

In this chapter you will learn:

- To understand and properly complete the HCFA-1500 claim form.
- To gain speed and accuracy in completing the HCFA-1500 claim form.

The HCFA-1500 claim form is a standardized form approved by the American Medical Association for use as a "universal" form for billing professional services (see Figure 18-1). This is the only form acceptable for billing Medicare for services. (The UB-92 is allowed for use when billing hospital services.)

As you use this form, you'll become familiar with the various boxes and know where to obtain the information required for completing and processing claim forms. The following list will assist in explaining the uses of the various fields. It contains the field number along with the name of the field and a brief description of the information needed. The word "same" refers to a description that is the same as the title of the box. Explanations that are too lengthy to be included here are expanded upon after this brief listing.

Field #	Field Name/Description
1	*Medicare, Medicaid, CHAMPUS, CHAMPVA, Feca Black Lung or Other.* Check the box of the organization to which you are submitting this claim for payment if you are submitting the form to one of the organizations listed.
1A	*Insured's ID Number.* Social Security number of insured.
2	*Patient's Name.* Same.
3	*Patient's Birth Date and Sex.* All dates should be recorded as Month/Day/Year. Check the box for the appropriate sex.
4	*Insured's Name.* Subscriber's name.
5	*Patient's Address and Phone Number.* Same.
6	*Patient's Relationship to Insured.* Same.
7	*Insured's Address and Phone Number.* Same.
8	*Patient's Status.* Check applicable boxes.
9	*Other Insured's Name.* Other insured whose coverage may be responsible, in whole or in part, for the payment of this claim.
9A	*Other Insured's Policy or Group Number.* Same.
9B	*Other Insured's Date of Birth and Sex.* Same.
9C	*Employer's Name or School Name.* Employer or School Name of other insured party.
9D	*Insurance Plan Name or Program Name.* Name of insurance company and/or group plan for other insured.
10A	*Was Condition Related to: Employment?* If YES is marked, there is Worker's Compensation Insurance involved. If NO is marked, Worker's Compensation is not involved. Circle whether employment is current or previous.
10B	*Was Condition Related to: Auto Accident?* If YES is marked, check for an injury date (Block 14) and an injury diagnosis (Block 23). The state the accident occurred in should also be indicated. If NO is marked, the claim may not be for an injury.
10C	*Was Condition Related to: Other Accident?* If YES is marked, check for an injury date (Block 14) and an injury diagnosis (Block 23). If NO is marked then the claim may not be for an injury.
10D	*Reserved for Local Use.* Same.
11	*Insured's Policy Group or FECA Number.* Subscriber's Group Number. This information refers to primary insured listed in 1a above.
11A	*Insured's Date of Birth.* Same.
11B	*Employer's Name or School Name.* Employer or School Name of insured party.
11C	*Insurance Plan Name or Program Name.* Name of insurance company and/or group plan.

PLEASE DO NOT STAPLE IN THIS AREA

APPROVED OMB-0938-0008

CARRIER

PICA

HEALTH INSURANCE CLAIM FORM

PICA

1. MEDICARE (Medicare #) MEDICAID (Medicaid #) CHAMPUS (Sponsor's SSN) CHAMPVA (VA File #) GROUP HEALTH PLAN (SSN or ID) FECA BLK LUNG (SSN) OTHER (ID)

1a. INSURED'S I.D. NUMBER (FOR PROGRAM IN ITEM 1)

2. PATIENT'S NAME (Last Name, First Name, Middle Initial)

3. PATIENT'S BIRTH DATE MM DD YY SEX M F

4. INSURED'S NAME (Last Name, First Name, Middle Initial)

5. PATIENT'S ADDRESS (No., Street)

6. PATIENT RELATIONSHIP TO INSURED Self Spouse Child Other

7. INSURED'S ADDRESS (No., Street)

CITY STATE

8. PATIENT STATUS Single Married Other

CITY STATE

ZIP CODE TELEPHONE (Include Area Code) ( )

Employed Full-Time Student Part-Time Student

ZIP CODE TELEPHONE (INCLUDE AREA CODE) ( )

9. OTHER INSURED'S NAME (Last Name, First Name, Middle Initial)

10. IS PATIENT'S CONDITION RELATED TO:

11. INSURED'S POLICY GROUP OR FECA NUMBER

a. OTHER INSURED'S POLICY OR GROUP NUMBER

a. EMPLOYMENT? (CURRENT OR PREVIOUS) YES NO

a. INSURED'S DATE OF BIRTH MM DD YY SEX M F

b. OTHER INSURED'S DATE OF BIRTH MM DD YY SEX M F

b. AUTO ACCIDENT? PLACE (State) YES NO

b. EMPLOYER'S NAME OR SCHOOL NAME

c. EMPLOYER'S NAME OR SCHOOL NAME

c. OTHER ACCIDENT? YES NO

c. INSURANCE PLAN NAME OR PROGRAM NAME

d. INSURANCE PLAN NAME OR PROGRAM NAME

10d. RESERVED FOR LOCAL USE

d. IS THERE ANOTHER HEALTH BENEFIT PLAN? YES NO *If yes,* return to and complete item 9 a-d.

READ BACK OF FORM BEFORE COMPLETING & SIGNING THIS FORM.

12. PATIENT'S OR AUTHORIZED PERSON'S SIGNATURE I authorize the release of any medical or other information necessary to process this claim. I also request payment of government benefits either to myself or to the party who accepts assignment below.

SIGNED DATE

13. INSURED'S OR AUTHORIZED PERSON'S SIGNATURE I authorize payment of medical benefits to the undersigned physician or supplier for services described below.

SIGNED

PATIENT AND INSURED INFORMATION

14. DATE OF CURRENT: MM DD YY ILLNESS (First symptom) OR INJURY (Accident) OR PREGNANCY(LMP)

15. IF PATIENT HAS HAD SAME OR SIMILAR ILLNESS. GIVE FIRST DATE MM DD YY

16. DATES PATIENT UNABLE TO WORK IN CURRENT OCCUPATION FROM MM DD YY TO MM DD YY

17. NAME OF REFERRING PHYSICIAN OR OTHER SOURCE

17a. I.D. NUMBER OF REFERRING PHYSICIAN

18. HOSPITALIZATION DATES RELATED TO CURRENT SERVICES FROM MM DD YY TO MM DD YY

19. RESERVED FOR LOCAL USE

20. OUTSIDE LAB? YES NO $ CHARGES

21. DIAGNOSIS OR NATURE OF ILLNESS OR INJURY. (RELATE ITEMS 1,2,3 OR 4 TO ITEM 24E BY LINE)

1. ___ . __
2. ___ . __
3. ___ . __
4. ___ . __

22. MEDICAID RESUBMISSION CODE ORIGINAL REF. NO.

23. PRIOR AUTHORIZATION NUMBER

24. A DATE(S) OF SERVICE From MM DD YY To MM DD YY	B Place of Service	C Type of Service	D PROCEDURES, SERVICES, OR SUPPLIES (Explain Unusual Circumstances) CPT/HCPCS MODIFIER	E DIAGNOSIS CODE	F $ CHARGES	G DAYS OR UNITS	H EPSDT Family Plan	I EMG	J COB	K RESERVED FOR LOCAL USE
1										
2										
3										
4										
5										
6										

25. FEDERAL TAX I.D. NUMBER SSN EIN

26. PATIENT'S ACCOUNT NO.

27. ACCEPT ASSIGNMENT? (For govt. claims, see back) YES NO

28. TOTAL CHARGE $

29. AMOUNT PAID $

30. BALANCE DUE $

31. SIGNATURE OF PHYSICIAN OR SUPPLIER INCLUDING DEGREES OR CREDENTIALS (I certify that the statements on the reverse apply to this bill and are made a part thereof.)

SIGNED DATE

32. NAME AND ADDRESS OF FACILITY WHERE SERVICES WERE RENDERED (If other than home or office)

33. PHYSICIAN'S, SUPPLIER'S BILLING NAME, ADDRESS, ZIP CODE & PHONE #

PIN# GRP#

PHYSICIAN OR SUPPLIER INFORMATION

(APPROVED BY AMA COUNCIL ON MEDICAL SERVICE 8/88)

PLEASE PRINT OR TYPE

FORM HCFA-1500 (12-90)
FORM OWCP-1500 FORM RRB-1500
FORM AMA OP050591

Figure 18-1: Front of HCFA-1500

BECAUSE THIS FORM IS USED BY VARIOUS GOVERNMENT AND PRIVATE HEALTH PROGRAMS, SEE SEPARATE INSTRUCTIONS ISSUED BY APPLICABLE PROGRAMS.

NOTICE: Any person who knowingly files a statement of claim containing any misrepresentation or any false, incomplete or misleading information may be guilty of a criminal act punishable under law and may be subject to civil penalties.

REFERS TO GOVERNMENT PROGRAMS ONLY

MEDICARE AND CHAMPUS PAYMENTS: A patient's signature requests that payment be made and authorizes release of any information necessary to process the claim and certifies that the information provided in Blocks 1 through 12 is true, accurate and complete. In the case of a Medicare claim, the patient's signature authorizes any entity to release to Medicare medical and nonmedical information, including employment status, and whether the person has employer group health insurance, liability, no-fault, worker's compensation or other insurance which is responsible to pay for the services for which the Medicare claim is made. See 42 CFR 411.24(a). If item 9 is completed, the patient's signature authorizes release of the information to the health plan or agency shown. In Medicare assigned or CHAMPUS participation cases, the physician agrees to accept the charge determination of the Medicare carrier or CHAMPUS fiscal intermediary as the full charge, and the patient is responsible only for the deductible, coinsurance and noncovered services. Coinsurance and the deductible are based upon the charge determination of the Medicare carrier or CHAMPUS fiscal intermediary if this is less than the charge submitted. CHAMPUS is not a health insurance program but makes payment for health benefits provided through certain affiliations with the Uniformed Services. Information on the patient's sponsor should be provided in those items captioned in "Insured"; i.e., items 1a, 4, 6, 7, 9, and 11.

BLACK LUNG AND FECA CLAIMS

The provider agrees to accept the amount paid by the Government as payment in full. See Black Lung and FECA instructions regarding required procedure and diagnosis coding systems.

SIGNATURE OF PHYSICIAN OR SUPPLIER (MEDICARE, CHAMPUS, FECA AND BLACK LUNG)

I certify that the services shown on this form were medically indicated and necessary for the health of the patient and were personally furnished by me or were furnished incident to my professional service by my employee under my immediate personal supervision, except as otherwise expressly permitted by Medicare or CHAMPUS regulations.

For services to be considered as "incident" to a physician's professional service, 1) they must be rendered under the physician's immediate personal supervision by his/her employee, 2) they must be an integral, although incidental part of a covered physician's service, 3) they must be of kinds commonly furnished in physician's offices, and 4) the services of nonphysicians must be included on the physician's bills.

For CHAMPUS claims, I further certify that I (or any employee) who rendered services am not an active duty member of the Uniformed Services or a civilian employee of the United States Government or a contract employee of the United States Government, either civilian or military (refer to 5 USC 5536). For Black-Lung claims, I further certify that the services performed were for a Black Lung-related disorder.

No Part B Medicare benefits may be paid unless this form is received as required by existing law and regulations (42 CFR 424.32).

NOTICE: Any one who misrepresents or falsifies essential information to receive payment from Federal funds requested by this form may upon conviction be subject to fine and imprisonment under applicable Federal laws.

NOTICE TO PATIENT ABOUT THE COLLECTION AND USE OF MEDICARE, CHAMPUS, FECA, AND BLACK LUNG INFORMATION
(PRIVACY ACT STATEMENT)

We are authorized by HCFA, CHAMPUS and OWCP to ask you for information needed in the administration of the Medicare, CHAMPUS, FECA, and Black Lung programs. Authority to collect information is in section 205(a), 1862, 1872 and 1874 of the Social Security Act as amended, 42 CFR 411.24(a) and 424.5(a) (6), and 44 USC 3101;41 CFR 101 et seq and 10 USC 1079 and 1086; 5 USC 8101 et seq; and 30 USC 901 et seq; 38 USC 613; E.O. 9397.

The information we obtain to complete claims under these programs is used to identify you and to determine your eligibility. It is also used to decide if the services and supplies you received are covered by these programs and to insure that proper payment is made.

The information may also be given to other providers of services, carriers, intermediaries, medical review boards, health plans, and other organizations or Federal agencies, for the effective administration of Federal provisions that require other third parties payers to pay primary to Federal program, and as otherwise necessary to administer these programs. For example, it may be necessary to disclose information about the benefits you have used to a hospital or doctor. Additional disclosures are made through routine uses for information contained in systems of records.

FOR MEDICARE CLAIMS: See the notice modifying system No. 09-70-0501, titled, 'Carrier Medicare Claims Record,' published in the Federal Register, Vol. 55 No. 177, page 37549, Wed. Sept. 12, 1990, or as updated and republished.

FOR OWCP CLAIMS: Department of Labor, Privacy Act of 1974, "Republication of Notice of Systems of Records," Federal Register Vol. 55 No. 40, Wed Feb. 28, 1990, See ESA-5, ESA-6, ESA-12, ESA-13, ESA-30, or as updated and republished.

FOR CHAMPUS CLAIMS: PRINCIPLE PURPOSE(S): To evaluate eligibility for medical care provided by civilian sources and to issue payment upon establishment of eligibility and determination that the services/supplies received are authorized by law.

ROUTINE USE(S): Information from claims and related documents may be given to the Dept. of Veterans Affairs, the Dept. of Health and Human Services and/or the Dept. of Transportation consistent with their statutory administrative responsibilities under CHAMPUS/CHAMPVA; to the Dept. of Justice for representation of the Secretary of Defense in civil actions; to the Internal Revenue Service, private collection agencies, and consumer reporting agencies in connection with recoupment claims; and to Congressional Offices in response to inquiries made at the request of the person to whom a record pertains. Appropriate disclosures may be made to other federal, state, local, foreign government agencies, private business entities, and individual providers of care, on matters relating to entitlement, claims adjudication, fraud, program abuse, utilization review, quality assurance, peer review, program integrity, third-party liability, coordination of benefits, and civil and criminal litigation related to the operation of CHAMPUS.

DISCLOSURES: Voluntary; however, failure to provide information will result in delay in payment or may result in denial of claim. With the one exception discussed below, there are no penalties under these programs for refusing to supply information. However, failure to furnish information regarding the medical services rendered or the amount charged would prevent payment of claims under these programs. Failure to furnish any other information, such as name or claim number, would delay payment of the claim. Failure to provide medical information under FECA could be deemed an obstruction.

It is mandatory that you tell us if you know that another party is responsible for paying for your treatment. Section 1128B of the Social Security Act and 31 USC 3801-3812 provide penalties for withholding this information.

You should be aware that P.L. 100-503, the "Computer Matching and Privacy Protection Act of 1988", permits the government to verify information by way of computer matches.

MEDICAID PAYMENTS (PROVIDER CERTIFICATION)

I hereby agree to keep such records as are necessary to disclose fully the extent of services provided to individuals under the State's Title XIX plan and to furnish information regarding any payments claimed for providing such services as the State Agency or Dept. of Health and Humans Services may request.

I further agree to accept, as payment in full, the amount paid by the Medicaid program for those claims submitted for payment under that program, with the exception of authorized deductible, coinsurance, co-payment or similar cost-sharing charge.

SIGNATURE OF PHYSICIAN (OR SUPPLIER): I certify that the services listed above were medically indicated and necessary to the health of this patient and were personally furnished by me or my employee under my personal direction.

NOTICE: This is to certify that the foregoing information is true, accurate and complete. I understand that payment and satisfaction of this claim will be from Federal and State funds, and that any false claims, statements, or documents, or concealment of a material fact, may be prosecuted under applicable Federal or State laws.

Public reporting burden for this collection of information is estimated to average 15 minutes per response, including time for reviewing instructions, searching existing date sources, gathering and maintaining data needed, and completing and reviewing the collection of information. Send comments regarding this burden estimate or any other aspect of this collection of information, including suggestions for reducing the burden, to HCFA, Office of Financial Management, P.O. Box 26684, Baltimore, MD 21207; and to the Office of Management and Budget, Paperwork Reduction Project (OMB-0938-0008), Washington, D.C. 20503.

Figure 18-1: Back of HCFA-1500

11D *Is There Another Health Benefit Plan?* Check appropriate box. If YES is checked, then items 9A–D must be completed.

12 *Patient's or Authorized Person's Signature.* Patient's release of medical information.

13 *Assignment of Benefits.* This box should always be signed by the patient to allow the insurer to pay the physician directly instead of paying the patient and waiting for the patient to pay the provider.

14 *Date of Illness, Injury, Accident or Pregnancy.* All injury claims (ie, injury diagnosis) must have an injury or accident date. If the patient's condition is a pregnancy, the date of the last menstrual period should be indicated.

15 *If Patient Has Had Same or Similar Illness, Give First Date.* Same.

16 *Dates Patient Unable to Work in Current Occupation.* Same.

17 *Name of Referring Physician or Other Source.* If this patient was referred to the current physician by another physician, a hospital, or clinic, the referring party should be listed here.

17A *ID Number of Referring Physician.* Same.

18 *Hospitalization Dates Relating to Current Services.* Same.

19 *Reserved for Local Use.* Same.

20 *Outside Lab.* Was laboratory work performed outside your office? If so, check the YES box and indicate the total of the charges.

21 *Diagnosis or Nature of Illness or Injury.* The diagnosis states why the patient went to see the provider. This should be indicated by the proper ICD-9 Code.

22 *Medicaid Resubmission Code.* Leave blank.

23 *Prior Authorization Number.* Authorization number for services that were approved prior to being rendered.

24A *Date of Service.* The date service was rendered by the provider. A complete date must be given.

24B *Place of Service.* The location where the services were performed. (See following section for further information.)

24C *Type of Service.* Leave blank.

24D *Procedure Code.* The 5-digit procedure code as found in the CPT/RVS and HCPC manuals.

24D *Modifier Code.* The two-digit modifier from the CPT/RVS further describing the procedure code.

24E *Diagnosis Code.* This is used in conjunction with Field 21. The number placed in Field 24E (ie, 1, 2, 3, 4) refers to diagnosis 1, 2, 3, 4 in Block 21. In other words, the doctor can perform different services for different illnesses or injuries on different dates and submit them all on one claim form.

24F *Charges.* The charge per line of service.

24G *Days or Units.* The number of times a service was performed.

24H *EPSDT Family Plan.* Leave blank.

24I *EMG.* If service was rendered in the hospital emergency room, this should match the service code in Item 24B.

24J *COB.* Coordination of Benefits. Are there other insurance policies or plans that may be responsible for payment on this claim? Indicate a Y for yes, an N for no.

24K *Reserved for Local Use.* Leave blank.

25 *Federal Tax ID Number.* If the provider of service is a physician or an individual, his/her Social Security number should be used. If the provider of service is a facility, an Employer ID Number should be used.

26 *Patient's Account Number.* Same.

27 *Accept Assignment for Government Claims.* Refers only to CHAMPUS or Medicare. Do not use to assign pay-

ment on this claim to the provider. Use Item 13 only for your assignment of payment.

28 *Total Charge.* The total charge of the claim.

29 *Amount Paid.* The amount paid by the patient or subscriber.

30 *Balance Due.* The difference between the total charge and the amount paid by the patient or subscriber (if any).

31 *Signature of Physician or Supplier of Service.* Must be signed by the provider indicating that the said services have indeed been rendered. Degrees or credentials (eg, MD, DO) should follow the name.

32 *Name and Address of Facility Where Services Rendered.* If this information is the same as Item 33, it may be left blank.

33 *Physician's/Supplier's Billing Name, Address, Zip Code and Phone Number.* The name, address and phone number of the physician or supplier of service. This is the address to which payments will be addressed if assignment of benefits has been signed for in Field 13.

HCFA-1500 Item 24B, Place of Service

This item needs further description, for which space was not available in the above text. Please study before completing any billing forms.

This requires a numerical code to indicate the place where the service was rendered.

00–10 Unassigned

11 Office (Location other than a hospital, Skilled Nursing Facility [SNF], Military Treatment Facility, Community Health Center, State or Local Public Health Clinic or Intermediate Care Facility [ICF], where the health professional routinely provides health examinations, diagnosis and treatment of illness or injury on an ambulatory basis)

12 Home (Location other than a hospital or other facility where the patient receives care in a private residence)

13–20 Unassigned

21 Inpatient hospital (A facility other than psychiatric, which primarily provides diagnostic, therapeutic [both surgical and nonsurgical] and rehabilitation services by, or under the supervision of, physicians to patients admitted for a variety of medical conditions)

22 Outpatient hospital (A portion of a hospital which provides diagnostic, therapeutic [both surgical and nonsurgical] and rehabilitation services to sick and injured persons who do not require hospitalization or institutionalization.) A patient who is not admitted to a hospital (eg, one who is under 24-hour supervision) is an outpatient.

23 Emergency Room (ER)–Hospital (A portion of a hospital where emergency diagnosis and treatment of illness or injury are provided.) Patients in the ER are considered to be facility outpatients. (Remember to also complete box 24I.)

24 Ambulatory Surgical Center (A free-standing facility, other than a physician's office, where surgical and diagnostic services are provided on an ambulatory basis.) When this code is used, the facility must be an HCFA-approved ASC.

25 Birthing Center (A facility, other than a hospital's maternity facilities or a physician's office, which provides a setting for labor, delivery and immediate post-partum care as well as immediate care of newborn infants)

26 Military Treatment Facility (MTF) (A

	medical facility operated by one or more of the Uniformed Services.) MTF also refers to certain former U.S. Public Health Service facilities now designated as Uniformed Service Treatment Facilities (USTF).
27–30	Unassigned
31	Skilled Nursing Facility (A facility that primarily provides inpatient skilled nursing care and related services to patients who require medical, nursing, or rehabilitative services and that does not provide the level of care or treatment available in a hospital)
32	Nursing Facility (A facility that provides skilled nursing care and related services for the rehabilitation of injured, disabled, or sick persons or on a regular basis health-related care services above the level of custodial care to other than mentally retarded individuals)
33	Custodial Care Facility (A facility that provides room, board, and personal assistance services, generally on a long-term basis, and that does not include a medical component)
34	Hospice (A facility, other than a patient's home, in which palliative and supportive care for terminally ill patients and their families are provided)
35–40	Unassigned
41	Ambulance—Land (A land vehicle specifically designed, equipped and staffed for lifesaving and transporting the sick or injured)
42	Ambulance—Air or Water (An air or water vehicle specifically designed, equipped, and staffed for lifesaving and transporting the sick or injured)
43–50	Unassigned
51	Inpatient Psychiatric Facility (A facility that provides inpatient psychiatric services for the diagnosis and treatment of mental illness on a 24-hour basis, by or under the supervision of a physician)
52	Psychiatric Facility Partial Hospitalization (A facility for the diagnosis and treatment of mental illness that provides a planned therapeutic program for patients who do not need full-time hospitalization, but who need broader programs than are possible from outpatient visits in a hospital-based or hospital-affiliated facility)
53	Community Mental Health Center (A facility that provides comprehensive mental health services on an ambulatory basis primarily to individuals residing or employed in a defined area.) Includes a physician-directed mental health facility.
54	Intermediate Care Facility/Mentally Retarded (A facility that primarily provides health-related care and services above the level of custodial care of mentally retarded individuals but does not provide the level of care or treatment available in a hospital or SNF)
55	Residential Substance Abuse Treatment Facility (A facility that provides treatment for substance [alcohol and drug] abuse to live-in residents who do not require acute medical care). Services include individual and group therapy and counseling, family counseling, laboratory tests, drugs and supplies, psychological testing, and room and board.
56	Psychiatric Residential Treatment Center (A facility or distinct part of a facility for psychiatric care, which provides a total 24-hour therapeutically planned and professionally staffed group living and learning environment)
57–60	Unassigned
61	Comprehensive Inpatient Rehabilitation Facility (A facility that provides comprehensive rehabilitation services under the supervision of a physician to inpa-

tients with physical disabilities.) Services include rehabilitation nursing, physical therapy, occupational therapy, speech pathology, social or psychological services, and orthotics and prosthetics services. There are specific licensing requirements for these facilities.

62	Comprehensive Outpatient Rehabilitation Facility (A facility that provides comprehensive rehabilitation services under the supervision of a physician to inpatients with physical disabilities.) Services include physical therapy, occupational therapy, and speech pathology services. There are specific licensing requirements for these facilities.
63–64	Unassigned
65	End-Stage Renal Disease Treatment Facility (A facility other than a hospital, which provides dialysis treatment, maintenance and/or training to patients or care givers on an ambulatory or home-care basis)
66–70	Unassigned
71	State or Local Public Health Clinic (A facility maintained by either state or local health departments that provides ambulatory primary medical care under the general direction of a physician.) Such facilities must be physician-directed.
72	Rural Health Clinic (A certified facility that is located in a rural medically underserved area that provides ambulatory primary medical care under the general direction of a physician.) Qualified facilities do not bill Part B of Medicare for items or services except for DME and orthotics and prosthetics.
73–80	Unassigned
81	Independent Laboratory (A laboratory certified to perform diagnostic and/or clinical tests independent of an institution or a physician's office) With the exception of hospital inpatients, the place of service for lab tests will be based on where "drawn" instead of where the test is actually performed. If the physician is billing for a lab service performed in his/her own office, then use the appropriate code for doctor's office. If an independent laboratory is billing, show the place where the sample is drawn. An independent laboratory drawing a sample in its laboratory shows the code for independent laboratory as the place of service. If an independent laboratory is billing for a test on a sample drawn on a hospital inpatient, then the appropriate code for hospital inpatient is entered as the place of service. If the independent laboratory is billing for a test on a sample drawn in a physician's office, then the appropriate code is for doctor's office.
82–98	Unassigned
99	Other Unlisted Facility (Other service facilities not identified above)

Summary

The HCFA-1500 is the most accepted form for billing professional services. It is vital that the correct information be inserted in each field to allow the claim to be processed quickly and accurately. Although the completion may seem simple, it takes practice to be able to fill out the form completely, quickly and accurately.

Assignments

Complete the Questions for Review.

Properly complete a billing form for the first five Physicians Services claims (Claims 3-1 to 3-5) in the student exercise manual. Once you are certain you are billing the claims correctly, move on to the first five claims in each of the remaining chapters, excluding Chapter 9.

Questions for Review

Directions: Answer the following questions without looking back into the material just covered. Write your answers in the space provided.

1. What is the HCFA-1500 billing form used for? ______________________________
____
2. If the provider of service is an individual, what should be placed in the box entitled Federal Tax ID Number? ______________________________
3. Which box denotes that Worker's Compensation is involved in the claim? ______________________________
____
4. How would you indicate that the place where services were rendered was an office? ______________________________
____
5. What are the boxes at the top of the HCFA-1500 form, labeled "Medicare, Medicaid, CHAMPUS, CHAMPVA, Feca Black Lung, and Other" for?______________________________
____
6. What does the term "Assignment of Benefits" mean?______________________________
____
7. On the HCFA-1500, what is Item 24I "EMG" for?______________________________
____
8. On the HCFA-1500, what does Item 24J "COB" stand for, and what does the term mean?______________________________
____
9. When a physician or provider of service signs a medical billing form, he/she is legally stating that the service(s) that he/she is seeking payment for have actually been performed. (True or false) ______________________________
10. What is a "Unit of service"? ______________________________
____

If you were unable to answer any of the questions, refer back to the section and then fill in the answers.

19

UB-92 Hospital Billing Form

In this chapter you will learn:

- To understand the UB-92 billing form and to properly complete it.
- To identify hospital revenue codes.
- To complete a UB-92 billing form from itemized hospital bills.

The Uniform Bill UB-92 is intended to be used by hospitals or other hospital-type facilities for inpatient and outpatient billing. The data elements and the design of the form were determined by the National Uniform Billing Committee. This form was designed to provide the basic data needed by most payors to adjudicate a large majority of their claims. The objective was to accommodate a wide range of needs while eliminating the need for attachments.

As you use this form (see Figure 19-1), you will become familiar with the various boxes and know where to obtain the information required for completing and processing claim forms. The following list will assist in explaining the uses of the various fields. It contains the field number along with the name of the field and a brief description of the information needed. The word "same" refers to a description that is the same as the title of the box. Explanations that are too lengthy to be included here have been expanded on after this brief listing.

Field #	Field Name/Description
1	*Provider Name, Address, and Telephone Number.* Name, address, and telephone number of hospital or clinic where services were rendered.
2	*Reserved (untitled).* All unlabeled fields are reserved for state or national use. Their use may be assigned by either the state or National Uniform Billing Committee.
3	*Patient Control Number.* Patient's account number.
4	*Type of Bill.* Three-digit code providing information regarding what type of bill is being submitted. (See following section for further information.)
5	*Federal Tax Number.* Provider's Identification Number or Social Security Number.
6	*Statement Covers Period.* The dates of service that this billing statement represents. Dates should match those on the itemized billing statement. For services rendered on the same day, both dates should be the same.
7	*Covered Days.* Number of days services covered by primary payor.
8	*Noncovered Days* (inpatient only). Number of days services not covered by primary payor. For Medicare, the reason for noncoverage should be explained by occurrence codes, PSRO fields, or in remarks.
9	*Coinsurance Days.* Number of days for which the patient must pay a portion of the costs of services. For Medicare, the inpatient Medicare days occurring after the 60th and before the 91st day in a single spell of illness.
10	*Lifetime Reserve Days.* Under Medicare, each beneficiary has a lifetime reserve of 60 additional days of inpatient hospital services after using 90 days of inpatient hospital services during a spell of illness.
11	*Reserved for State Assignment.*
12	*Patient's Name.* Same.
13	*Patient's Address.* Same.
14	*Birth Date.* Patient's date of birth.
15	*Sex.* Patient's sex.
16	*Marital Status.* Patient's marital status (S = Single, M = Married, X = Legally Separated, D = Divorced, W = Widowed, U = Unknown).
17	*Date of Admission.* Date patient was admitted to hospital.
18	*Hour of Admission.* Hour patient admitted to hospital according to a 24-hour clock (eg, 10:10 PM would be written 22:10). 99 = unknown.
19	*Type of Admission.* Numerical code denoting the priority of this admission. (See following section for further information.)

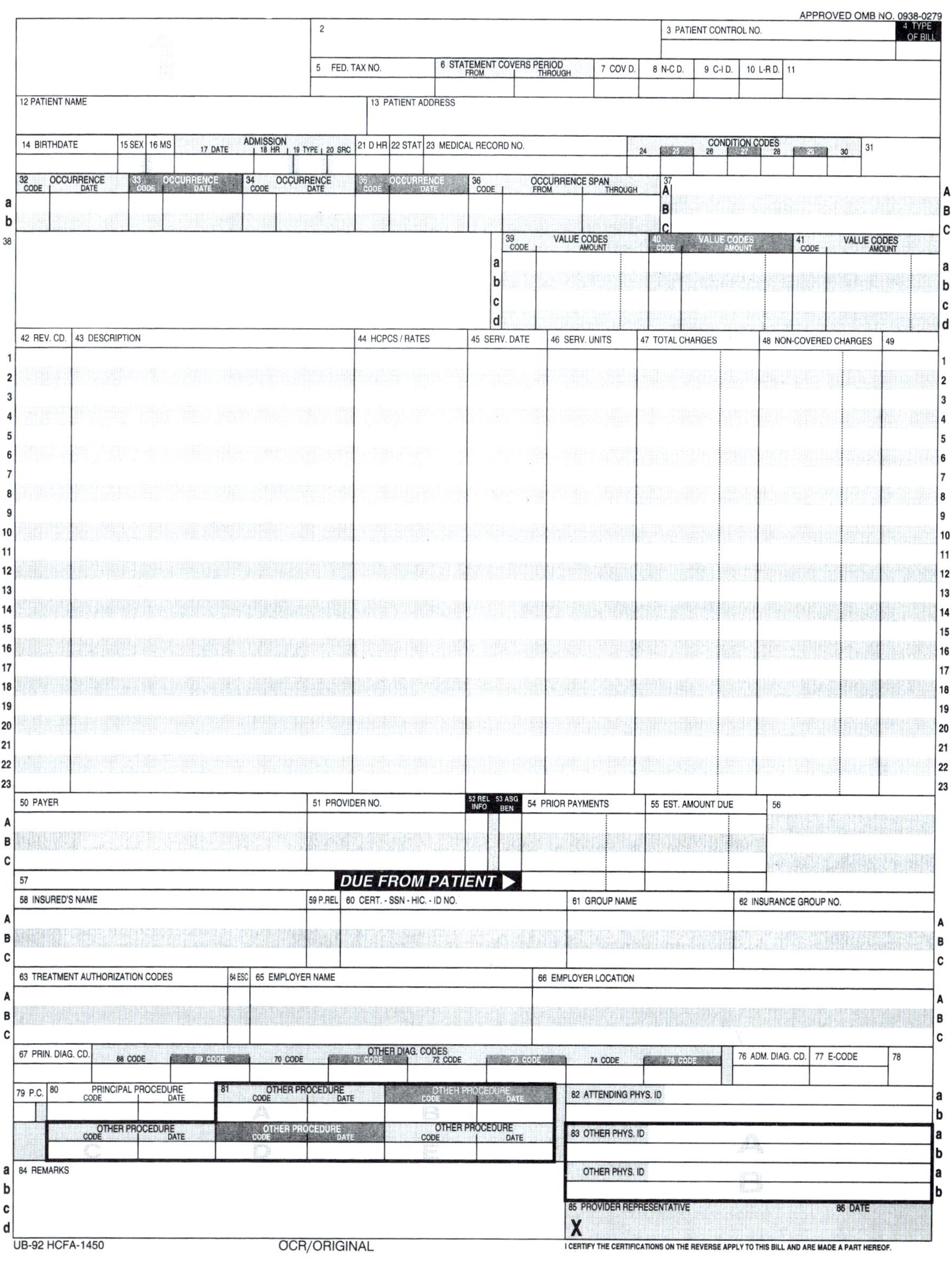

APPROVED OMB NO. 0938-0279

2
3 PATIENT CONTROL NO.
4 TYPE OF BILL
5 FED. TAX NO.
6 STATEMENT COVERS PERIOD FROM THROUGH
7 COV D.
8 N-C D.
9 C-I D.
10 L-R D.
11
12 PATIENT NAME
13 PATIENT ADDRESS
14 BIRTHDATE
15 SEX
16 MS
ADMISSION 17 DATE 18 HR 19 TYPE 20 SRC
21 D HR
22 STAT
23 MEDICAL RECORD NO.
CONDITION CODES 24 25 26 27 28 29 30
31
32 OCCURRENCE CODE DATE
33 OCCURRENCE CODE DATE
34 OCCURRENCE CODE DATE
35 OCCURRENCE CODE DATE
36 OCCURRENCE SPAN CODE FROM THROUGH
37 A B C
a b
38
39 VALUE CODES CODE AMOUNT
40 VALUE CODES CODE AMOUNT
41 VALUE CODES CODE AMOUNT
a b c d
42 REV. CD.
43 DESCRIPTION
44 HCPCS / RATES
45 SERV. DATE
46 SERV. UNITS
47 TOTAL CHARGES
48 NON-COVERED CHARGES
49
1 2 3 4 5 6 7 8 9 10 11 12 13 14 15 16 17 18 19 20 21 22 23
50 PAYER
51 PROVIDER NO.
52 REL INFO
53 ASG BEN
54 PRIOR PAYMENTS
55 EST. AMOUNT DUE
56
A B C
57
DUE FROM PATIENT ▶
58 INSURED'S NAME
59 P.REL
60 CERT. - SSN - HIC. - ID NO.
61 GROUP NAME
62 INSURANCE GROUP NO.
A B C
63 TREATMENT AUTHORIZATION CODES
64 ESC
65 EMPLOYER NAME
66 EMPLOYER LOCATION
A B C
67 PRIN. DIAG. CD.
OTHER DIAG. CODES 68 CODE 69 CODE 70 CODE 71 CODE 72 CODE 73 CODE 74 CODE 75 CODE
76 ADM. DIAG. CD.
77 E-CODE
78
79 P.C.
80 PRINCIPAL PROCEDURE CODE DATE
81 OTHER PROCEDURE CODE DATE (A)
OTHER PROCEDURE CODE DATE (B)
82 ATTENDING PHYS. ID a b
OTHER PROCEDURE CODE DATE (C)
OTHER PROCEDURE CODE DATE (D)
OTHER PROCEDURE CODE DATE (E)
83 OTHER PHYS. ID a b (A)
OTHER PHYS. ID a b (B)
84 REMARKS a b c d
85 PROVIDER REPRESENTATIVE X
86 DATE
UB-92 HCFA-1450
OCR/ORIGINAL
I CERTIFY THE CERTIFICATIONS ON THE REVERSE APPLY TO THIS BILL AND ARE MADE A PART HEREOF.

Figure 19-1: Front of the Uniform Bill (UB-92) Form

UNIFORM BILL: **NOTICE: ANYONE WHO MISREPRESENTS OR FALSIFIES ESSENTIAL INFORMATION REQUESTED BY THIS FORM MAY UPON CONVICTION BE SUBJECT TO FINE AND IMPRISONMENT UNDER FEDERAL AND OR STATE LAW.**

Certifications relevant to the Bill and Information Shown on the Face Hereof: Signatures on the face hereot incorporate the following certifications or verifications where pertinent to this Bill:

1. If third party benefits are indicated as being assigned or in participation status, on the face thereof, appropriate assignments by the insured/beneficiary and signature of patient or parent or legal guardian covering authorization to release information are on file. Determinations as to the release of medical and financial information should be guided by the particular terms of the release forms that were executed by the patient or the patient's legal representative. The hospital agrees to save harmless, indemnify and defend any insurer who makes payment in reliance upon this certification, from and against any claim to the insurance proceeds when in fact no valid assignment of benefits to the hospital was made.

2. If patient occupied a private room or required private nursing for medical necessity, any required certifications are on file.

3. Physician's certifications and re-certifications, if required by contract or Federal regulations, are on file.

4. For Christian Science Sanitoriums, verifications and if necessary re-verifications of the patient's need for sanitorium services are on file.

5. Signature of patient or his representative on certifications, authorization to release information, and payment request, as required by Federal law and regulations (42 USC 1935f, 42 CFR 424.36, 10 USC 1071 thru 1086, 32 CFR 199) and, any other applicable contract regulations, is on file.

6. This claim, to the best of my knowledge, is correct and complete and is in conformance with the Civil Rights Act of 1964 as amended. Records adequately disclosing services will be maintained and necessary information will be furnished to such governmental agencies as required by applicable law.

7. For Medicare purposes:

   If the patient has indicated that other health insurance or a state medical assistance agency will pay part of his medical expenses and he wants information about his claim released to them upon their request, necessary authorization is on file. The patient's signature on the provider's request to bill Medicare authorizes any holder of medical and other information to release to Medicare medical and non-medical information, including employment status, and whether the person has employer group health insurance, liability, no-fault, workers' compensation, or other insurance which is responsible to pay for the services for which this Medicare claim is made.

8. For Medicaid purposes:

   This is to certify that the foregoing information is true, accurate, and complete.

   I understand that payment and satisfaction of this claim will be from Federal and State funds, and that any false claims, statements, or documents, or concealment of a material fact, may be prosecuted under applicable Federal or State Laws.

9. For CHAMPUS purposes:

   This is to certify that:

   (a) the information submitted as a part of this claim is true, accurate and complete, and, the services shown on this form were medically indicated and necessary for the health of the patient;

   (b) the patient has represented that by a reported residential address outside a military treatment center catchment area he or she does not live within the catchment area of a U.S. military or U.S. Public Health Service medical facility, or if the patient resides within a catchment area of such a facility, a copy of a Non-Availability Statement (DD Form 1251) is on file, or the physician has certified to a medical emergency in any instance where a copy of a Non-Availability Statement is not on file;

   (c) the patient or the patient's parent or guardian has responded directly to the provider's request to identify all health insurance coverages, and that all such coverages are identified on the face of the claim except those that are exclusively supplemental payments to CHAMPUS-determined benefits;

   (d) the amount billed to CHAMPUS has been billed after all such coverages have been billed and paid, excluding Medicaid, and the amount billed to CHAMPUS is that remaining claimed against CHAMPUS benefits;

   (e) the beneficiary's cost share has not been waived by consent or failure to exercise generally accepted billing and collection efforts; and,

   (f) any hospital-based physician under contract, the cost of whose services are allocated in the charges included in this bill, is not an employee or member of the Uniformed Services. For purposes of this certification, an employee of the Uniformed Services is an employee, appointed in civil service (refer to 5 USC 2105), including part-time or intermittent but excluding contract surgeons or other personnel employed by the Uniformed Services through personal service contracts. Similarly, member of the Uniformed Services does not apply to reserve members of the Uniformed Services not on active duty.

   (g) based on the Consolidated Omnibus Budget Reconciliation Act of 1986, all providers participating in Medicare must also participate in CHAMPUS for inpatient hospital services provided pursuant to admissions to hospitals occurring on or after January 1, 1987.

   (h) if CHAMPUS benefits are to be paid in a participating status, I agree to submit this claim to the appropriate CHAMPUS claims processor as a participating provider. I agree to accept the CHAMPUS-determined reasonable charge as the total charge for the medical services or supplies listed on the claim form. I will accept the CHAMPUS-determined reasonable charge even if it is less than the billed amount, and also agree to accept the amount paid by CHAMPUS, combined with the cost-share amount and deductible amount, if any, paid by or on behalf of the patient as full payment for the listed medical services or supplies. I will make no attempt to collect from the patient (or his or her parent or guardian) amounts over the CHAMPUS-determined reasonable charge. CHAMPUS will make any benefits payable directly to me, if I submit this claim as a participating provider.

ESTIMATED CONTRACT BENEFITS

Figure 19-2: Back of the Uniform Bill (UB-92) Form

20 *Source of Admission.* Numerical code denoting the source of this admission. (See following section for further information.)

21 *Discharge Hour.* Time patient was discharged from inpatient care. Time should be written according to a 24-hour clock. 99 = unknown. This element is not necessary for outpatient care.

22 *Patient Status.* Numerical code denoting the status of the patient as of the statement-through date. This element is necessary only for inpatient care. (See following section for further information.)

23 *Medical Record Number.* Number assigned by the provider to the medical record.

24-30 *Condition Codes.* Codes used to identify conditions relating to the claim that may affect payor processing. (See following section for further information.) No specific date is associated with this code.

31 *Reserved for National Assignment.*

32-35 *Occurrence Codes.* The code and associated date defining a significant event relating to this bill that may effect payor processing. (See following section for further information.)

36 *Occurrence Span.* The code and the related dates that identify an event that relates to the payment of the claim. These codes identify occurrences that happened over a span of time. (See following section for further information.)

37 *Internal Control Number.* The control number assigned to the original bill by the payor or the payor's intermediary.

38 *Responsible Party Name and Address.* Name and address of person ultimately responsible for insuring payment of the bill. This is usually the patient, or the parent or legal guardian if the patient is a minor.

39-41 *Value Codes and Amounts.* Codes and the related dollar amount that identify data of a monetary nature that is necessary for the processing of this claim. (See following section for further information.)

42 *Revenue Code.* Revenue code referencing the type of services provided. (See following section for further information.)

43 *Revenue Description.* A description of the services provided. Abbreviations may be used. Accommodation (room) descriptions must be entered first on the bill and must be in chronologic order of appearance (eg, 03/01/89 ICU, 03/02/89 Semiprivate room).

44 *HCPCS/Rates.* The accommodation rate for inpatient bills, or the CPT or HCPCS code for ancillary or outpatient services. Outpatient Worker's Compensation and Medicaid require CPT-4/HCPCS coding in this space.

45 *Service Date.* The date the service was provided if this is a series bill where the date of service differs from the from/through date on the bill.

46 *Units of Service.* Quantitative measure of services, days, miles, pints of blood, units, or treatments (eg, if a patient was hospitalized for 3 days, a 3 would be placed here).

47 *Total Charges.* Total charges for that line of services.

48 *Noncovered Charges.* The amount per line of service that is not covered by the primary payor.

49 *Reserved for National Assignment.*

50 *Payor Identification.* Name of Insurer(s) covered by the patient who may be responsible for payment on this bill. Insurers should be listed in order of Primary Payor, Secondary Payor, Tertiary

Payor(s). If required, numbers identifying each payor organization should be listed.

51 *Provider Number.* The number assigned to the provider by the listed payor.

52 *Release Information.* A Y (yes) or N (no) designation stating whether or not patient's signature is on file authorizing the release of information. An R may also be entered to show that a hospital has restricted authorization to release information. In such a case the authorization should be attached.

53 *Assignment of Benefits.* A Y (yes) or N (no) designation stating whether or not patient's signature is on file authorizing the insurer to pay the provider of service directly instead of the patient. If a Y is placed in this box, you must have an assignment of benefits, signed by the insured, on file in your office. (See following section for further information.)

54 *Prior Payments.* The amount that has been paid toward this bill prior to the current billing date. These can include payments by the patient, other payors, and so on.

55 *Estimated Amount Due.* The amount estimated by the provider to be due from the indicated payor. This is usually the total amount due minus any previous payments.

56 *Reserved for State Assignment.*

57 *Reserved for National Assignment.*

58 *Insured's Name.* Name of the person listed on the insurance forms (subscriber's name). This may be a spouse or parent of the patient.

59 *Patient's Relationship to Insured.* Numerical code designation indicating the relationship between the patient and the insured. (See following section for further information.)

60 *Subscriber's Certificate Number.* The policy number under which the insured is covered if it is an individual policy. If the insured is covered under a group policy (such as one offered by his/her employer), often the insured's Social Security number is used as the subscriber number.

61 *Insured Group Name.* The name of the group or company that holds the insured's policy. Often this is the employer of the insured. This information is required by Medicare when Medicare is not the primary payor.

62 *Insurance Group Number.* The group number denoting the group policy or plan under which the insured is covered.

63 *Treatment Authorization Code.* A number indicating that the treatment described by this bill has been authorized by the payor.

64 *Employment Status Code.* A code denoting whether or not the employee is currently employed part- or full-time, is retired or is in active military service. (See following section for further information.)

65 *Employer Name.* Name of the employer of the insured person.

66 *Employer Location.* Address of the employer of the insured or responsible party.

67 *Principal Diagnosis Code.* ICD-9 code for the diagnosis of the patient's condition. The diagnosis shown should reflect the information contained in the patient's medical record for the dates indicated in Item 6 even if the diagnosis is changed at a later date.

68—75 *Other Diagnosis Codes.* ICD-9, V, and E Codes for any additional diagnosis of the patient's condition.

76 *Admitting Diagnosis.* The ICD-9 code

provided at the time of admission.

77 *External Cause of Injury Code (E Code).* The ICD-9 code for an external cause of injury, poisoning or adverse effect.

78 *Reserved for State Assignment.*

79 *Procedure Coding Method Used.* An indicator code that identifies the coding method used for procedure coding on the claim.

1-3 Reserved for State Assignment.
4 CPT-4
5 HCPCS
6-8 Reserved for National Assignment.
9 ICD-9C

80 *Principal Procedure Codes and Date.* CPT code for principal procedure rendered and the date that procedure was rendered. For Medicare, ICD-9 codes must be entered here and on Item 81.

81 *Other Procedure Codes and Dates.* CPT code for additional procedures rendered and the dates of those procedures.

82 *Attending Physician ID.* Name and license number of the physician who is primarily responsible for the patient.

83 *Other Physician ID.* Name and license number of secondary physician, assistant surgeon, and so on.

84 *Remarks.* Pertinent data for which there are no other specific places on the form. Often this space is used to record the nature of an accident (eg, fell and hit head on concrete, 06/09/93). For Medicaid, required for abortion certification when the attending physician is an employee of the hospital and does not submit a separate bill. Also, multiple visits to the ER on the same day should be recorded.

85 *Provider Representative Signature.* Signature of provider representative. In the case of a hospital billing, it is not necessary for the attending physician to sign, as long as a representative of the hospital signs the form certifying that the information entered is in conformance with the certifications specified on the reverse of the bill. Billers should make sure that the physician's certification is contained in the hospital records.

86 *Date Bill Submitted.* Date the bill was signed and submitted for payment.

The following items needed further description for which space was not available in the above text. Please study the following before completing the billing forms.

Item 4, Type of Bill

The following code structure is used to classify the type of bill. Each claim should have a 3-digit code entered in this space that corresponds with the following information.

First Digit—Type of Facility

1 Hospital
2 Skilled Nursing
3 Home Health
4 Christian Science (Hospital)
5 Christian Science (Extended Care)
6 Intermediate Care
7 Clinic*
8 Special Facility*
9 Reserved For National Use

* If Type of Facility is a Clinic (Code 7), then the Bill Classifications for Clinics Only must be used. If Type of Facility is a Special Facility (Code 8), then the Bill Classifications for Special Facilities Only must be used.

Second Digit—Bill Classification

For All Except Clinics

1 Inpatient (including Medicare Part A)
2 Inpatient (Medicare Part B only)

3 Outpatient
4 Other (for hospital-referenced diagnostic procedures or home health not under plan of treatment. This is to be further defined at the state level.)
5-7 Reserved For National use
8 Swing Beds
9 Reserved For National Use

Clinics Only
1 Rural Health
2 Hospital-based or Independent Renal Dialysis Center
3 Free Standing
4 Outpatient Rehabilitation Facility (ORF)
5 Comprehensive Outpatient Rehabilitation Facility (CORF)
6-8 Reserved For National Use
9 Other

Special Facilities Only
1 Hospice (non-hospital-based)
2 Hospice (hospital-based)
3 Ambulatory Surgery Center
4 Free-Standing Birthing Center
5-8 Reserved for National Use
9 Other

Third Digit—Frequency of Billing

0 Nonpayment/Zero Claim (Claim is being submitted for information purposes only. Provider does not anticipate payment on this claim.)
1 Admit through Discharge Claim (This claim is expected to be the only bill submitted for this course of treatment.)
2 Interim—First Claim (This is the first claim in a series for the same course of treatment.)
3 Interim—Continuing Claim (A prior claim has been submitted for this course of treatment or confinement, and a subsequent bill is also expected to be issued.)
4 Interim—Last Claim (A prior claim has been submitted for this course of treatment or confinement and this is expected to be the last bill issued.)
5 Late Charge(s) Only Claim (A prior claim or complete set of claims has been submitted to the provider and late charges are being added to the prior billing(s).)
6 Adjustment of Prior Claim (This claim adjusts a prior claim. Adjustments should be made by altering the prior claim with the addition of an explanation and a credit or additional charge added to the claim.)
7 Replacement of Prior Claim (This claim replaces a prior claim and the prior claim should be considered null and void.)
8 Void/Cancel Prior Claim (This bill voids the prior bill that was submitted with the same information. In effect, submitting a bill with this code is the same as submitting a duplicate copy of the claim with the word VOID written across the front. This bill may be followed by a subsequent replacement claim.)
9 Reserved for National Assignment

For example:

Claims for the following types of bills would be coded the following way:

Hospital, admit through discharge inpatient claim 111
Hospital, inpatient, replacement of prior claim 117
Hospital Emergency Room outpatient claim, only bill 131
Rural Clinic, outpatient, adjustment of prior claim 716

Item 19, Type of Admission

This is a 1-digit code indicating the priority of this admission according to the following structure:

1 Emergency. The patient requires immediate medical intervention as a result of severe, life-threatening, or potentially disabling conditions. Generally, the patient is admitted through the ER.
2 Urgent. The patient requires immediate attention for the care and treatment of a physical or mental disorder. Generally, the patient is admitted to the first available and suitable accommodation.
3 Elective. The patient's condition permits adequate time to schedule the availability of a suit-

able accommodation.

4 Newborn. A baby born within this facility. Use of this code necessitates the use of special Source of Admission Codes (Item 20).

5-8 Reserved for National Assignment.

9 Information Not Available.

Item 20, Source of Admission

This is a 1-digit code indicating the source of the admission according to the following structure:

For Emergency, Elective, or Other Types of Admissions

1 Physician Referral. The patient was admitted or referred to this facility upon the recommendation of his or her personal physician. If outpatient, the patient may request services (self-referral).

2 Clinic Referral. The patient was admitted or referred to this facility upon recommendation of this facility's clinic physician.

3 HMO Referral. The patient was admitted or referred to this facility upon the recommendation of a Health Maintenance Organization physician.

4 Transfer from a Hospital. The patient was admitted or referred to this facility as a transfer from an acute care facility where he/she was an inpatient.

5 Transfer from a Skilled Nursing Facility. The patient was admitted or referred to this facility as a transfer from a skilled nursing facility where he/she was an inpatient.

6 Transfer from Another Health Care Facility. The patient was admitted or referred to this facility as a transfer from a health care facility other than an acute care facility or a skilled nursing facility.

7 Emergency Room. The patient was admitted or referred to this facility upon the recommendation of this facility's ER physician.

8 Court/Law Enforcement. The patient was admitted or referred to this facility upon the direction of a court of law, or upon the request of a law enforcement agency representative.

9 Information Not Available. The means by which the patient was admitted or referred to this hospital, clinic, and so on, is not known.

A-Z Reserved for National Assignment.

For Newborns

1 Normal Delivery. A baby delivered without complications.

2 Premature Delivery. A baby delivered with time and/or weight factors qualifying it for premature status.

3 Sick Baby. A baby delivered with medical complications, other than those relating to premature status.

4 Extramural Birth. A newborn baby born in a nonsterile environment.

5-8 Reserved for National Assignment.

9 Information Not Available.

Item 22, Patient Status

This is a 2-digit code indicating the status of the patient at the last date covered by this billing statement.

01 Discharged to home or self-care (routine discharge)

02 Discharged/transferred to another short-term general hospital (inpatient)

03 Discharged/transferred to skilled nursing facility (SNF)

04 Discharged/transferred to an intermediate care facility (ICF)

05 Discharged/transferred to another type of institution (either inpatient or outpatient)

06 Discharged/transferred to home under care of organized home health service organization

07 Left or discontinued care against medical advice

08 Discharged/transferred to home under care of a home IV provider

09 Admitted as an inpatient to this hospital. This code is for use on outpatient Medicare claims.

10-19 Discharge to be defined at state level, if necessary

20 Expired
21-29 Expired to be defined at state level, if necessary
30 Still a patient or expected to return for outpatient services
31-39 Still a patient to be defined at state level, if necessary
40* Expired at home
41* Expired in a medical facility (hospital, freestanding clinic, hospice)
42* Expired, place unknown
43-99 Reserved for National Assignment
*NOTE: Codes marked with an asterisk are for use only on Medicare claims for hospice care.

Items 24-30, Condition Codes

This is a 2-digit code used to identify conditions relating to this bill that may affect payor processing. There is no specific date associated with this code as there is in Items 32-36. Condition codes should be entered in numeric sequence.

Insurance Codes

01 Military Service-Related. Medical condition incurred during military service.
02 Condition is Employment-Related. Patient alleges that medical condition is due to environment/events resulting from employment.
03 Patient Covered By Insurance Not Reflected Here. Indicates that patient/patient representative has stated that coverage may exist beyond that reflected on this bill.
04 HMO Enrollee. Indicates Medicare beneficiary is enrolled in an HMO and provider expects to receive payment from the HMO.
05 Lien Has Been Filed. Provider has filed legal claim for recovery of funds potentially due a patient as a result of legal action initiated by or on behalf of the patient.
06 ESRD Patient in First 18 Months of Entitlement Covered by Employer Group Health Insurance. Code indicates Medicare may be a secondary insurer if the patient is also covered by employer group health insurance during the first 18 months of end-stage renal disease entitlement.
07 Treatment of Nonterminal Condition for Hospice Patient. The patient is a hospice enrollee, but the provider is not treating his/her terminal condition and is requesting regular Medicare reimbursement.
08 Beneficiary Would Not Provide Information Concerning Other Insurance Coverage. Same.
09 Neither Patient Nor Spouse is Employed. Same.
10 Patient and/or Spouse is Employed But No Employer Group Health Plan Exists. Same.
11 Disabled Beneficiary But No Large Group Health Plan. Patient is disabled (therefore no longer an employee) and is not covered by a large group health plan. A large group health plan is a health plan composed of a large group of individuals with a common bond (ie, a national or state organization).
12-16 Payor Codes. These codes are reserved for payor processing.

Special Conditions

17 Reserved for National Assignment.
18 Maiden Name Retained. A dependent spouse entitled to benefits who does not use her husband's last name.
19 Child Retains Mother's Name. A patient who is a dependent child entitled to benefits that does not have his or her father's last name.
20 Beneficiary Requested Billing. Provider understands services are not covered or excluded, but beneficiary requests determination by payor.
21 Billing for Denial Notice. Provider understands services are not covered or excluded, but requests denial notice from payor.
22-25 Reserved for National Assignment.
26 VA-Eligible Patient Chooses to Receive Ser-

vices in a Medicare-Certified Facility. Patient has chosen a Medicare-certified facility rather than a VA-certified facility.

27 Patient Referred to a Sole Community Hospital for a Diagnostic Laboratory Test. This code is for use by Sole Community hospitals only. It indicates patient was referred for a diagnostic laboratory test. Payment is generally made at 62%. This code should not be used when a specimen only is referred to a hospital.

28 Patient and/or Spouse's Employee Health Plan is Secondary to Medicare. Patient has indicated that there is employer group coverage through either the patient or the patient's spouse, however the employer health plan is under a single employer that has fewer than 20 full- and part-time employees or the employer health plan is a multi or multiple employer plan that has elected to pay secondary to Medicare for employees and their spouses aged 65 or older for those employers who have fewer than 20 employees.

29 Disabled Beneficiary and/or Family Member's Large Group Health Plan is Secondary to Medicare. Patient or family members have indicated that one or more is employed and covered by a large group health plan or other employer sponsored health plan, but the large group health plan is a single employer plan and the employer has less than 100 full- and part-time employees or the large group health plan is a multi- or multiple employer plan and that all employers participating in the plan have fewer than 100 full- and part-time employees.

30 Reserved for National Assignment.

Student Status

This information is required when the patient is a dependent child over age 18. (Use only one of the following codes. The one with the lowest numerical value should take precedence.)

31 Patient is Student (full-time—day). Patient declares that he or she is enrolled as a full-time day student.

32 Patient is Student (cooperative/work study program). Same.

33 Patient is Student (full-time—night). Patient declares that he or she is enrolled as a full-time night student.

34 Patient is Student (part-time). Patient declares that he or she is enrolled as a part-time student.

35 Reserved for National Assignment.

Accomodations

36 General Care Patient in a Special Unit. Patient temporarily placed in special care unit bed because no general care beds available.

37 Ward Accommodation at Patient Request. Patient assigned to ward accommodations at patient's request.

38 Semiprivate Room Not Available. Indicates that either private or ward accommodations were assigned because semiprivate accommodations were not available.

39 Private Room Medically Necessary. Patient needs a private room for medical requirements.

40 Same Day Transfer. Patient transferred to another facility before midnight on the day of admission.

41 Partial Hospitalization. Indicates claim is for partial hospitalization services. For outpatient Medicare this may include some psychiatric services such as drug and alcohol rehabilitation.

42-45 Reserved for National Assignment.

CHAMPUS Information

46 Nonavailability Certificate On File. Any CHAMPUS beneficiary who lives within 40 miles of a military or public health service hospital has provided to the treating facility a certificate of nonavailability (DD1251) certifying the fact that medical care was not obtainable from a military or public health hospital.

47 Reserved for CHAMPUS.

48 Psychiatric Residential Treatment Centers for Children and Adolescents. Indicates the claim is submitted by a CHAMPUS authorized residential psychiatric treatment center for children and adolescents.

49-54 Reserved for National Assignment.

SNF Information

55 SNF Bed Not Available. Patient's SNF admission was delayed more than 30 days after hospital discharge because a SNF bed was not available.

56 Medical Appropriateness. Patient's SNF admission was delayed more than 30 days after discharge from a hospital because his/her condition made it inappropriate to begin active care within that period.

57 SNF Readmission. Patient was previously receiving Medicare covered SNF care within 30 days of this readmission.

58-59 Reserved for National Assignment.

Prospective Payment

60 Day Outlier. A hospital being paid under a prospective payment system is reporting this stay as a day outlier. This entry may be made by either the provider or the payor.

61 Cost Outlier. A hospital being paid under a prospective payment system is requesting additional payment for this stay as a cost outlier.

62 Payor Code. This code indicates the claim was paid under a DRG. This code is for use by payors, not providers.

63-65 Payor Codes. These codes are set aside for payor use.

66 Provider Does Not Wish Cost Outlier Payment. A hospital being paid under a prospective payment system is not requesting additional payment for this stay as an outlier.

67-69 Reserved for National Assignment.

Renal Dialysis Setting

70 Self-Administered Erythropoietin (EPO). Home dialysis patient who self-administers EPO.

71 Full Care in Unit. Patient who received staff-assisted dialysis services in a hospital or renal dialysis facility.

72 Self-Care in Unit. Patient who managed his own dialysis services without staff assistance in a hospital or renal dialysis facility.

73 Self-Care Training. For special dialysis services where a patient and his helper (if necessary) were learning to perform dialysis.

74 Home. Patient who received dialysis services at home, but where condition code 75 does not apply.

75 Home 100% Reimbursement. Patient received dialysis services at home, using a dialysis machine that was purchased by Medicare under the 100% program.

76 Back-up in Facility Dialysis. Home dialysis patient who received back-up.

77 Provider Accepts or is Obligated to Accept Payment by a Primary Payor as Payment in Full. Provider has accepted or is obligated (by a contractual arrangement or by law) to accept payment as payment in full.

78 New Coverage Not Implemented by HMO. A Medicare newly dialysis services in a facility covered service for which the HMO does not pay.

79 CORF Services Provided Off-Site. Physical therapy, occupational therapy, or speech pathology services were provided off-site.

80-99 Reserved for State Assignment.

Special Program Indicator Codes

This is a code indicating that the services on this claim are related to a special program.

A0 CHAMPUS External Partnership Program. Identifies CHAMPUS claims submitted under the External Partnership Program.

A1 EPSDT-CHAP. Early and Periodic Screening Diagnosis and Treatment.

A2 Physically Handicapped Children's Program. Services provided under this program receive special funding through Title 8 of the Social Security Act or the CHAMPUS Program for the handicapped.

A3 Special Federal Funding. This code has been designed for uniform use by state uniform billing committees.

A4 Family Planning. This code has been designed for uniform use by state uniform billing committees.

A5 Disability. This code has been designed for uniform use by state uniform billing committees.

A6 PPV/Medicare 100% Payment. This code identifies that pneumococcal pneumonia vaccine (PPV) services given should be reimbursed under a special Medicare program provision.

A7 Induced Abortion—Danger to Life. Abortion was performed to avoid danger to the woman's life.

A8 Induced Abortion Victim Rape/Incest. Same.

A9 Second Opinion—Surgery. Services requested to support second opinion on surgery. Part B deductible and coinsurance do not apply.

B0-B9 Reserved for National Assignment.

PRO Approval Indicator Services

Peer Review Organizations (PRO) periodically review inpatient hospital stays for medical necessity of length of stay, procedures, or other services. This review is conducted by the organization that will ultimately be responsible for payment of the incurred hospital stay. PRO is occasionally referred to as Utilization Review (UR).

C0 Reserved for National Assignment.

C1 Approved as Billed. Approved by the PRO/UR as billed (only for cases that have actually been approved).

C2 Automatic Approval as Billed Based on Focused Review. Include categories of cases that the PRO/UR has determined it need not review under a focused review program.

C3 Partial Approval. PRO/UR approved of some services but disapproved others.

C4 Admission/Services Denied. All services denied by the PRO/UR.

C5 Postponement Review Applicable. PRO/UR review will take place after payment.

C6 Admission Preauthorization. The PRO/UR authorized the admission but not the services.

C7 Extended Authorization. The PRO/UR has authorized these services for an extended period of time but has not reviewed the services provided.

C8-C9 Reserved for National Assignment.

Claim Change Reasons

Enter only one of the following claim change reasons. The codes have been prioritized. Use the first claim change reason that applies.

D0 Changes to Service Dates. Same.

D1 Changes to Charges. Same.

D2 Changes in Revenue Codes/HCPCS. Same.

D3 Second or Subsequent Interim PPS Bill. Same.

D4 Change in GROUPER Input. Same.

D5 Cancel to Correct HICN or Provider ID. Same.

D6 Cancel Only to Repay a Duplicate or OIG Overpayment. Includes cancellation of an outpatient bill containing services required to be included on the inpatient bill.

D7 Change to Make Medicare the Secondary Payor. Same.

D8 Change to Make Medicare the Primary Payor. Same.

D9 Any Other Change. Same.

E0 Change in Patient Status. Same.

E1-W9 Reserved for National Assignment.

X1-Z9 Reserved for State Assignment.

Items 32-35, Occurrence Codes

The Occurrence Code is a code and associated date defining a significant event relating to this bill that may affect payor processing.

Due to the varied nature of occurrence and occurrence span codes, provisions have been made to allow the use of both types of codes within each. The occurrence span code can contain an occurrence code where the "through" date would not contain an entry. This allows as many as 10 occurrence codes to be used.

When reporting occurrence span codes, Items 32a through 35a should be used before using Items 32b through 35b. If these spaces have been filled, you may use Items 36a and 36b to report additional occurrence span codes. In such a case, the beginning date is entered and the through date is left off.

Likewise, if there are more than two occurrence codes to report, additional codes may be entered in Items 32a through 36b.

Accident-Related

01 Auto Accident. Code indicating the date of an auto accident.

02 No Fault Insurance Involved. Code indicating the date of an accident (either auto or other) where the state has applicable no fault liability laws (eg, legal basis for settlement without admission or proof of guilt).

03 Accident/Tort Liability. Code indicating the date of an accident resulting from a third party's action that may involve a civil court process in an attempt to require payment by the third party, other than no fault liability.

04 Accident/Employment-Related. Code indicating the date of an accident relating to the patient's employment.

05 Other Accident. Code indicating the date of an accident not described by the above codes.

06 Crime Victim. Code indicating the date on which a medical condition resulted from allegedly criminal action committed by one or more parties.

07-08 Reserved for National Assignment.

Medical Condition

09 Start of Infertility Treatment Cycle. The date of the start of infertility treatment cycle.

10 Last Menstrual Period. Code indicating the date of the last menstrual period; ONLY applies when patient is being treated for a maternity-related condition.

11 Onset of Symptoms/Illness. Code indicating the date the patient first became aware of symptoms/illness.

12 Date of Onset for a Chronically Dependent Individual. The date the patient/beneficiary became or becomes a Chronically Dependent Individual. This date begins the first month of the 3-month period prior to eligibility for respite care benefits.

13-16 Reserved for National Assignment.

Insurance-Related

17 Date Outpatient Occupational Therapy Plan Established or Last Reviewed. Same.

18 Date of Retirement Patient/Beneficiary. The beneficiary or patient's date of retirement.

19 Date of Retirement Spouse. The date of retirement of the spouse of the patient.

20 Guarantee of Payment Began. Code indicating the date on which the provider began claiming Medicare payment under the guarantee of payment provision (HIM 10, 402.1, Item 21).

21 UR Notice Received. Code indicating the date of receipt by the hospital of the UR Committee's (PSRO or other responsible group's) finding that an admission for further stay was not medically necessary.

22 Date Active Care Ended. Code indicating the date on which a covered level of care ended in a general hospital, or date on which active care ended in a psychiatric or tuberculosis hospital. (HIM 10, 402.1, Item 23). Code not required when PSRO/UR approval is completed.

23 Reserved for National Assignment.

24 Date Insurance Denied. Code indicating the date the denial of coverage was received by the hospital from any insurer.

25 Date Benefits Terminated By Primary Payor. Code indicating the date on which coverage (including Worker's Compensation benefits or no-fault coverage) is no longer available to the patient.

26 Date SNF Bed Available. Code indicating the date on which an SNF bed became available to hospital inpatient who requires only SNF-level care (HIM 10, 405C).

27 Date Home Health Plan Established or Last Reviewed. The date a home plan of treatment was established (this code is only to be used by Home Health providers), (HIM 11 402, Item 13).

28 Date CORF Plan Established or Last Reviewed. The date a comprehensive outpatient rehabilitation plan (CORF) was established or last reviewed.
NOTE: Codes 27 and 28 should only be used by hospitals with a Home Health (27) or Comprehensive Outpatient Rehabilitation facility (28).

29 Date Outpatient Physical Therapy Plan Established or Last Reviewed. Same.

30 Date Outpatient Speech Pathology Plan Established or Last Reviewed. Same.

31 Date Beneficiary Notified of Intent to Bill Accommodations. The date notice was provided to the beneficiary by the hospital to the patient that inpatient care is no longer required. Beyond this date the patient will be billed for accommodations.

32 Date Beneficiary Notified of Intent to Bill Procedures or Treatments. The date notice was provided to the beneficiary that requested procedures or treatments are not reasonable or necessary under Medicare or CHAMPUS. Beyond this date the patient will be billed for all procedures and services.

33 First Day of the Medicare Coordination Period for ESRD Beneficiaries Covered by an Employee Group Health Plan. The first day of the Medicare coordination period during which Medicare or CHAMPUS benefits are secondary to benefits payable under an employee group health plan. This is required only for ESRD patients.

34 Date of Election of Extended Care Facilities. The date the patient elected to receive extended care services. This code is used by Christian Science Sanitoria only.

35 Date Treatment Started for Physical Therapy. Same.

36 Date of Inpatient Hospital Discharge for Covered Transplant Patient. The date of discharge for a hospital stay during which the patient received a covered transplant procedure and the hospital is billing for immunosuppressive drugs. If the patient received both a covered and a noncovered transplant, the covered transplant would take precedence.

37 Date of Inpatient Hospital Discharge for Noncovered Transplant Patient. The date of discharge for a hospital stay during which the patient received a noncovered transplant procedure and the hospital is billing for immunosuppressive drugs.

38-39 Reserved for National Assignment.

40 Scheduled Date of Admission. The date on which a patient will be admitted as an inpatient to the hospital. This code is for use on an outpatient claim.

41 Date of First Test for Pre-Admission. The date on which the first outpatient diagnostic test was performed as part of a pre-admission testing program. This code should be used only if a date of admission was scheduled prior to the administration of the test(s).

Service-Related Codes

42 Date of Discharge. Only to be used when "through" date in Item 6 is not the actual discharge date and the frequency code in Item 4 is that of a final bill.

43 Scheduled Date of Canceled Surgery. The date for which ambulatory surgery was scheduled.

44 Date Occupational Therapy Treatment Started. Same.

45 Date Speech Therapy Treatment Started. Same.

46 Date Cardiac Rehabilitative Treatment Started. Same.

47-49 Payor Codes. These codes are reserved for use by the payor.

50-69 Reserved for State Assignment.

70-99 Occurrence Span Codes and Dates. See following section.

A0 Reserved for National Assignment.

A1 Birth Date—Insured A. The birth date of the insured individual covered by insurance considered as primary payor.

A2 Effective Date—Insured A Policy. The date insurance coverage under the primary payor began.

A3 Benefits Exhausted—Payor A. The last date for which benefits are available. No payments will be made after this date by the primary payor. This code is to be used by the payor, not the provider of services.

A4-A9 Reserved for National Assignment.

B0 Reserved for National Assignment.

B1 Birth Date—Insured B. The birth date of the insured individual covered by insurance considered as secondary payor.

B2 Effective Date—Insured B Policy. The date insurance coverage under the secondary payor began.

B3 Benefits Exhausted—Payor B. The last date for which benefits are available. No payments will be made after this date by the secondary payor. This code is to be used by the payor, not the provider of services.

B4-B9 Reserved for National Assignment.

C0 Reserved for National Assignment.

C1 Birth Date—Insured C. The birth date of the insured individual covered by insurance considered as tertiary payor.

C2 Effective Date—Insured C Policy. The date insurance coverage under the tertiary payor began.

C3 Benefits Exhausted—Payor C. The last date for which benefits are available. No payments will be made after this date by the tertiary payor. This code is to be used by the payor, not the provider of services.

C4-I9 Reserved for National Assignment.

J0-L9 Reserved for State Assignment.

M0-Z9 Occurrence Span Codes and Dates. See following section.

Item 36, Occurrence Span Codes and Dates

Occurrence span codes and dates refers to the code and the related dates that identify an event that relates to the payment of the claim. These codes identify occurrences that happened over a span of time. Therefore, they have both a beginning and an ending date. See the information contained under the heading for Occurrence Codes for further information.

70 Qualifying Stay Dates. The beginning and ending dates of a hospital stay of at least 3 days that qualifies the patient for Medicare payment of SNF services billed. This code may only be used by skilled nursing facilities.

70 Payor Code—Nonutilization Dates. The beginning and ending dates during a PPS inlier stay for which the beneficiary had exhausted all full and/or coinsurance days, but which is covered on the cost report. This code is for payor use only.

71 Prior Stay Dates. The beginning and ending dates given by the patient of any hospital, SNF, or nursing home stay that ended within 60 days of this hospital or SNF admission (HIM 10, 310.1, Item 12).

72 First/Last Visit. The beginning and ending dates of outpatient services. This code is for use on outpatient bills only where the entire billing period is not represented by the billing statement dates reflected in Item 4.

73 Benefit Eligibility Period (Primary Payor). The inclusive dates during which CHAMPUS medical benefits are available to a sponsor's beneficiary as shown on the beneficiary's ID card.

74 Noncovered Level of Care. The beginning and ending dates of noncovered care in an otherwise covered hospital stay. This should exclude any days reported with the use of occurrence span code 76, 77, or 79.

75 SNF Level of Care. The beginning and ending dates of a hospital stay for which SNF care was

provided. This code should be used only when the payor has given approval for the patient to remain in the hospital due to a SNF bed not being available. This code should not be used for swing-bed cases. For hospitals under prospective payment, this code is needed in day outlier cases only.

76 Patient Liability. The beginning and ending dates of a Medicare patient's hospital stay for which the hospital is allowed to charge the Medicare beneficiary. This charge may be used only when prior approval for the stay has been received from the PRO or Medicare intermediary and the patient has been notified in writing at least 3 days prior to the beginning stay date.

77 Provider Liability Period. The beginning and ending dates of noncovered care for which the provider is liable. Utilization is charged.

78 SNF Prior Stay Dates. The beginning and ending dates given by the patient of a SNF or nursing home stay that ended within 60 days of this hospital or SNF admission.

79 Payor Code. The code is for payor use only.

80-99 Reserved for State Assignment.

M0 PRO/UR Approved Stay Dates. The beginning and ending dates of a hospital stay that were approved when the entire stay was not approved. Condition code 3 should be used in Items 24-30.

M1-W9 Reserved for National Assignment.

X0-Z9 Reserved for State Assignment.

Items 39-41, Value Codes and Amounts

These spaces are for codes and their related dollar amounts that identify data of a monetary nature that is necessary for processing the claim. The value code structure is intended to provide reporting capability for those data elements that are widely used but do not warrant dedicated fields. The codes should be written in numerical sequence. Negative numbers are not allowed except in Item 41.

01 Most Common Semiprivate Rate. To provide for the recording of the hospital's most common semiprivate rate.

02 Hospital Has No Semiprivate Rooms. Entering this code requires entering a dollar amount.

03 Reserved for National Assignment.

04 Inpatient Professional Component. The amount shown is the total inpatient professional component charges combined together. For use on Medicare inpatient bills in which there is no Part A eligibility or Part A benefits have been exhausted. Medicare uses the information for internal processing procedures and also for HCFA notice of utilization, which is sent to the patient to explain the Part B coinsurance portion that applies to the patient.

05 Outpatient Professional Component included in Charges and also Billed Separately to Carrier. For use on Medicare OP bills and all Medicaid bills if State specifies the need for this information.

06 Medicare Blood Deductible. Total cash blood deductible, if appropriate. Enter the Part A blood deductible amount.

07 Reserved for National Assignment.

08 Medicare Lifetime Reserve Amount. Medicare lifetime reserve charged in the year of admission.

09 Medicare Coinsurance Amount. Medicare coinsurance amounts charged in the year of admission. This code is to be used only if 08 is used.

10 Lifetime Reserve Amount in the Second Calendar Year. The amount of the Medicare lifetime reserve in the year of discharge. This code is used only when the bill's beginning and ending dates fall into 2 different years.

11 Coinsurance Amount in the Second Calendar Year. The amount of the Medicare coinsurance

in the year of discharge. This code is used only when the bill's beginning and ending dates fall into 2 different years.

12 Working Aged Beneficiary/Spouse with Employer Group Health Plan. The dollar amount shown is the amount that was paid by a employer group health plan whose payments were primary to Medicare. The provider signifies this amount is being applied toward Medicare-covered services on this bill.

13 ESRD Beneficiary in a Medicare Coordination Period with an Employer Group Health Plan. The dollar amount shown is the amount that was paid on behalf of an ESRD beneficiary by a employer group health plan whose payments were primary to Medicare. The provider signifies this amount is being applied toward Medicare-covered services on this bill.

14 No Fault Auto/Other. The dollar amount shown is the amount that was paid by no-fault insurance (including auto and other) whose payments were primary to Medicare. The provider signifies this amount is being applied toward Medicare covered services for a Medicare beneficiary on this bill.

15 Worker's Compensation. The dollar amount shown is the amount that was paid by workers' compensation insurance whose payments were primary to Medicare. The provider signifies this amount is being applied toward Medicare-covered services for a Medicare beneficiary on this bill.

NOTE: If benefits were reduced due to the failure to file a proper claim, the provider should indicate the amount for codes 12-15 that would have been paid had the claim been properly completed.

16 PHS, or Other Federal Agency. The dollar amount shown is the amount that was paid by a Public Health Service or the Federal Agency whose payments were primary to Medicare. The provider signifies this amount is being applied toward Medicare-covered services for a Medicare beneficiary on this bill.

NOTE: If the provider is claiming conditional payment from Medicare on codes 12-16, six zeros should be entered in the amount field. Conditional payment signifies that no amount has been collected from the other insurance as yet and the provider will repay to Medicare any amounts that are subsequently paid by the other insurance (see TPL in the General Plan Provisions section in Volume II).

17-20 Payor Codes. These codes are for payor use only.

Medicaid-Specific Codes

21-24 Reserved for State Assignment.

25-29 Reserved for National Assignment—Medicaid.

Code Structure

30 Pre-admission Testing. The amount indicated is the charge for outpatient pre-admission testing. Hospital admission should have been previously scheduled.

31 Patient Liability Amount. The amount indicated is the amount approved for the provider to charge the beneficiary for noncovered diagnostic services, accommodations or procedures.

32-36 Reserved for National Assignment.

37 Pints of Blood Furnished. Total number of pints of whole blood or units of packed red cells furnished to the patient.

38 Blood Deductible Pints. The number of unreplaced blood units furnished for which the patient is responsible.

39 Pints of Blood Replaced. The number of blood pints or packed blood cells that have been replaced by and on behalf of the patient.

40 New Coverage not Implemented by HMO. The amount indicated is for inpatient charges covered by the HMO. This code is used when the bill includes inpatient charges for newly covered services that are not paid by the HMO. It should only be utilized for inpatient service. Condition codes 4 and 78 should also be reported.

41 Black Lung. The dollar amount shown is the

amount that was paid on behalf of a Medicare beneficiary by a Black Lung payment, which payment was primary to Medicare. The provider signifies this amount is being applied toward Medicare-covered services on this bill.

42 VA. The dollar amount shown is the amount that was paid on behalf of a Medicare beneficiary by a VA payment, which payment was primary to Medicare. The provider signifies this amount is being applied toward Medicare-covered services on this bill.

43 Disabled Beneficiary Under Age 65 with Large Group Health Plan. The dollar amount shown is the amount that was paid on behalf of a Medicare beneficiary by a large group health plan whose payments were primary to Medicare. The provider signifies this amount is being applied toward Medicare-covered services on this bill.
NOTE: If benefits were reduced due to the failure to file a proper claim, the provider should indicate the amount for codes 41 and 43 that would have been paid had the claim been properly completed.

44 Amount Provider Agreed to Accept from Primary Payor, which Amount is Less than Charges but Higher than Payment Received and a Medicare Secondary Payment is Due. The amount indicated is the amount the provider was required to accept from a primary payor. When this amount is less than the charges, a Medicare secondary payment is due.

45 Accident Hour. Medical treatment is the result of an accident. The time of the accident should be indicated in the amount column. Times should be written according to a 24-hour clock. 99 = unknown.

46 Number of Grace Days. The number of days necessary to arrange for postdischarge care for the patient. This number is determined by PRO/UR review.

47 Any Liability Insurance. The dollar amount shown is the amount that was paid by liability insurance whose payments were primary to Medicare. The provider signifies this amount is being applied toward Medicare-covered services for a Medicare beneficiary on this bill. If the provider is claiming conditional payment from Medicare, six zeros should be entered in the amount field. Conditional payment signifies that no amount has been collected from the other insurance as yet and the provider will repay to Medicare any amounts that are subsequently paid by the other insurance (see TPL in the General Plan Provisions section in Volume II).

48 Hemoglobin Reading. The latest hemoglobin reading taken during this billing cycle.

49 Hematocrit Reading. The hematocrit reading taken prior to the last administration of erythropoietin that was given during this billing cycle.

50 Physical Therapy Visits. The number of physical therapy visits given by this provider from the outset of the illness until the last date indicated in the billing period.

51 Occupational Therapy Visits. The number of occupational therapy visits given by this provider from the outset of the illness until the last date indicated in the billing period.

52 Speech Therapy Visits. The number of speech therapy visits given by this provider from the outset of the illness until the last date indicated in the billing period.

53 Cardiac Rehabilitation Visits. The number of cardiac rehabilitation visits given by this provider from the outset of the illness until the last date indicated in the billing period.
NOTE: Whole numbers for Items 48-53 should be reported in the dollar portion of the item.

54-55 Reserved for National Assignment.

56 Skilled Nurse—Home Visit Hours. The number of skilled nursing hours provided during the billing period. This code should be used only by Home Health Aides. Only hours spent in the home are counted. This excludes travel time. Round out to the nearest whole hour.

57 Home Health Aide—Home Visit Hours. The number of home health aide services and home services hours provided during the billing period. This code should be used only by Home Health Aides. Only hours spent in the home are counted. This excludes travel time. Round out to the nearest whole hour.

58 Arterial Blood Gas (Po_2/PA_2). The arterial blood gas value at the beginning of each reporting period for oxygen therapy.

59 Oxygen Saturation (O_2 SAT/Oximetry). The oxygen saturation count at the beginning of each reporting period for oxygen therapy. NOTE: Either code 58 or 59 is required on the initial bill and the fourth-month bill for oxygen therapy. The value should be rounded out to the nearest whole number and entered in the dollar area to the right of the code.

60 HHA Branch MSA. Metropolitan Statistical Area in which the Home Health Agency is located. If the branch location is different than the HHA location, report the MSA in which the branch is located. The MSA number should be entered into the dollar column to the right of the code.

61-67 Reserved for National Assignment.

68 EPO-Drug. Number of units of erythropoietin administered or supplied during the billing period. Report amount in whole units.

69 Reserved for National Assignment.

70-72 Payor Codes. These codes are provided for payor use only.

73-74 Reserved for National Assignment.

75-79 Payor Codes. These codes are provided for payor use only.

80 Most Common Ward Rate. The amount indicated is the hospital's most common ward rate.

81-99 Reserved for State Assignment.

A0 Reserved for National Assignment.

A1 Deductible Payor A. The amount indicated is the amount assumed by the provider to be applied toward the deductible amount for the indicated payor.

A2 Coinsurance Payor A. The amount indicated is the amount assumed by the provider to be applied toward the coinsurance amount for the indicated payor.

A3 Estimated Responsibility Payor A. The amount indicated is the amount assumed by the provider to be the estimated responsibility for the indicated payor.

A4-A9 Reserved for National Assignment.

B0 Reserved for National Assignment.

B1 Deductible Payor B. The amount indicated is the amount assumed by the provider to be applied toward the deductible amount for the indicated payor.

B2 Coinsurance Payor B. The amount indicated is the amount assumed by the provider to be applied toward the coinsurance amount for the indicated payor.

B3 Estimated Responsibility Payor B. The amount indicated is the amount assumed by the provider to be the estimated responsibility for the indicated payor.

B4-B9 Reserved for National Assignment.

C0 Reserved for National Assignment.

C1 Deductible Payor C. The amount indicated is the amount assumed by the provider to be applied toward the deductible amount for the indicated payor.

C2 Coinsurance Payor C. The amount indicated is the amount assumed by the provider to be applied toward the coinsurance amount for the indicated payor.

C3 Estimated Responsibility Payor C. The amount indicated is the amount assumed by the provider to be the estimated responsibility for the indicated payor.

C4-C9 Reserved for National Assignment.

D0-D2 Reserved for National Assignment.

D3 Estimated Responsibility Patient. The amount indicated is the amount assumed by the provider to be the estimated responsibility for the patient.

D4-W9 Reserved for National Assignment.

X0-Z9 Reserved for State Assignment.

Item 42, Hospital Revenue Codes

Revenue codes identify a specific accommodation, ancillary service, or billing calculation. The correct subcategory classification should be added to the major category number to create a 3-digit number. The use of a fourth digit has been approved by the NUBC for possible future needs. These 4-digit numbers are thus far unassigned and therefore not in use.

Major Category

001 **Total Charges.** To reflect the total of all charges on this bill.

01X **Reserved for internal payor use.**

02X-06X **Reserved for National Assignment.**

07X-09X **Reserved for State Assignment.**

10X **All-Inclusive Rate.** Flat fee charge incurred on either a daily basis or total stay basis for services rendered. Charge may cover room and board plus ancillary services or room and board only.

Subcategory (Standard Abbreviation)

0 All-inclusive room and board plus ancillary (ALL-INCL R&B/ANC)
1 All-inclusive room and board (ALL INCL R&B)

11X **Room and Board—Private (Medical or General).** Routine service charges for single-bed rooms.

Subcategory (Standard Abbreviation)

0 General Classification (ROOM-BOARD/PVT)
1 Medical/Surgical/Gyn (MED-SUR-GY/PVT)
2 OB (OB/PVT)
3 Pediatric (PEDS/PVT)
4 Psychiatric (PSYCH/PVT)
5 Hospice (HOSPICE/PVT)
6 Detoxification (DETOX/PVT)
7 Oncology (ONCOLOGY/PVT)
8 Rehabilitation (REHAB/PVT)
9 Other (OTHER/PVT)

12X **Room and Board—Semiprivate Two-Bed (Medical or General).** Routine service charges incurred for accommodations with two beds.

Subcategory (Standard Abbreviation)

0 General Classification (ROOM-BOARD/SEMI)
1 Medical/Surgical/Gyn (MED-SUR-GY/2 Bed)
2 OB (OB/2 Bed)
3 Pediatric (PEDS/2 Bed)
4 Psychiatric (PSYCH/2 Bed)
5 Hospice (HOSPICE/2 Bed)
6 Detoxification (DETOX/2 Bed)
7 Oncology (ONCOLOGY/2 Bed)
8 Rehabilitation (REHAB/2 Bed)
9 Other (OTHER/2 Bed)

13X **Semiprivate—Three and Four Beds.** Routine service charges incurred for accommodations with three and four beds.

Subcategory (Standard Abbreviation)

0 General Classification (ROOM-BOARD/3&4 Bed)
1 Medical/Surgical/Gyn (MED-SUR-GY/3&4 Bed)
2 OB (OB/3&4 Bed)
3 Pediatric (PEDS/3&4 Bed)
4 Psychiatric (PSYCH/3&4 Bed)
5 Hospice (HOSPICE/3&4 Bed)
6 Detoxification (DETOX/3&4 Bed)
7 Oncology (ONCOLOGY/3&4 Bed)
8 Rehabilitation (REHAB/3&4 Bed)
9 Other (OTHER/3&4 Bed)

14X **Private (Deluxe).** Deluxe rooms are accommodations with amenities substantially in excess of those provided to other patients.

Subcategory (Standard Abbreviation)

0 General Classification (ROOM-BOARD/PVT/DLX)
1 Medical/Surgical/Gyn (MED-SUR-GY/DLX)

2 OB (OB/DLX)
3 Pediatric (PEDS/DLX)
4 Psychiatric (PSYCH/DLX)
5 Hospice (HOSPICE/DLX)
6 Detoxification (DETOX/DLX)
7 Oncology (ONCOLOGY/DLX)
8 Rehabilitation (REHAB/DLX)
9 Other (OTHER/DLX)

15X **Room and Board—Ward (Medical or General).** Routine service charge for accommodations with five or more beds.

Subcategory (Standard Abbreviation)
0 General Classification (ROOM-BOARD/WARD)
1 Medical/Surgical/Gyn (MED-SUR-GY/WARD)
2 OB (OB/WARD)
3 Pediatric (PEDS/WARD)
4 Psychiatric (PSYCH/WARD)
5 Hospice (HOSPICE/WARD)
6 Detoxification (DETOX/WARD)
7 Oncology (ONCOLOGY/WARD)
8 Rehabilitation (REHAB/WARD)
9 Other (OTHER/WARD)

16X **Other Room and Board.** Any routine service charges for accommodations that cannot be included in the more specific revenue center codes.

Subcategory (Standard Abbreviation)
0 General Classification (R&B)
4 Sterile Environment (R&B/STER-ILE)
7 Self-Care (R&B/SELF)
9 Other (R&B/Other)

17X **Nursery.** Charges for nursing care to new-born and premature infants in nurseries.

Subcategory (Standard Abbreviation)
0 General Classification (NURSERY)
1 Newborn (NURSERY/NEW-BORN)
2 Premature (NURSERY/PREMIE)
5 Neonatal ICU (NURSERY/ICU)
9 Other (NURSERY/OTHER)

18X **Leave of Absence.** Charges for holding a room while the patient is temporarily away from the provider.

Subcategory (Standard Abbreviation)
0 General Classification (LEAVE OF ABSENCE OR LOA)
1 Reserved
2 Patient Convenience (LOA/PT CONV)
3 Therapeutic Leave (LOA THERA-PEUTIC)
4 ICF/MR—any reason (LOA/ICF/MR)
5 Nursing Home (for hospitaliza-tion) (LOA/ NURS HOME)
9 Other Leave of Absence (LOA/OTHER)

19X **Not Assigned.**

20X **Intensive Care.** Routine service charge for medical or surgical care provided to patients who require a more intensive level of care than is rendered with the general medical or surgical unit.

Subcategory (Standard Abbreviation)
0 General Classification (INTEN-SIVE CARE or ICU)
1 Surgical (ICU/SURGICAL)
2 Medical (ICU/MEDICAL)
3 Pediatric (ICU/PEDS)
4 Psychiatric (ICU/PSTAY)
6 Post-ICU (POST ICU)
7 Burn Care (ICU/BURN CARE)
8 Trauma (ICU/TRAUMA)
9 Other Intensive Care (ICU/OTHER)

21X **Coronary Care.** Routine service charge for medical care provided to patients with coronary illness who require a more intensive level of care than is rendered in the general medical care unit.

Subcategory (Standard Abbreviation)
0 General Classification (CORONARY CARE or CCU)
1 Myocardial Infarction (CCU/MYO INFARC)
2 Pulmonary Care (CCU/PULMONARY)
3 Heart Transplant (CCU/TRANSPLANT)
4 Post-CCU (POST CCU)
9 Other Coronary Care (CCU/OTHER)

22X **Special Charges.** Charges incurred during an inpatient stay or on a daily basis for certain services.

Subcategory (Standard Abbreviation)
0 General Classification (SPECIAL CHARGES)
1 Admission Charge (ADMIT CHARGE)
2 Technical Support Charge (TECH SUPPT CHG)
3 UR Service Charge (UR CHARGE)
4 Late Discharge, Medically Necessary (LATE DISCH/MED NEC)
9 Other Special Charges (OTHER SPEC CHG)

23X **Incremental Nursing Charge Rate.** Charge for nursing service assessed in addition to room and board.

Subcategory (Standard Abbreviation)
0 General Classification (NURSING INCREM)
1 Nursery (NUR INCR/NURSERY)
2 OB (NUR INCR/OB)
3 ICU (NUR INCR/ICU)
4 CCU (NUR INCR/CCU)
5 Hospice (NUR INCR/HOSPICE)
9 Other (NUR INCR/OTHER)

24X **All-Inclusive Ancillary.** A flat-rate charge incurred on either a daily basis or total stay basis for ancillary services only.

Subcategory (Standard Abbreviation)
0 General Classification (ALL INCL ANCIL)
9 Other Inclusive Ancillary (ALL INCL ANCIL/OTHER)

25X **Pharmacy.** Charges for medication produced, manufactured, packaged, controlled, assayed, dispensed, and distributed under the direction of licensed pharmacist. This category includes blood plasma, other components of blood, and IV solutions.

Subcategory (Standard Abbreviation)
0 General Classification (PHARMACY)
1 Generic Drugs (DRUGS/GENERIC)
2 Nongeneric Drugs (DRUGS/NONGENERIC)
3 Take Home Drugs (DRUGS/TAKEHOME)
4 Drugs Incident to Other Diagnostic Services (DRUGS/INCIDENT OTHER DX)
5 Drugs Incident to Radiology (DRUGS/INCIDENT RAD)
6 Experimental Drugs (DRUGS/EXPERIMT)
7 Nonprescription (DRUGS/NONSCRPT)
8 IV Solutions (IV SOLUTIONS)
9 Other Pharmacy (DRGS/OTHER)

26X **IV Therapy.** Administration of intravenous solution by specially trained personnel to individuals requiring such treatment.

Subcategory (Standard Abbreviation)
0 General Classification (IV THERAPY)
1 Infusion Pump (IV THER/INFSN PUMP)
2 IV Therapy—Pharmacy Services (IV THER/PHARM/SVC)
3 IV Therapy/Drug/Supply Delivery

(IV THER/DRUG/SUPPLY DELV)
4 IV Therapy/Supplies (IV THER/SUPPLIES)
9 Other IV Therapy (IV THERP/OTHER)
NOTE: Providers billing for home IV therapy should use the HCPCS code that describes the pump in Item 44.

27X **Medical/Surgical Supplies and Devices.** Charges for supply items required for patient care.

Subcategory (Standard Abbreviation)
0 General Classification (MED-SUR SUPPLIES)
1 Nonsterile Supply (NON-STER SUPPLY)
2 Sterile Supply (STERILE SUPPLY)
3 Take Home Supplies (TAKE HOME SUPPLY)
4 Prosthetic/Orthotic Devices (PROSTH/ORTH DEV)
5 Pacemaker (PACE MAKER)
6 Intraocular Lens (INTRA OC LENS)
7 Oxygen-Take Home (O2/TAKE-HOME)
8 Other Implants (SUPPLY/IMPLANTS)
9 Other Supplies/Devices (SUPPLY/OTHER)

28X **Oncology.** Charges for the treatment of tumors and related diseases.

Subcategory (Standard Abbreviation)
0 General Classification (ONCOLOGY
9 Other Oncology (ONCOLOGY/OTHER)

29X **Durable Medical Equipment (Other Than Renal).** Charge for medical equipment that can withstand repeated use (excluding renal equipment).

Subcategory (Standard Abbreviation)
0 General Classification (MED EQUIP/DURAB)
1 Rental (MED EQUIP/RENT)
2 Purchase of new DME (MED EQUIP/NEW)
3 Purchase of used DME (MED EQUIP/USED)
4 Supplies/Drugs for DME Effectiveness (Home Health Agency Only) (MED EQUIP/SUPPLIES/DRUGS)
9 Other Equipment (MED EQUIP/OTHER)

30X **Laboratory.** Charges for the performance of diagnostic and routine clinical laboratory tests.

Subcategory (Standard Abbreviation)
0 General Classification (LABORATORY or LAB)
1 Chemistry (LAB/CHEMISTRY)
2 Immunology (LAB/IMMUNOLOGY)
3 Renal Patient (Home) (LAB/RENAL HOME)
4 Nonroutine Dialysis (LAB/NR DIALYSIS)
5 Hematology (LAB/HEMATOLOGY)
6 Bacteriology & Microbiology (LAB/BACT-MICRO)
7 Urology (LAB/UROLOGY)
9 Other Laboratory (LAB/OTHER)

31X **Laboratory Pathological.** Charges for diagnostic and routine laboratory tests on tissues and culture.

Subcategory (Standard Abbreviation)
0 General Classification (PATHOLOGY LAB or PATH LAB)
1 Cytology (PATHOL/CYTOLOGY)
2 Histology (PATHOL/HYSTOL)
4 Biopsy (PATHOL/BIOPSY)
9 Other (PATHOL/OTHER)

32X **Radiology—Diagnostic.** Charges for diagnostic radiology services provided for the examination and care of patients. Includes taking, processing, examining, and interpreting radiographs and fluorographs.

Subcategory (Standard Abbreviation)

0 General Classification (DX X-RAY)
1 Angiocardiography (DX X-RAY/ANGIO)
2 Arthrography (DX X-RAY/ARTH)
3 Arteriography (DX X-RAY/ARTER)
4 Chest X-Ray (DX X-RAY/CHEST)
9 Other (DX X-RAY/OTHER)

33X **Radiology—Therapeutic.** Charges for therapeutic radiology services and chemotherapy are required for care and treatment of patients. Included therapy by injection or ingestion of radioactive substances.

Subcategory (Standard Abbreviation)

0 General Classification (RX X-RAY)
1 Chemotherapy—Injected (CHEMOTHER/INJ)
2 Chemotherapy—Oral (CHEMOTHER/ORAL)
3 Radiation Therapy (RADIATION RX)
5 Chemotherapy—IV (CHEMOTHERP-IV)
9 Other (RX X-RAY/OTHER)

34X **Nuclear Medicine.** Charges for procedures and tests performed by a radioisotope laboratory utilizing radioactive materials as required for diagnosis and treatment of patients.

Subcategory (Standard Abbreviation)

0 General Classification (NUCLEAR MEDICINE or NUC MED)
1 Diagnostic (NUC MED/DX)
2 Therapeutic (NUC MED/RX)
9 Other (NUC MED/OTHER)

35X **CT Scan.** Charges for computed tomographic scans of the head and other parts of the body.

Subcategory (Standard Abbreviation)

0 General Classification (CT SCAN)
1 Head Scan (CT SCAN/HEAD)
2 Body Scan (CT SCAN/BODY)
9 Other CT Scans (CT SCAN/OTHER)

36X **Operating Room Services.** Charges for services provided to patients in the performance of surgical and related procedures during and immediately following surgery.

Subcategory (Standard Abbreviation)

0 General Classification (OR SERVICES)
1 Minor Surgery (OR/MINOR)
2 Organ Transplant—Other than kidney (OR/ORGAN TRANS)
7 Kidney Transplant (OR/KIDNEY TRANS)
9 Other Operating Room Services (OR/OTHER)

37X **Anesthesia.** Charges for anesthesia services in the hospital.

Subcategory (Standard Abbreviation)

0 General Classification (ANESTHESIA)
1 Anesthesia Incident to Radiology (ANESTHE/INCIDENT RAD)
2 Anesthesia Incident to Other Diagnostic Services (ANESTHE/INCDNT OTHER DX)
4 Acupuncture (ANESTHE/ACUPUNC)
9 Other Anesthesia (ANESTHE/OTHER)

38X **Blood**

Subcategory (Standard Abbreviation)

0 General Classification (BLOOD)
1 Packed Red Cells (BLOOD/PKD RED)
2 Whole Blood (BLOOD/WHOLE)
3 Plasma (BLOOD/PLASMA)

4 Platelets (BLOOD PLATELETS)
5 Leucocytes (BLOOD/LEUCOCYTES)
6 Other Components (BLOOD/COMPONENTS)
7 Other Derivatives (Cryoprecipitates) (BLOOD/DERIVATIVES)
9 Other Blood (BLOOD/OTHER)

39X **Blood Storage and Processing.** Charges for the storage and processing of whole blood.

Subcategory (Standard Abbreviation)
0 General Classification (BLOOD/STOR-PROC)
1 Blood Administration (BLOOD/ADMIN)
9 Other Blood Storage and Processing (BLOOD/OTHER STOR)

40X **Other Imaging Services**

Subcategory (Standard Abbreviation)
0 General Classification (IMAGE SERVICES)
1 Diagnostic Mammography (DIAG MAMMOGRAPHY)
2 Ultrasound (ULTRASOUND)
3 Screening Mammography (SCRN MAMMOGRAPHY)
4 Positron Emission Tomography (PET SCAN)
9 Other Imaging Services (OTHER IMAGE SVS)
NOTE: High-risk beneficiaries should be noted by the inclusion of one of the following ICD-9 diagnosis codes:
V10.3 Personal History—Malignant neoplasm breast cancer
V16.3 Family History—Malignant neoplasm breast cancer (mother, sister or daughter with breast cancer)
V15.89 Other specified personal history representing hazards to health (not given birth prior to 30, a personal history of biopsy proven benign breast disease). Must be coded to the appropriate 4th or 5th digit.

41X **Respiratory Services.** Charges for administration of oxygen and certain potent drugs through inhalation or positive pressure and other forms of rehabilitative therapy through measurement of inhaled and exhaled gases and analysis of blood and evaluation of the patient's ability to exchange oxygen and other gases.

Subcategory (Standard Abbreviation)
0 General Classification (RESPIRATORY SVC)
2 Inhalation Services (INHALATION SVC)
3 Hyperbaric Oxygen Therapy (HYPERBARIC O2)
9 Other Respiratory Services (OTHER RESPIR SVS)

42X **Physical Therapy.** Charges for therapeutic exercises, massage, and utilization of effective properties of light, heat, cold, water, electricity, and assistive devices for diagnosis and rehabilitation of patients who have neuromuscular, orthopedic, and other disabilities.

Subcategory (Standard Abbreviation)
0 General Classification (PHYSICAL THERP)
1 Visit Charge (PHYS THERP/VISIT)
2 Hourly Charge (PHYS THERP/HOUR)
3 Group Rate (PHYS THERP/GROUP)
4 Evaluation or Reevaluation (PHYS THERP/EVAL)
9 Other Physical Therapy (OTHER PHYS THERP)

43X **Occupational Therapy.** Charges for teaching manual skills and independence in personal care to stimulate mental and emotional activity on the part of patients.

Subcategory (Standard Abbreviation)

0 General Classification (OCCUPATION THERP)
1 Visit Charge (OCCUP THERP/VISIT)
2 Hourly Charge (OCCUP THERP/HOUR)
3 Group Rate (OCCUP THERP/GROUP)
4 Evaluation or Reevaluation (OCCUP THER/EVAL)
9 Other Occupational Therapy (OTHER OCCUP THERP)

44X **Speech-Language Pathology.** Charges for services provided to persons with impaired functional communications skills.

Subcategory (Standard Abbreviation)

0 General Classification (SPEECH PATHOL)
1 Visit Charge (SPEECH PATH/VISIT)
2 Hourly Charge (SPEECH PATH/HOUR)
3 Group Rate (SPEECH PATH/GROUP)
4 Evaluation or Reevaluation (SPEECH PATH/EVAL)
9 Other Speech-Language Pathology (OTHER SPEECH PAT)

45X **Emergency Room.** Charges for emergency treatment to those ill and injured persons who require immediate unscheduled medical or surgical care.

Subcategory (Standard Abbreviation)

0 General Classification (EMERG ROOM)
9 Other Emergency Room (OTHER EMER ROOM)

46X **Pulmonary Function.** Charges for tests that measure inhaled and exhaled gases and analysis of blood and for tests that evaluate the patient's ability to exchange oxygen and other gases.

Subcategory (Standard Abbreviation)

0 General Classification (PULMONARY FUNC)
9 Other Pulmonary Function (OTHER PULMON FUNC)

47X **Audiology.** Charges for the detection and management of communication handicaps centering in whole or in part on the hearing function.

Subcategory (Standard Abbreviation)

0 General Classification (AUDIOLOGY)
1 Diagnostic (AUDIOLOGY/DX)
2 Treatment (AUDIOLOGY/RX)
9 Other Audiology (OTHER AUDIOL)

48X **Cardiology.** Charges for cardiac procedures rendered in a separate unit within the hospital. Such procedures include but are not limited to heart catheterization, coronary angiography, Swan-Ganz catheterization, and exercise stress test.

Subcategory (Standard Abbreviation)

0 General Classification (CARDIOLOGY)
1 Cardiac Cath Lab (CARDIAC CATH LAB)
2 Stress Test (STRESS TEST)
9 Other Cardiology (OTHER CARDIOL)

49X **Ambulatory Surgical Care**

Subcategory (Standard Abbreviation)

0 General Classification (AMBUL SURG)
9 Other Ambulatory Surgical Care (OTHER AMBL SURG)

50X **Outpatient Services.** Outpatient charges for services rendered to an outpatient who is admitted as an inpatient before midnight of the day following the date of service. These charges are incorporated on the inpatient bill of Medicare patients.

Subcategory (Standard Abbreviation)

0 General Classification (OUTPATIENT SVS)
9 Other Outpatient Services (OUTPATIENT/ OTHER)

51X **Clinic.** Clinic (non-emergency/scheduled outpatient visit) charges for providing diagnostic, preventive, curative, rehabilitative, and education services on a scheduled basis to ambulatory patients.

Subcategory (Standard Abbreviation)

0 General Classification (CLINIC)
1 Chronic Pain Center (CHRONIC PAIN CL)
2 Dental Clinic (DENTAL CLINIC)
3 Psychiatric Clinic (PSYCH CLINIC)
4 OB-GYN Clinic (OB-GYN CLINIC)
5 Pediatric Clinic (PEDS CLINIC)
9 Other Clinic (OTHER CLINIC)

52X **Freestanding Clinic.**

Subcategory (Standard Abbreviation)

0 General Classification (FREESTAND CLINIC)
1 Rural Health—Clinic (RURAL/CLINIC)
2 Rural Health—Home (RURAL/HOME)
3 Family Practice (FAMILY PRACTICE)
9 Other Freestanding Clinic (OTHER FR/STD CLINIC)

53X **Osteopathic Services.** Charges for a structural evaluation of the cranium, entire cervical, dorsal, and lumbar spine by a doctor of osteopathy.

Subcategory (Standard Abbreviation)

0 General Classification (OSTEOPATH SVS)
1 Osteopathic Therapy (OSTEOPATH RX)
9 Other Osteopathic Services (OTHER OSTEOPATH)

54X **Ambulance.** Charges for ambulance service, usually on an unscheduled basis, to the ill and injured who require immediate medical attention.

Subcategory (Standard Abbreviation)

0 General Classification (AMBULANCE)
1 Supplies (AMBUL/SUPPLY)
2 Medical Transport (AMBUL/MED TRANS)
3 Heart Mobile (AMBUL/HEARTMOBL)
4 Oxygen (AMBUL/OXY)
5 Air Ambulance (AIR AMBULANCE)
6 Neonatal Ambulance Services (AMBUL/NEONAT)
7 Pharmacy (AMBUL/PHARMACY)
8 Telephone Transmission EKG (AMBUL/TELEPHONIC EKG)
9 Other Ambulance (OTHER AMBULANCE)
NOTE: Units may be either miles or trips.

55X **Skilled Nursing.** Charges for nursing services that must be provided under the direct supervision of a licensed nurse to ensure the safety of the patient and to achieve the medically desired result. This code may be used for nursing home services, CORFS, or a service charge for home health billing.

Subcategory (Standard Abbreviation)

0 General Classification (SKILLED

NURSING)
1 Visit Charge (SKILLED NURS/VISIT)
2 Hourly Charge (SKILLED NURS/HOUR)
9 Other Skilled Nursing (SKILLED NURS/OTHER)
NOTE: Charges should be reported to the nearest hour.

56X **Medical Social Services.** Charges for services such as counseling patients, interviewing patients, and interpreting problems of social situation rendered to patients on any basis.

Subcategory (Standard Abbreviation)
0 General Classification (MED SOCIAL SVS)
1 Visit Charge (MED SOC SERVS/VISIT)
2 Hourly Charge (MED SOC SERVS/HOUR)
9 Other Medical Social Services (MED SOCIAL SERVS/OTHER)
NOTE: Charges should be reported to the nearest hour.

57X **Home Health Aide (Home Health).** Charges made by a home health agency for personnel that are primarily responsible for the personal care of the patient.

Subcategory (Standard Abbreviation)
0 General Classification (AIDE/HOME HEALTH)
1 Visit Charge (AIDE/HOME HLTH/VISIT)
2 Hourly Charge (AIDE/HOME HLTH/HOUR)
9 Other Home Health Aide (AIDE/HOME HLTH/OTHER)
NOTE: Charges should be reported to the nearest hour.

58X **Other Visits (Home Health).** Charges by a home health agency for visits other than physical therapy, occupational therapy or speech therapy, which must be specifically identified.

Subcategory (Standard Abbreviation)
0 General Classification (VISIT/HOME HEALTH)
1 Visit Charge (VISIT/HOME HLTH/VISIT)
2 Hourly Charge (VISIT/HOME HLTH/HOUR)
9 Other Home Health (VISIT/HOME HLTH/OTHER)
NOTE: Charges should be reported to the nearest hour.

59X **Units of Service (Home Health).** Revenue code used by a home health agency that bills on the basis of units of service.

Subcategory (Standard Abbreviation)
0 General Classification (UNIT/HOME HEALTH)
9 Home Health Other Units (UNIT/HOME HLTH/OTHER)

60X **Oxygen Home Health.** Charges by a home health agency for oxygen equipment supplies, or contents, excluding purchased equipment. If a beneficiary has purchased a stationary oxygen system, an oxygen concentrator or portable equipment, current revenue codes 292 or 293 apply. DME other than oxygen systems is billed under current revenue codes 291, 292, or 293.

Subcategory (Standard Abbreviation)
0 General Classification (O2/HOME HEALTH)
1 Oxygen—Stationary Equipment, Supplies or Contents (O2/STAT EQUIP/SUPPL/CONT)
2 Oxygen—Stationary Equipment or Supplies Under 1 LPM (O2/STAT EQUIP/UNDER 1 LPM)
3 Oxygen—Stationary Equipment

Over 4 LPM (O2/STAT EQUIP/OVER 4 LPM)
4 Oxygen—Portable Add-on (O2/PORTABLE ADD-ON)

61X **MRI.** Charges for Magnetic Resonance Imaging of the brain and other parts of the body.

Subcategory (Standard Abbreviation)

0 General Classification (MRI)
1 Brain (including brainstem) (MRI-BRAIN)
2 Spinal Cord (including spine) (MRI-SPINE)
9 Other MRI (MRI-OTHER)

62X **Medical/Surgical Supplies.** Charges for supplies required for patient care. This code is an extension of code 27X and allows for the reporting of additional breakdown, if needed. Subcategory 1 is for providers who are not able to bill supplies used for radiology procedures under radiology. Subcategory 2 is for providers who are not able to bill supplies used for other diagnostic procedures under diagnostic procedures.

Subcategory (Standard Abbreviation)

1 Supplies Incident to Radiology (MED-SUR SUPP/INCDNT RAD)
2 Supplies Incident to Other Diagnostic Services (MED-SUR SUP/INCDNT ODX)

63X **Drugs Requiring Specific Identification.** Charges for drugs and biologicals requiring specific identification required by the payor. If you are using HCPCS to identify the drug, the HCPCS code should be entered in Item 44.

Subcategory (Standard Abbreviation)

0 General Classification (DRUGS)
1 Single Source Drug (DRUG/SNGLE)
2 Multiple Source Drug (DRUG/MULT)
3 Restrictive Prescription (DRUG/RSTR)
4 Erythropoietin (EPO) less than 10,000 units (DRUG/EPO≤10,000 Units)
5 Erythropoietin (EPO) more than 10,000 units (DRUG/EPO≥10,000 Units)
6 Drugs requiring Detailed Coding (DRUGS/DETAIL CODE) NOTE: Revenue Code 636 relates to a HCPCS code. Therefore, the appropriate HCPCS code should be entered in Item 44. The specific units of service to be reported should be in hundreds (100s) rounded to the nearest hundred.

64X **Home IV Therapy Services.** Charge for IV drug therapy services that are done in the patient's home. For Home IV providers, the appropriate HCPCS code must be entered for all equipment and all covered therapy.

Subcategory (Standard Abbreviation)

0 General Classification (IV THERAPY SVC)
1 Nonroutine Nursing, Central Line (NON RT NURSING/CENTRAL)
2 IV Site Care, Central Line (relates to HCPCS code) (IV SITE CARE/CENTRAL)
3 IV Start/Change Peripheral Line (IV STRT/CHNG/PERIPHRL)
4 Nonroutine Nursing Peripheral Line (NON RT NURSING/PERIPHRL)
5 Training Patient/Caregiver, Central Line (TRNG PT/CAREGVR/CENTRAL)
6 Training Disabled Patient, Central Line (TRNG DSBLPT/CENTRAL)
7 Training Patient/Caregiver, Peripheral Line (TRNG

PT/CAREGVR/PERIPHRL)
8 Training Disabled Patient, Peripheral Line (TRNG DSBLPT/PERIPHRL)
9 Other IV Therapy Services (OTHER IV THERAPY SVC)
NOTE: Units need to be reported in 1-hour increments.

65X **Hospice Service.** Charges for hospice care services for a terminally ill patient. The patient would need to elect these services in lieu of other services for a terminal condition.

Subcategory (Standard Abbreviation)
0 General Classification (HOSPICE)
1 Routine Home Care (HOSPICE/RTN HOME)
2 Continuous Home Care (HOSPICE/CTNS HOME)
3 RESERVED
4 RESERVED
5 Inpatient Respite Care (HOSPICE/IP RESPITE)
6 General Inpatient Care (Non-respite) (HOSPICE/IP NON-RESPITE)
7 Physician Services (HOSPICE/PHYSICIAN)
9 Other Hospice (HOSPICE/OTHER)
NOTE: There must be a minimum of 8 hours of care (not necessarily continuous) during a 24-hour period to receive the Continuous Home Care rate from Medicare under code 652. If less than 8 hours of care are provided, code 651 should be used. Any portion of an hour counts as an hour. When billing Medicare under code 657, a physician procedure code must be entered in Item 44. Code 657 is used by the hospice to bill for physician's services furnished to hospice patients when the physician is employed by the hospice or receives payment from the hospice for services rendered.

66X **Respite Care.** Charges for hours of service under the Respite Care Benefit for homemaker or home health aide, personal care services, and nursing care provided by a licensed professional nurse.

Subcategory (Standard Abbreviation)
0 General Classification (RESPITE CARE)
1 Hourly Charge/Skilled Nursing (RESPITE/SKILLED NURSE)
2 Hourly Charge/Home Health Aide/ Homemaker (RESPITE/HMEAID/HMEMKR)

67X **Not Assigned**

68X **Not Assigned**

69X **Not Assigned**

70X **Cast Room.** Charges for services related to the application, maintenance, and removal of casts.

Subcategory (Standard Abbreviation)
0 General Classification (CAST ROOM)
9 Other Cast Room (OTHER CAST ROOM)

71X **Recovery Room**

Subcategory (Standard Abbreviation)
0 General Classification (RECOVERY ROOM)
9 Other Recovery Room (OTHER RECOV RM)

72X **Labor Room/Delivery.** Charges for labor and delivery room services provided by specially trained nursing personnel to patients, including prenatal care during labor, assistance during delivery, postnatal care in the recovery room, and minor gynecological procedures if they are performed in the delivery suite.

Subcategory (Standard Abbreviation)

0 General Classification (DELIV-ROOM/LABOR)
1 Labor (LABOR)
2 Delivery (DELIVERY ROOM)
3 Circumcision (CIRCUMCISION)
4 Birthing Center (BIRTHING CENTER)
9 Other Labor Room/Delivery (OTHER/DELIV-LABOR)

73X **EKG/ECG (Electrocardiogram).** Charges for operation of specialized equipment to record electromotive variations in actions of the heart muscle on an electrocardiograph for diagnosis of heart ailments.

Subcategory (Standard Abbreviation)

0 General Classification (EKG/ECG)
1 Holter Monitor (HOLTER MON)
2 Telemetry (TELEMETRY)
9 Other EKG/ECG (OTHER EKG-ECG)

74X **EEG (Electroencephalogram).** Charges for operation of specialized equipment to measure impulse frequencies and differences in electrical potential in various areas of the brain to obtain data for use in diagnosing brain disorders.

Subcategory (Standard Abbreviation)

0 General Classification (EEG)
9 Other EEG (OTHER EEG)

75X **Gastrointestinal Services**

Subcategory (Standard Abbreviation)

0 General Classification (GASTR-INTS SVS)
9 Other Gastrointestinal (OTHER GASTROINTS)
NOTE: Use 759 with the procedure code for endoscopic procedure.

76X **Treatment/Observation Room.** Charges for the use of a treatment room, or observation room charges for outpatient observation services.

Subcategory (Standard Abbreviation)

0 General Classification (TREAT-MENT/ OBSERVATION RM)
1 Treatment Room (TREATMENT RM)
2 Observation Room (OBSERVA-TION RM)
9 Other Treatment/Observation Room (OTHER TREAT/OBSERV RM)

77X **Not Assigned**

78X **Not Assigned**

79X **Lithotripsy.** Charges for the use of lithotripsy in the treatment of kidney stones.

Subcategory (Standard Abbreviation)

0 General Classification (LITHOTRIPSY)
9 Other Lithotripsy (LITHOTRIP-SY/OTHER)

80X **Inpatient Renal Dialysis.** A waste removal process performed in an inpatient setting that uses an artificial kidney when the body's own kidneys have failed. The waste may be removed directly from the blood (hemodialysis) or indirectly from the blood by flushing a special solution between the abdominal covering and the tissue (peritoneal dialysis). In-unit lab nonroutine tests are medically necessary tests in addition to or at greater frequency than routine tests that are performed in the dialysis unit.

Subcategory (Standard Abbreviation)

0 General Classification (RENAL DIALYSIS)

1 Inpatient Hemodialysis (DIALY/INPT)

2 Inpatient Peritoneal (Non-CAPD) (DIALY/INPT/PER)

3 Inpatient Continuous Ambulatory Peritoneal Dialysis (DIALY/INPT/CAPD)

4 Inpatient Continuous Cycling Peritoneal Dialysis (DIALY/INPT/CCPD)

9 Other Inpatient Dialysis (DIALY/INPT/ OTHER)

81X **Organ Acquisition.** The acquisition of a kidney, liver, or heart for use in transplantation. Organs other than these are included in category 89X. Living donor is a living person from whom kidney is obtained for transplantation. Cadaver is an individual who has been pronounced dead according to medical and legal criteria from whom organs have been obtained for transplantation.

Subcategory (Standard Abbreviation)

0 General Classification (ORGAN ACQUISIT)

1 Living Donor—Kidney (KIDNEY/LIVE)

2 Cadaver Donor—Kidney (KIDNEY/ CADAVER)

3 Unknown Donor—Kidney (KIDNEY/ UNKNOWN)

4 Other Kidney Acquisition (KIDNEY/OTHER)

5 Cadaver Donor—Heart (HEART/CADAVER)

6 Other Heart Acquisition (HEART/OTHER)

7 Donor—Liver (LIVER ACQUISIT)

9 Other Organ Acquisition (ORGAN/OTHER)

82X **Hemodialysis—Outpatient or Home.** A program under which a patient performs hemodialysis away from the facility using his or her own equipment and supplies. The process of hemodialysis is the removal of waste directly from the blood.

Subcategory (Standard Abbreviation)

0 General Classification (HEMO/OP OR HOME)

1 Hemodialysis/Composite or Other Rate (HEMO/COMPOSITE)

2 Home Supplies (HEMO/HOME/SUPPL)

3 Home Equipment (HEMO/HOME/EQUIP)

4 Maintenance 100% (HEMO/HOME/100%)

5 Support Services (HEMO/HOME/SUPSERV)

9 Other Outpatient Hemodialysis (HEMO/HOME/OTHER)

83X **Peritoneal Dialysis—Outpatient or Home.** A program under which a patient performs peritoneal dialysis away from the facility using his or her own equipment and supplies. Waste is removed by flushing a special solution between the tissue and the abdominal covering.

Subcategory (Standard Abbreviation)

0 General Classification (PERITONEAL/OP OR HOME)

1 Peritoneal/Composite or Other Rate (PERTNL/COMPOSITE)

2 Home Supplies (PERTNL/HOME/SUPPL)

3 Home Equipment (PERTNL/HOME/EQUIP)

4 Maintenance 100% (PERTNL/HOME/100%)
5 Support Services (PERTNL/HOME/ SUPSERV)
9 Other Outpatient Peritoneal Dialysis (PERTNL/HOME/OTHER)

84X **Continuous Ambulatory Peritoneal Dialysis (CAPD)—Outpatient or Home.** A program under which a patient performs continual dialysis away from the facility using his or her own equipment and supplies. The patient's peritoneal membrane is used as a dialyzer.

Subcategory (Standard Abbreviation)
0 General Classification (CAPD/OP OR HOME)
1 CAPD/Composite or Other Rate (CAPD/ COMPOSITE)
2 Home Supplies (CAPD/HOME/SUPPL)
3 Home Equipment (CAPD/HOME/EQUIP)
4 Maintenance 100% (CAPD/HOME/100%)
5 Support Services (CAPD/HOME/SUPSERV)
9 Other Outpatient CAPD (CAPD/HOME/ OTHER)

85X **Continuous Cycling Peritoneal Dialysis (CCPD)—Outpatient or Home.** A program under which a patient performs continual dialysis away from the facility using his or her own equipment and supplies. A machine is used to make automatic exchanges at night.

Subcategory (Standard Abbreviation)
0 General Classification (CCPD/OP OR HOME)
1 CCPD/Composite or Other Rate (CCPD/ COMPOSITE)
2 Home Supplies (CCPD/HOME/SUPPL)
3 Home Equipment (CCPD/HOME/EQUIP)
4 Maintenance 100% (CCPD/HOME/100%)
5 Support Services (CCPD/HOME/SUPSERV)
9 Other Outpatient CCPD (CCPD/HOME/ OTHER)

86X **Reserved for Dialysis (National Assignment)**

87X **Reserved for Dialysis (National Assignment)**

88X **Miscellaneous Dialysis.** Charges for dialysis services not identified elsewhere. Ultrafiltration is the process of removing excess fluid from the blood of dialysis patients by using a dialysis machine but without the dialysis solution. The designation is only used when the procedure is not performed as a part of a normal dialysis session.

Subcategory (Standard Abbreviation)
0 General Classification (DIALY/MISC)
1 Ultrafiltration (DIALY/ULTRA-FILT)
2 Home Dialysis Aid Visit (HOME DIALYSIS AID VISIT)
9 Miscellaneous Dialysis Other (DIALY/MISC/ OTHER)

89X **Other Donor Bank.** Charges for the acquisition, storage, and preservation of all human organs (excluding kidneys, livers and hearts—See 81X).

Subcategory (Standard Abbreviation)
0 General Classification (DONOR BANK)
1 Bone (DONOR BANK/BONE)
2 Organ (other than kidney) (DONOR BANK/ ORGN)
3 Skin (DONOR BANK/SKIN)
9 Other Donor Bank (OTHER DONOR BANK)

90X **Psychiatric/Psychological Treatments.** Charges for providing treatment for emotionally disturbed patients, including patients admitted for diagnosis and for treatment.

Subcategory (Standard Abbreviation)

0 General Classification (PSYCH TREATMENT)
1 Electroshock Treatment (ELECTRO SHOCK)
2 Milieu Therapy (MILIEU THERAPY)
3 Play Therapy (PLAY THERAPY)
9 Other (OTHER PSYCH RX)

91X **Psychiatric/Psychological Services.** Charges for providing nursing care and employee, professional services for emotionally disturbed patients, including patients admitted for diagnosis and those admitted for treatment.

Subcategory (Standard Abbreviation)

0 General Classification (PSYCH SERVICES)
1 Rehabilitation (PSYCH/REHAB)
2 Day Care (PSYCH/DAYCARE)
3 Night Care (PSYCH/NIGHTCARE)
4 Individual Therapy (PSYCH/INDIV RX)
5 Group Therapy (PSYCH/GROUP RX)
6 Family Therapy (PSYCH/FAMILY RX)
7 Biofeedback (PSYCH/BIOFEED)
8 Testing (PSYCH/TESTING)
9 Other (PSYCH/OTHER)

92X **Other Diagnostic Services.** Charges for other diagnostic services not otherwise categorized.

Subcategory (Standard Abbreviation)

0 General Classification (OTHER DX SVS)
1 Peripheral Vascular Lab (PERIVASCUL LAB)
2 Electromyogram (EMG)
3 Pap Smear (PAP SMEAR)
4 Allergy Test (ALLERGY TEST)
5 Pregnancy Test (PREG TEST)
9 Other Diagnostic Service (ADDL DX SVS)

93X **Not Assigned**

94X **Other Therapeutic Services.** Charges for other therapeutic services not otherwise categorized.

Subcategory (Standard Abbreviation)

0 General Classification (OTHER RX SVS)
1 Recreational Therapy (RECREATION RX)
2 Education/Training (EDUC/TRAINING)
3 Cardiac Rehabilitation (CARDIAC REHAB)
4 Drug Rehabilitation (DRUG REHAB)
5 Alcohol Rehabilitation (ALCOHOL REHAB)
6 Complex Medical Equipment—Routine (CMPLX MED EQUIP-ROUT)
7 Complex Medical Equipment—Ancillary (CMPLX MED EQUIP-ANC)
9 Other Therapeutic Services (ADDITIONAL RX SVS)
NOTE: Use 930 with a procedure code for plasmapheresis. Use 932 for dietary therapy and diabetes-related services, education, and training.

95X **Not Assigned**

96X **Professional Fees.** Charges for medical professionals that the hospitals or third-party payors require to be separately identified.

Subcategory (Standard Abbreviation)

0 General Classification (PRO FEE)
1 Psychiatric (PRO FEE/PSYCH)
2 Ophthalmology (PRO FEE/EYE)
3 Anesthesiologist (MD) (PRO FEE/ANES MD)
4 Anesthetist (CRNA) (PRO FEE/ANES CRNA)
9 Other Professional Fees (OTHER PRO FEE)

97X **Professional Fees (continued)**

Subcategory (Standard Abbreviation)

1 Laboratory (PRO FEE/LAB)
2 Radiology—Diagnostic (PRO FEE/RAD/DX)
3 Radiology—Therapeutic (PRO FEE/RAD/RX)
4 Radiology—Nuclear Medicine (PRO FEE/NUC MED)
5 Operating Room (PRO FEE/OR)
6 Respiratory Therapy (PRO FEE/RESPIR)
7 Physical Therapy (PRO FEE/PHYSI)
8 Occupational Therapy (PRO FEE/OCUPA)
9 Speech Pathology (PRO FEE/SPEECH)

98X **Professional Fees (continued)**

Subcategory (Standard Abbreviation)

1 Emergency Room (PRO FEE/ER)
2 Outpatient Services (PRO FEE/OUTPT)
3 Clinic (PRO FEE/CLINIC)
4 Medical Social Services (PRO FEE/SOC SVC)
5 EKG (PRO FEE/EKG)
6 EEG (PRO FEE/EEG)
7 Hospital Visit (PRO FEE/HOS VIS)
8 Consultation (PRO FEE/CONSULT)
9 Private Duty Nurse (FEE/PVT NURSE)

99X **Patient Convenience Items.** Charges for items that are generally considered by the third-party payors to be strictly convenience items and, as such, are not covered.

Subcategory (Standard Abbreviation)

0 General Classification (PT CONVENIENCE)
1 Cafeteria/Guest Tray (CAFETERIA)
2 Private Linen Service (LINEN)
3 Telephone/Telegraph (TELEPHONE)
4 TV/Radio (TV/RADIO)
5 Nonpatient Room Rentals (NONPT ROOM RENT)
6 Late Discharge Charge (LATE DISCHARGE)
7 Admission Kits (ADMIT KITS)
8 Beauty Shop/Barber (BARBER/BEAUTY)
9 Other Patient Convenience Items (PT CONVENCE/OTH)

ITEM 53, Assignment of Benefits

This assignment of benefits will not allow you to release information regarding the patient. A written authorization to release information, signed by the patient or patient representative, is needed (see Item 53). Please note the certification procedure on the back of the UB-92 before completing this item.

Although the UB-92 eliminates the need to send an assignment of benefits to accident and health insurers, hospitals may wish to be extremely careful in the way in which they handle claims involving property and casualty insurers. Property and casualty insurers may not be familiar with the UB-92 and may not be aware that the wording on the back of the UB-92 is sufficient notification of assignment of benefits. Hospitals may wish to send a copy of the assignment on auto accident and similar non-health-oriented insurance carrier claims.

Item 59, Relationship

Numerical code designation indicating that the patient is related to the insured in the following manner:

01 Insured party
02 Spouse of insured
03 Child of insured
04 Natural child/insured does not have financial responsibility for child
05 Stepchild of insured
06 Foster child of insured
07 Ward of the Court (patient is a ward of the insured as a result of court order)
08 Employee (patient is employed by the insured)
09 Unknown (patient's relationship to the insured is unknown)
10 Handicapped Dependent (dependent child whose coverage extends beyond normal termination age limits as a result of laws or agreement extending coverage)
11 Organ Donor (used in cases where bill is submitted for care given to organ donor where such care is paid for by the receiving patient's insurance coverage)
12 Cadaver Donor (used in cases where bill is submitted for procedures performed on a cadaver (deceased) donor where such procedures are paid for by the receiving patient's insurance coverage)
13 Grandchild of insured
14 Niece/nephew of insured
15 Injured Plaintiff (used when patient claims insurance as a result of injury covered by insured)
16 Sponsored Dependent (individual not normally covered by insurance coverage, but coverage has been specially arranged to include relationships such as grandparent or former spouse that would require further investigation by the payor)
17 Minor Dependent of a Minor Dependent. This code is used when the patient is a dependent minor of a dependent minor (though not a child) of the insured.
18 Parent of insured
19 Grandparent
20-99 Reserved

ITEM 64, Employment Status Code

Employment Status Code is used to define the employment status of the individual in Item 58.

1 Employed Full-Time
2 Employed Part-Time
3 Not Employed
4 Self-Employed
5 Retired
6 On Active Military Duty
7-8 Reserved for National Assignment
9 Employment Status Unknown

Summary

The UB-92 is the claim form used when billing for hospital services. It was created by the National Uniform Billing Committee to allow for the necessary information to be inserted on a single form, thus eliminating the need for attachments.

You should familiarize yourself with the form and know the necessary information. Completely and accurately filling out the UB-92 will help to ensure proper claim payments without unnecessary delays.

Assignments

Complete the Questions for Review.
Properly complete a billing form for Claims 9-1 to 9-25, 10-4, 10-8, 10-10, 10-11, 10-14, 11-9, 11-10, and 11-14 in the student exercise manual.

Questions for Review

Directions: Answer the following questions without looking back into the material just covered. Write your answers in the space provided.

1. What is the purpose of the UB-92 billing form? ______________________

2. What does Item 17 indicate? ______________________

3. What are occurrence codes and occurrence span codes and what is the difference between them? ______________________

4. What would the code 20 indicate in Item 22 on the UB-92? ______________________

5. What would the code 3 indicate in Item 59 on the UB-92? ______________________

6. What are coinsurance days? ______________________

7. How would you write the following times on a UB-92?

a.	9:55 A.M.	________	f.	2:48 P.M.	________
b.	10:25 P.M.	________	g.	5:56 P.M.	________
c.	1:18 A.M.	________	h.	Noon	________
d.	8:01 P.M.	________	i.	Midnight	________
e.	12:23 A.M.	________	j.	6:06 P.M.	________

8. What does a "Y" in the "Release Information?" box denote? ______________________

9. A patient entered the hospital on 12/01/93 complaining of chest pains. He was diagnosed as having a heart attack and admitted. On 12/05/93 the patient developed pneumonia. On 12/10/93 the patient expired due to causes associated with pneumonia. You are billing the insurance company for services rendered through 12/04/93. What is the proper diagnosis for the patient? ______________________

10. Are the source of admission codes the same for a newborn baby as they are for an adult? ______________________

If you were unable to answer any of the questions, refer back to the section and then fill in the answers.

20

Medical Reports

In this chapter you will learn:

- To understand medical reports and how they relate to billing forms.
- To recognize a triage report, an operative report, a diagnostic report and a medical history report.

Medical reports are required to be prepared for virtually every procedure and for all laboratory and x-ray examinations. Often medical billers use medical reports to extract the information needed to complete the billing forms. Virtually all information needed on a claim form is included in the medical reports and the patient's medical record.

Of the numerous types of medical reports, the most common that are used by medical billers include triage reports, operative reports, and diagnostic testing reports.

Triage Reports

Triage is the process of sorting and allocating treatment to patients on the basis of need. It is designed to maximize the number of survivors. Therefore, triage reports are reports generated at the scene of an accident or in the emergency room of a hospital.

These reports are usually handwritten rather than typed, since often speed and accuracy of accumulating the information is more important than appearance.

Five triage reports are included in the following pages.

Operative Reports

Operative reports are required to be generated for any surgical procedure that is performed. The information contained in these reports is often the sole means of information for medical billers regarding the procedures performed. Therefore, it is important that the medical biller understand the basics of an operative report and how to use it to perform medical billing.

Health claims examiners seldom have the laboratory and x-ray reports submitted with a claim. However, operative reports are required by examining personnel when there is a question as to what procedure(s) were actually performed. Most frequently, an examiner will utilize such reports in the following circumstances:

- when multiple procedures are performed during the same operative session
- when the fee for a single procedure significantly exceeds UCR
- when a BR or RNE procedure is performed.

As a rule, an examiner is not required to read and interpret operative reports. When a report is received, it is usually matched with the claim and then referred to a supervisor, technical assistant, or medical consultant for interpretation and evaluation. However, the examiner should always be able to perform a cursory evaluation. Sometimes, this evaluation is all that is required to answer a simple evaluation. A referral to other personnel may not be necessary. Therefore, it is important for the examiner to learn the basics of this procedure.

Diagnostic Testing Reports

Often diagnostic testing is done by an independent laboratory, pathologist, or radiologist. Diagnostic testing reports are the "readings" or the interpretation of the test performed.

Medical billers need to familiarize themselves with the terminology contained within the reports to understand the procedures that were rendered.

Health claims examiners will find that diagnostic testing reports assist in identifying what procedure(s) should actually be billed for and whether expenses should be bundled together or not. However, diagnostic testing reports often do not contain a beginning diagnosis or symptoms for which treatment is sought. Therefore, although these reports are helpful in identifying the final diagnosis and proper bundling of charges, they do not assist in verifying whether the patient had a complaint or illness when he or she first went to see the physician.

Medical History Reports

Whenever a patient is examined by a physician, a brief history of that exam is kept as part of the patient's permanent file. This history should include the following:

- date of service
- symptoms and complaints
- medications prescribed
- diagnosis
- laboratory and x-ray examinations ordered or other referrals
- other miscellaneous medical data.

The physician is allowed to bill for the service of compiling a medical history report on a patient. This code would be considered an E/M (Evaluation and Management) code, since it is not a surgical procedure.

Physicians who have a propensity for excessive charges and ordering of worthless, expensive testing are routinely put on special audit by payors. Each claim received by the payor is pended and a copy of the patient's medical record is requested. Tests not substantiated by the reported symptoms would not be covered. Additionally, questionable tests, those of little diagnostic value, will not be covered either. Unfortunately, although it is illegal to falsify medical records, some establishments do so to get insurance to pay the bills. This is considered fraud and severe punishments are enacted on those who are found guilty of doing these things.

Summary

The four most common types of medical reports that medical billers use are triage, operative, diagnostic, and medical history reports. Medical billers should familiarize themselves with these reports and how the information relates to the standard medical billing forms.

Assignments

Complete the Questions for Review.

Complete medical report exercises 20-1 through 20-20.* Use the information from each of the following reports and the patient chart that was completed in Exercise 1-1 to complete a claim for each report. The physician's patient information sheet will not necessarily be in the hospital; however, the hospital will have a very similar form. For simplicity purposes, we will use the former.

Only after completing the forms should you look at the interpretive information contained in the chapter appendix. Interpretive information is not given for all reports, so that they may be assigned as a class or homework exercise. After the exercises have been completed, the student should continue billing the claims contained in the student exercise manual.

*Each report follows each patient through a single episode of care.

Questions for Review

Directions: Answer the following questions without looking back into the material just covered. Write your answers in the space provided.

1. What are triage reports? ______________________________

2. What are operative reports? ______________________________

3. What are diagnostic reports? ______________________________

4. What six things should be included on a patient history?
   a. ______________________________
   b. ______________________________
   c. ______________________________
   d. ______________________________
   e. ______________________________
   f. ______________________________

5. In what way does a medical biller use the above reports? ______________________________

If you were unable to answer any of the questions, refer back to the section and then fill in the answers.

Exercise 20-1

Triage Report 1

EMERGENCY SERVICE REPORT

Abby Addison.
5678 Any Avenue.
Alverville, AK 99087.
(765) 890-4321.

DATE: 1-13-94.

ALLERGIES: NKA

CURRENT MEDS: None.

LAST TET. TOX. DATE

ARRIVED VIA: Ambulance. ACCOMPANIED BY: Friend

P.M.D. NAME TEL. # NOTIFIED ☐

TRIAGE TIME 14:09 T 98 P 110 R 23 BP 115/82

TIME T P R BP

SIGN:

25 y/o Ⓦ c̄. severe abd pain & nausea⁺ beginning 1-12-94. Hematemesis this am. Pt was hospitalized 1-6-94 c̄ epigastric pain & gallbladder disease. Pt underwent ERCP 1-10-94 stone removed. D/C home 1-11-94

⊕ dizzyness & lightheadedness
⊖ chest pain, dyspnea
⊖ dysuria
⊖ Jt disturbances.
⊖ preg.

DOCTORS ORDERS

TIME	INIT	RESULTS
		RUA:
		CBC: HGB/HCT 10.2/30.
		WBC OTHER 14.4
		DIFF: P B M
		E B L
		LYTES:
		Na 140 K 4.5
		CO2 CL
		GLU: 126
		BUN: 23
		CREAT: 0.6
		OTHER LAB
		Chl 100
		HCO_3 25
		ABG:
		FIO2 BE
		PCO2 PO2
		% SAT pH
		X-RAY:
		Ultra: Gall & Up Abd.
		EKG:

COMMUNICATION LOG

CONSULT	CALLED	COMMENTS

DISCHARGE IMPRESSION	DR. ORDERS	TIME	SITE	SIGNATURE
	Admit			

DRAW WOUND IN DIAGRAM
WOUND LENGTH ______
☐ COMPLEX ☐ SIMPLE
☐ PLASTIC DEPTH ______

INVOLVEMENT
DISTAL ROM ______ OK
DISTAL SENS ______ OK
DISTAL CIRC ______ OK
TENDONS ______ OK

TREATMENT
☐ Y ☐ N BET. PREP
☐ Y ☐ N ANESTH. 1% XYLOC.
☐ Y ☐ N SUTURES (*TYPE) ___

TIME OUT:
☐ Y ☐ N IRRIG
DRESSING ______
☐ Y ☐ N SPLINT

☐ CHARGES
☐ VALUABLES LISTED
☐ NURSES NOTES
☐ AFTER CARE INSTRUCTIONS GIVEN

PLAN Esophagogastroduodenoscopy.

CONDITION: ☐ GOOD ☒ FAIR ☐ POOR
DISPOSITION: ☐ HOME ☐ LEFT WITHOUT BEING SEEN ☒ ADMIT
☐ LEFT AGAINST MEDICAL ADVICE ☐ EXPIRED
☐ TRANSFER TO ______ RET TO WORK ______

Ann Anderson MD ______ MD Adrian Adams. RN

PRINT NAME Ann Anderson PRINT NAME ______ PRINT NAME Adrian Adams

Exercise 20-2

Triage Report 2

EMERGENCY SERVICE REPORT

Bobby Bumble
93485 Bumpkiss Court
Barkingville, DC 23456
(210)938-4756

DATE: 6-19-93.

ALLERGIES: NKA

CURRENT MEDS: None

LAST TET. TOX. DATE

ARRIVED VIA: Ambulance ACCOMPANIED BY: Wife

P.M.D. NAME TEL. # NOTIFIED ☐

TRIAGE TIME 9:37 T 97.5 P 83 R 23 BP 122/81

TIME T P R BP

SIGN:

(49) ♂ w/injury to R wrist.
Pt states he was running to catch a bus when his R ankle gave way. Pt fell to pavement injuring R wrist.
⊖ L.O.C. ⊖ head trauma
⊖ dizzyness or lightheadedness.

DOCTORS ORDERS

TIME	INIT	RESULTS
		RUA:
		CBC: HGB/HCT
		WBC OTHER
		DIFF: P B M
		E B L
		LYTES:
		Na K
		CO2 CL
		GLU:
		BUN:
		CREAT:
		OTHER LAB
		ABG:
		FIO2 BE
		PCO2 PO2
		% SAT pH
		X-RAY:
		R wrist AP&L ⊖
		R ankle AP&L ⊖
		EKG:

COMMUNICATION LOG

CONSULT	CALLED	COMMENTS

DISCHARGE IMPRESSION	DR. ORDERS	TIME	SITE	SIGNATURE
Sprain, R wrist	F/U c̄ Bill Blake re: wrist injury			

DRAW WOUND IN DIAGRAM
WOUND LENGTH ______
☐ COMPLEX ☐ SIMPLE
☐ PLASTIC DEPTH ______

INVOLVEMENT
DISTAL ROM ______ OK
DISTAL SENS ______ OK
DISTAL CIRC ______ OK
TENDONS ______ OK

TREATMENT
☐ Y ☐ N BET. PREP
☐ Y ☐ N ANESTH. 1% XYLOC.
☐ Y ☐ N SUTURES (*TYPE) ___

TIME OUT: 13:01
☐ Y ☐ N IRRIG
DRESSING ______
☐ Y ☐ N SPLINT

☐ CHARGES
☐ VALUABLES LISTED
☐ NURSES NOTES
☐ AFTER CARE INSTRUCTIONS GIVEN

PLAN Splint applied.

CONDITION: ☒ GOOD ☐ FAIR ☐ POOR
DISPOSITION: ☒ HOME ☐ LEFT WITHOUT BEING SEEN ☐ ADMIT
☐ LEFT AGAINST MEDICAL ADVICE ☐ EXPIRED
☐ TRANSFER TO ______ RET TO WORK ______

Bruno Ball. MD — PRINT NAME Bruno Ball

MD — PRINT NAME

Benny Baker. RN — PRINT NAME Benny Baker.

Exercise 20-3

Triage Report 3

EMERGENCY SERVICE REPORT

Cathy Crenshaw
9876 Cranbury Lane
Crabapple, CT 06192
(086) 421-3579.

DATE: 11-1-93.

ALLERGIES: NKDA

CURRENT MEDS: NPH insulin; 50U, Rocaltrol 0.5 mcg PO
Capozide 25/25 PO
Eskalith (lithium) 450 mg PO unknown others

LAST TET. TOX. DATE

ARRIVED VIA: Car ACCOMPANIED BY: Self.

P.M.D. NAME TEL. # NOTIFIED ☐

TRIAGE TIME 7:00 T 98 P 84 R 24 BP 170/90

TIME T P R BP

SIGN:

C/O Pt (50) w nausea c̄ vom
x 1.5 wk+

(−) dizzyness
(+) lightheadedness.
(−) L.O.C.

DOCTORS ORDERS

TIME	INIT	RESULTS
		RUA:
		CBC: HGB/HCT
		WBC OTHER
		DIFF: P B M E B L
		LYTES:
		Na K
		CO2 CL
		GLU:
		BUN:
		CREAT:
		OTHER LAB
		ABG:
		FIO2 BE
		PCO2 PO2
		% SAT pH
		X-RAY: Ultra Gal & Up Abd.
		EKG:

COMMUNICATION LOG

CONSULT	CALLED	COMMENTS

DISCHARGE IMPRESSION	DR. ORDERS	TIME	SITE	SIGNATURE
Jaundice RO Bile Duct obstruction.	F/U c̄ Dr. Carl Callahan.			

DRAW WOUND IN DIAGRAM
WOUND LENGTH ______
☐ COMPLEX ☐ SIMPLE
☐ PLASTIC DEPTH ______

INVOLVEMENT
DISTAL ROM ______ OK
DISTAL SENS ______ OK
DISTAL CIRC ______ OK
TENDONS ______ OK

TREATMENT
☐ Y ☐ N BET. PREP
☐ Y ☐ N ANESTH. 1% XYLOC.
☐ Y ☐ N SUTURES (*TYPE) ___

TIME OUT: 14:22
☐ Y ☐ N IRRIG
DRESSING ______
☐ Y ☐ N SPLINT

☐ CHARGES
☐ VALUABLES LISTED
☐ NURSES NOTES
☐ AFTER CARE INSTRUCTIONS GIVEN

PLAN ______

CONDITION: ☐ GOOD ☒ FAIR ☐ POOR
DISPOSITION: ☒ HOME ☐ LEFT WITHOUT BEING SEEN ☐ ADMIT ☐ LEFT AGAINST MEDICAL ADVICE ☐ EXPIRED ☐ TRANSFER TO ______ RET TO WORK ______

Christopher Campbell, MD — PRINT NAME Christopher Campbell

PRINT NAME ______ MD

Cindy Carter, RN — PRINT NAME Cindy Carter.

Exercise 20-4

Triage Report 4

Daisy Doolittle.
2345 Daffy Lane.
Danbury, DE 19876
(098)765-4311

DATE: 11-26-93.

EMERGENCY SERVICE REPORT

ALLERGIES: NKA

CURRENT MEDS: Ø

LAST TET. TOX. DATE

ARRIVED VIA: Green Light Amb. ACCOMPANIED BY: Self

P.M.D. NAME TEL. # NOTIFIED ☐

TRIAGE TIME 7:03 T 97 P 92 R 25 BP 125/85

TIME T P R BP

SIGN:

34 y/o ♀ LMP= Feb 93.
c/o x 1 wk vag discharge c̄ bleeding.
Pt feels she is pregnant, but didn't pass tissue.
Last intercourse: Sunday (11/24)
⊖ dizzy, lightheaded.
Abdo: findings in palp.
Pelvic: white discharge.
No adnexal tenderness or masses, noted.

DOCTORS ORDERS

TIME	INIT	RESULTS
		RUA: 1.008 SG
		CBC: HGB/HCT
		WBC OTHER RBC
		1-2 1-2
		DIFF: P B M
		E B L
		LYTES:
		Na K
		CO2 CL
		GLU:
		BUN:
		CREAT:
		OTHER LAB GC Culture
		wet mount
		⊖, ⊖
		Gram stain
		ABG:
		FIO2 BE
		PCO2 PO2
		% SAT pH
		X-RAY: Low abd.
		EKG:

COMMUNICATION LOG

CONSULT	CALLED	COMMENTS

DISCHARGE IMPRESSION	DR. ORDERS	TIME	SITE	SIGNATURE
Dysfunctional uterine bleeding.				

DRAW WOUND IN DIAGRAM
WOUND LENGTH ______
☐ COMPLEX ☐ SIMPLE
☐ PLASTIC DEPTH ______

INVOLVEMENT
DISTAL ROM ______ OK
DISTAL SENS ______ OK
DISTAL CIRC ______ OK
TENDONS ______ OK

TREATMENT
☐ Y ☐ N BET. PREP
☐ Y ☐ N ANESTH. 1% XYLOC.
☐ Y ☐ N SUTURES (*TYPE) ___

TIME OUT: 9:38
☐ Y ☐ N IRRIG
DRESSING ______
☐ Y ☐ N SPLINT

☐ CHARGES
☐ VALUABLES LISTED
☐ NURSES NOTES
☐ AFTER CARE INSTRUCTIONS GIVEN

PLAN D/C home. 1. F/u c̄ Dr. David Day this week for w/u of Dys. ut. Bl. 2. Use condoms.

CONDITION: ☒ GOOD ☐ FAIR ☐ POOR
DISPOSITION: ☒ HOME ☐ LEFT WITHOUT BEING SEEN ☐ ADMIT
☐ LEFT AGAINST MEDICAL ADVICE ☐ EXPIRED
☐ TRANSFER TO ______ RET TO WORK ______

Doris Dean. MD   MD   D.C. D[signature] RN

PRINT NAME Doris Dean   PRINT NAME   PRINT NAME D.C. Davidson.

Exercise 20-5

Triage Report 5

EMERGENCY SERVICE REPORT

Edward Edmunds.
8888 Every Lane.
Evansville, CA 90012
(123) 456-7890.

DATE: 5-9-93.

ALLERGIES: Penicillin.

CURRENT MEDS: ⊖

LAST TET. TOX. DATE

ARRIVED VIA: Red Alert Amb. ACCOMPANIED BY: Self

P.M.D. NAME TEL. # NOTIFIED ☐

TRIAGE TIME 6:07 T 97 P 84 R 23 BP 120/80

TIME T P R BP

SIGN:

66 y/o ♂ gunshot wound to both knees.
Pt drove to store. While walking to entrance was struck by bullet which crossed L knee & entered R knee.
⊖ L.O.C, ⊖ head trauma
Minimal pain.
Minimal bleeding.

DOCTORS ORDERS

TIME	INIT	RESULTS
		RUA:
		CBC: HGB/HCT
		WBC OTHER
		DIFF: P B M
		E B L
		LYTES:
		Na K
		CO2 CL
		GLU:
		BUN:
		CREAT:
		OTHER LAB
		ABG:
		FIO2 BE
		PCO2 PO2
		% SAT pH
		X-RAY:
		L knee ⊖
		R knee ⊕ FB
		EKG:

COMMUNICATION LOG

CONSULT	CALLED	COMMENTS

DISCHARGE IMPRESSION	DR. ORDERS	TIME	SITE	SIGNATURE
Gunshot wound to both knees.	Cipro 7.50 mg	6:30		

DRAW WOUND IN DIAGRAM
WOUND LENGTH 1"
☐ COMPLEX ☒ SIMPLE
☐ PLASTIC DEPTH

INVOLVEMENT
DISTAL ROM ____ OK
DISTAL SENS ____ OK
DISTAL CIRC ____ OK
TENDONS ____ OK

TREATMENT
☐ Y ☐ N BET. PREP
☐ Y ☐ N ANESTH. 1% XYLOC.
☐ Y ☐ N SUTURES (*TYPE) ___

TIME OUT: 2:58
☐ Y ☐ N IRRIG
DRESSING ____
☐ Y ☐ N SPLINT

☐ CHARGES
☐ VALUABLES LISTED
☐ NURSES NOTES
☐ AFTER CARE INSTRUCTIONS GIVEN

PLAN D/C to Dr. Esther Edelman.

CONDITION: ☒ GOOD ☐ FAIR ☐ POOR
DISPOSITION: ☒ HOME ☐ LEFT WITHOUT BEING SEEN ☐ ADMIT
☐ LEFT AGAINST MEDICAL ADVICE ☐ EXPIRED
☐ TRANSFER TO ____ RET TO WORK ____

Eric Ericson. MD | MD | Emilio Evans RN

PRINT NAME Eric Ericson. | PRINT NAME | PRINT NAME Emilio Evans

Exercise 20-6

Operative Report 1

ARCADIA MEDICAL CENTER
8000 Another Street
Alverville, AK 99188

PATIENT NAME: Abby Addison
PATIENT NUMBER: 33299-08

SURGEON: Albert Adler, MD

DATE OF PROCEDURE: 1-13-94

PREOPERATIVE DIAGNOSIS:
Rule out cause of upper gastrointestinal bleed.

POSTOPERATIVE DIAGNOSIS:
Most likely cause of the patient's gastrointestinal bleeding was a Mallory-Weiss tear.

NAME OF PROCEDURE:
Upper gastrointestinal endoscopy because of patient with upper gastrointestinal bleed.

PROCEDURE IN BRIEF:
Status post informed consent, the patient was premedicated with Demerol 50 and Versed 2. At this point, an upper GI endoscope was advanced through the esophagus, stomach, and duodenum.

Findings included the following: Normal esophagus, normal stomach, normal duodenum. There was a slightly raised streak at the GE junction, which was exudative. This was approximately 1 mm × 3 mm. This was consistent with possible Mallory-Weiss tear. No other lesions were appreciated throughout the entire examination. It was noted also that the patient had some mild gastritis consistent with NG tube trauma but no evidence of bleeding.

The overall procedure was tolerated well. The patient was extubated.

ALBERT ADLER, MD

AA: AA443
d: 1-14-94
t: 1-14-94
Document: 448800.aaa

Exercise 20-7

Operative Report 2

BRONSON BROTHERS MEDICAL CENTER
9876 Bright Lane
Brighton, DC 23787

DATE: 8/20/93
PATIENT: Bobby Bumble
93485 Bumpkiss Court
Barkingville, DC 23456

PATIENT DOB: 1/1/44

SURGEON: Ben Bennett, MD
ASSISTANT: Brian Bradley, MD

PRE-OP DX: Chronic Anterior and Lateral Instability of the Right Ankle

POST-OP DX: Anterior Lateral Ligamentous Reconstruction of the Right Ankle Using the Peroneus Brevis Tendon

ANESTHESIOLOGIST: Bertha Blues, MD

ANESTHESIA: Epidural

OPERATIVE FINDINGS: Included a positive drawer test, a very positive inversion test with the preoperative x-ray showing at least 23° of Taylor tilt.

PROCEDURE: The patient was brought into the room and placed in the sitting position. Dr. Blues did an epidural anesthesia without difficulty. Patient was then placed in the supine position. A lift was placed under the right buttock and a sandbag was placed at the foot area when the knee was bent 90°. The entire right lower extremity was then prepped and draped in the usual fashion. A pneumatic tourniquet was used during the initial stages of the case for 22 minutes. This was during the isolation and dissection of the tissues. A long incision was made over the peroneal tendons halfway up the calf, carried behind the lateral malleolus down to the base of the fifth metatarsal. It was dissected through skin and subcutaneous tissue. The sural nerve was not visualized and was felt to be protected by the posterior skin flap. The sheath of the peroneal tendon was then incised its entire length. The peroneus brevis tendon was isolated from the peroneus longus tendon. The brevis tendon was quite small and therefore decision was made after surgery to use the entire tendon rather than the usual half of the tendon. Muscle tissue was dissected from the tendon at the proper length. After measurement for the eventual coursing of the graft, an incision was made across the tendon. The peroneal brevis tendon was then pulled distally and a Bunnell-type suture was placed into the tendon with a double armed 2-0 Ethibond suture. The needles were then cut and a tag was placed. The dissection of the anterior flap was done so that the anterior talofibular area was dissected free. There was a lot of scarring in this area. Hemostasis was obtained by means of cautery. The tourniquet was deflated at this point.

Further dissection was done into the ankle joint so that it was viewed. It was felt to be fairly normal. A small drill hole was placed on the anterior aspect of the fibula and drilled posteriorly. This was widened with a larger drill. The pin was passed through this tunnel from anterior to posterior and was held quite tightly with the foot in neutral position of dorsiflexion plantar flexion and just slight eversion. It was not maximally everted. Sutures were then placed in the tendon and through the bone with #2 Ethibond.

Once this was secured, sutures were placed into the posterior aspect of the tunnel also with 2-0 Ethibond. The peroneal brevis tendon was then further dissected from its sheath and dislodged from its normal groove and carried anterior so the dissection on the calcaneus could occur. The ridge of the calcaneus was identified, and periosteum was stripped using an elevator. The same drill holes were then made keeping the ridge between the two holes and the distance between the holes was approximately 1½ cm. The hole was then widened to the same hole as the fibular hole and the graft was passed from posterior to anterior in the calcaneal tunnel. This was done with the suture ligature passer. This was pulled in quite nicely. There was enough graft to suture the remaining part of the graft back into the position of the anterior talar fibular ligament which was done again with #2 Ethibond.

Once wound was all secured with proper sutures, the drawer sign was negative and patient had slight inversion and could be further everted.

The wound was then irrigated with copious amounts of antibiotic solution. Prior to any drill holes, the superior portion of the wound was closed so that the rest of the tendon that was exposed would not dry out. During the procedure, the tendons were kept constantly moistened with antibiotic irrigation fluid. 2-0 Vicryl was then used for the deep subcutaneous tissue, 3-0 Vicryl for the superficial subcutaneous tissue and staples for the skin. The limb was then dressed sterilely and placed into a Jones compression dressing using cotton and for and aft plaster splints with bias cut and Ace wrap.

The patient tolerated the procedure from an anesthetic standpoint and was transferred to the RR with stable vital signs under the direction of Dr. Blues. Time under anesthesia: 1 hour, 20 min.

Dictated and authenticated by: BEN BENNETT, MD

BB: BB77
DT: 8-20-93
T: 8-20-93
Job#: 8112.B

Exercise 20-8

Operative Report 3

CANYON CITY HOSPITAL
4440 Center Drive
Carson, CT 06001

PATIENT NAME: Cathy Crenshaw
PATIENT NUMBER: 8779-09

SURGEON: Chung Choi, MD

DATE OF PROCEDURE: 11/12/93

OPERATIVE REPORT

PREOPERATIVE DIAGNOSIS: Rule out cause of obstructive jaundice in this patient with a recent cholecystectomy in March 1993 and now with obvious jaundice.

POSTOPERATIVE DIAGNOSIS: No evidence of obvious stones. Stricture at the distal common bile duct, consistent with benign versus malignant disease. Stent placed without difficulty. The patient's pathology report will be reviewed to determine if this is a periampullary carcinoma versus a benign stricture.

NAME OF PROCEDURE:

1. Endoscopic retrograde cholangiopancreatography with biopsy of the ampulla
2. Cytologic specimens from the pancreatic duct
3. Sphincterotomy
4. Placement of an internal stent, common bile duct and the duodenum

PROCEDURE IN BRIEF:
Status post informed consent, the patient was premedicated with a total of 150 mg of Demerol, 9 mg of Versed, and 2.5 mg of Glucagon.

At this point, a Pentax upper GI endoscope was advanced through the esophagus into the duodenum and also into the ampulla. The ampulla appeared somewhat erythematous and consistent with the possibility of an infiltrating periampullary carcinoma. A cholangiogram was obtained showing dilatation of the common bile duct with a narrow stricture involving the distal common bile duct. A sphincterotomy was completed at this time and a pancreatogram was also obtained. The pancreatogram appeared normal without any pathology.

A cytologic brush was used to obtain specimens from the pancreatic duct, from the mid body to the ampulla. At this point, with a marked amount of difficulty, the common bile duct was recannulated and a guide wire was advanced into the secondary radicles and a one-step stent was advanced into the common bile duct. This stent was noted to lie between the common hepatic duct and the duodenum with good positioning and good drainage.

The patient also had a biopsy of the ampulla, which appeared abnormal, consistent with possible periampullary carcinoma.

CHUNG CHOI, MD

CC: cc33
d: 11-12-93
t: 11-12-93
Document: 777.ccc

Exercise 20-9

Operative Report 4

DUNCAN DAY HOSPITAL
4499 Door Way
Duncan, DE 15678

OPERATIVE REPORT

Doolittle, Daisy 2345 Daffy Lane Danbury, DE 19876	DOB: 08/01/59
Date of Surgery:	12/7/93
Surgeon: Assistant:	Donald Denny, MD Diana Dorman, MD
Pre-operative DX:	Carcinoma of the Cervix
Anesthesiologist:	Debbie Donovan, MD
Anesthesia:	General
Post-Op DX:	Same
Procedure:	Radical Hysterectomy, Partial Vaginectomy, Bilateral Salpingo-oophorectomy, Bilateral Pelvic Lymph Node Dissection, Supra-pubic Cystostomy, Sigmoidoscopy, Cystoscopy

Findings: On examination under anesthesia, the vaginal vault was clear. The cervix showed signs of cancer that was biopsied but it seemed to be confined to the cervix and not into the parametrium. Sigmoidoscopy to 20 cm was clear. The bladder was entirely normal with no evidence of problems with the bladder. Both urethral orifices were clear. The entire abdominal cavity was explored. Liver and gallbladder were normal. The appendix was absent. There was no evidence of any other diseases within the pelvis. No lymph nodes were palpable in the periaortic common iliac and pelvic lymph nodes. The uterus was anterior freely moveable. Both tubes and ovaries appeared normal. There was a corpus luteum cyst on the left ovary and no evidence of any disease once we opened up the parametrium, paracolpos, superior vesical space and perirectal spaces were clear.

Procedure: Routine prepping and draping of the perineum, inhalation anesthesia. First, examination was carried out using a disposable sigmoidoscope. We examined the rectum to 20 cm. Finding no disease in that area, the bladder was examined using 30° water cystoscopy unit. Finding no disease in that area, the Foley catheter was placed within the bladder and the abdomen was prepped and draped in the usual manner and opened through a transverse incision through skin and subcutaneous tissue and fascia, muscle and peritoneum. Once the peritoneum was opened, and bleeding was controlled with the Bovie, the above findings were noted.

Some peritoneal washings were obtained. The bowel was packed off by means of laparotomy sponges and Balfour retractor was placed within. The uterus was lifted by Carmalt clamps along the broad ligament. The round ligaments were bilaterally clamped, cut, and ligated with stick ties of 0 Vicryl suture. Retroperitoneal space was then opened exposing the ureter and the external iliac vessels. The ureter was dissected down to the tunnel. The infundibulopelvic ligaments were isolated, doubly ligated and cut. Posterior peritoneum was cut down to the ureter. Bladder flap was developed by sharp dissection to the middle third of the vagina. The tissue of this area was dissected off. Lymph node dissection was carried down to the common iliac, external iliac, obturator fossa and hypogastric vessels bilaterally. Lymph nodes on the right side were suspicious for tumor and so were obtained for frozen section.

The entire area was dissected out and bleeding was contained with the Bovie or with clips. The webb was then taken down by first clamping, cutting, and ligating the uterine vessels and part of the webb was taken down with large Weck clips. Once this was accomplished, our attention was directed to the ureter. The ureter was dissected out of its tunnel, the uterine vessels and parametria being taken over it until we could see the ureter from the pelvic brim down to the bladder. The entire webb was taken down with Bovie or hemoclips. Free ties of 2-0 silk suture.

At this point, the posterior peritoneum was cut. The uterosacral ligaments were taken as far laterally as possible. This was taken down with either large Weck clips or stick ties of 0 Vicryl suture until they were entirely free. The rectum was entirely separated from the vagina. The cardinal and uterosacral ligaments were clamped, cut, and ligated with stick ties of 0 Vicryl suture.

The vaginal vault was then entered and the upper third of the specimen was removed. The vaginal vault was closed with interrupted figure 8 of 0 Vicryl suture. Angles were placed with interrupted 0 Vicryl suture. No bleeding was noted from any of the pedicles. The entire pelvis was irrigated with saline. Retroperitoneal drains were then placed with Jackson-Pratts and these were stitched into the skin with 0 silk suture. Retroperitoneal space was closed with 0 Vicryl suture. Sponge and needle counts were reported as correct. The peritoneum was closed with running 0 Vicryl suture. The fascia was closed with interrupted 0 Vicryl suture. Estimated blood loss was 900 cc.

Total time under anesthesia, 2 hr, 15 min.

DONALD DENNY, MD

DD: DD333
d: 12/7/93
t: 12/7/93
Document: 5556.dd

Exercise 20-10

Operative Report 5

EASTWOOD COMMUNITY MEDICAL CENTER
7854 East Road
Eastwood, CA 98765

PATIENT NAME: Edward Edmunds
PATIENT NUMBER: 098-000-432EE

PHYSICIAN: Evelyn Elliot, MD

ASSISTANT: Ernie Escalante

DATE OF OPERATION: 5-10-93

OPERATIVE REPORT

PREOPERATIVE DIAGNOSIS: Punctate wounds L knee. FB embedded distal R femur, D/T gunshot wound.

POSTOPERATIVE DIAGNOSIS: Same.

NAME OF OPERATION: Diagnostic and operative arthroscopy, removal of loose and foreign bodies, right knee and partial lateral meniscectomy, right knee.

ANESTHESIA: General.

PROCEDURE: The patient was prepped and draped in the usual aseptic manner under adequate general anesthetic with the patient in the supine position on a flat operating table with a knee post in place. The arthroscope was introduced into the joint through the anteriolateral portal and the arthroscope was passed into the joint and visualization was started in the medial compartment of the joint. The medial meniscus appeared to be intact with ragged frayed edges but none of which appeared to be a significant tear of the meniscus. The intercondylar notch was found to have an intact anterior cruciate ligament. There was an attached loose body in the anterior portion of the intercondylar notch region along the medial eminence at the base of the anterior cruciate ligament. The lateral compartment was then visualized in its entirety and was found to have no loose bodies. The lateral meniscus was found to have a tear at its anterior to middle third junction. With the aid of basket forceps and motorized incisor shaver, this portion of the meniscus was carefully removed, taking care to leave behind a stable rim of meniscus for support of the patient's knee structures. Following this removal, the loose body in the anterior aspect of the knee was carefully removed with the aid of a pituitary rongeur, and a shaver also was used in this region. Visualization was then turned to the posterior compartments of the knee and in the lateroposterior compartment, there was found a penduculated attached loose body in this region, which was carefully removed in a piecemeal fashion with the pituitary rongeur and with a curved motorized suction incisor blade. Following complete removal of this loose body, a small portion was found to have been detached from the main body of this structure and this was carefully removed with the pituitary rongeur. Attention was then turned to the distal right femur. The foreign body was removed with the aid of a pituitary ronguer and a curved motorized suction incisor blade. Following this, all areas were copiously irrigated. Visualization was carried out in the suprapatellar pouch. There was found no loose bodies in this region. The patient's knee was then carefully flushed of all extraneous fragments and debris and then the puncture incisions were closed with 3-0 nylon suture. Following closure of these punctures, three in total, in the anteromedial, anterolateral as well as the suprapatellar area, the joint was then injected with 25 cc of Marcaine with epinephrine for post-op analgesia.

Attention was then turned to the left knee. The arthroscope was introduced into the joint through the anteriolateral portal and the arthroscope was passed into the joint and visualization was started in the medial compartment of the joint. The medial meniscus appeared to be intact with no significant damage. All areas were copiously irrigated, followed by closure of the punctate wounds, four in total. The joint was then injected with 25 cc of Marcaine with epinephrine for post-op analgesia.

Peripheral pulses were checked prior to removing the patient from the operating room. The pulses were adequate and commensurate with the level they were prior to surgery.

The patient tolerated this well and was removed from the operating room in satisfactory condition.

Evelyn Elliot, MD

EE: EE56
D: 5/10/93
T: 5/10/93
DOCUMENT: 77-997.ee

Exercise 20-11

Diagnostic Report 1

RADIATION ONCOLOGY

ARCADIA MEDICAL CENTER
8000 Another Street
Alverville, AK 99188
RADIOLOGY CENTER

Patient: Abby Addison

Referring MD: Ann Anderson, MD

Date: 1-13-94

Procedure: Ultrasound Upper Abdominal and Gallbladder

Scans of the upper abdomen were performed using 3.5 mHz transducer.

The liver is normal in size, contour, and echogenicity. The pancreatic head appears normal in size and echogenic texture. Both kidneys are normal in size, shape and position with a normal echogenic relationship to the liver. The common bile duct measures 4 mm in size, which is well within normal limits, but is inflamed.

Plan: Upper gastrointestinal endoscopy.

Al Alexander, MD

AAA: aa91
d: 1-13-94
t: 1-14-94
Document: 77738.aa

Exercise 20-12

Diagnostic Report 2

RADIATION
ONCOLOGY

BRONSON BROTHERS MEDICAL CENTER
9876 Bright Lane
Brighton, DC 23787

PATIENT'S NAME	HOSPITAL NUMBER
Bobby Bumble	9888-009
X-RAY NUMBER	ROOM NUMBER
80090	ER
REFERRING PHYSICIAN	DATE OF EXAM
Bruno Ball, MD	6-19-93

AP & LAT R ANKLE, AP & LAT R WRIST:

INDICATION:
Chronic instability R ankle, injury R wrist

FINDINGS:
R ankle: There is no evidence of fx or dislocation. Taylor tilt > 23 degrees.
R wrist: There is no evidence of fx or dislocation.

INTERPRETATION:
R ankle: Evidence of ligament damage, Taylor tilt.
R wrist: Sprain

Beth Brown, MD

BB: BB95
d: 6-19-93 1300
t: 6-19-93 1405
Document: 111122.bbb

Exercise 20-13

Diagnostic Report 3

CANYON CITY HOSPITAL
4440 Center Drive
Carson, CT 06001
RADIOLOGY CENTER

Patient: Cathy Crenshaw

Referring MD: Christopher Campbell, MD

Date: 11-1-93

Procedure: Gallbladder and Upper Abdominal Ultrasound

Scans of the upper abdomen were performed using 3.5 mHz transducer.

The liver is normal in size, contour, and echogenicity.

The pancreatic head appears normal in size and echogenic texture.

Both kidneys are consistent with renal failure. The common bile duct is inflamed.

Impressions:

1. Jaundice; rule out common bile duct obstruction, rule out pancreatic tumor.
2. Leukocytosis; possibly secondary to #1.
3. End-stage chronic renal failure with hemodialysis.
4. Adult-onset diabetes mellitus.
5. Peripheral vascular disease.
6. Left above-knee amputation, 4 months ago secondary to #5.
7. Hypertension.
8. Pregangrenous changes, right foot.
9. Status post aortofemoral bypass graft surgery, 2 years ago.
10. Pulmonary embolism during hospitalization.
11. History of asthma.
12. Surgical correction of small bowel obstruction, 10 years ago.
13. History of polio in childhood with bilateral foot deformities.
14. History of multiple podiatric procedures, secondary to #13.

15. History of recurrent perianal abscesses.
16. History of multiple hospitalization for psychiatric disorders.

Treatment plan:

1. Surgical evaluation and probable intervention for obstructive jaundice.
2. Laboratory profile.
3. Adjust insulin regimen.
4. Hemodialysis.

CHRISTINE CAPLAN, MD

CC: CC80
d: 11-1-93
t: 11-1-93
Document: 5566.cc

Exercise 20-14

Diagnostic Report 4

RADIATION
ONCOLOGY

DUNCAN DAY HOSPITAL
4499 Door Way
Duncan, DE 15678

PATIENT'S NAME	HOSPITAL NUMBER
Daisy Doolittle	88290499
X-RAY NUMBER	ROOM NUMBER
22097222	ER
REFERRING PHYSICIAN	DATE OF EXAM
Doris Dean, MD	11/26/93

ABDOMEN:

INDICATION: Dysfunctional uterine bleeding

FINDINGS: Numerous small masses uterus, cervix & vaginal canal

IMPRESSION: Carcinoma of the cervix

DAVE DAVIS, MD

DD: DD55
d: 11/26/93 1130
t: 11/26/93 1205
Document: 111122.ddd

Exercise 20-15

Diagnostic Report 5

RADIATION
ONCOLOGY

EASTWOOD COMMUNITY MEDICAL CENTER
7854 East Road
Eastwood, CA 98765

PATIENT'S NAME
Edward Edmunds

HOSPITAL NUMBER
512555655

X-RAY NUMBER
89898003876

ROOM NUMBER
ER

REFERRING PHYSICIAN
Evelyn Elliot, MD

DATE OF EXAM
5/9/93

AP & LAT R & L KNEES:

INDICATION:
Gunshot wound to both knees

FINDINGS:
L knee: No evidence of fracture, dislocation or other significant bone or joint pathology
R knee: FB embedded distal R femur, bone fragments in joint space

IMPRESSION:
Gunshot wound to both knees. Bullet in distal right femur.

Eve Ellis, MD

EE: EE66
d: 5/9/93
t: 5/9/93
Document: 333322.eee

Exercise 20-16

Medical History Report 1

ARCADIA MEDICAL CENTER
8000 Another Street
Alverville, AK 99188

PATIENT NAME: Abby Addison

PATIENT NUMBER: 778-922

PHYSICIAN: Alfred Ackerman, MD

DATE: 1-13-94

HISTORY AND PHYSICAL

CHIEF COMPLAINT: Nausea with hematemesis

HISTORY OR PRESENT ILLNESS: This 25-year-old female, who was discharged from Arcadia Medical Center 2 days ago, is readmitted after severe abdominal pain and nausea, followed by hematemesis today. The patient had been hospitalized on 1-6-94 with epigastric pain due to gallbladder disease. There was also evidence for common bile duct obstruction. The patient underwent a laparoscopic cholecystectomy without complications. A gallstone that was blocking the common bile duct could not be retrieved at that time. The patient underwent ERCP on 1-10-94 by Dr. Albert Adler, who successfully removed the obstructing stone. The patient felt relief of abdominal symptoms almost immediately. She was discharged home on 1-11-94. The next day the patient began to experience nausea. She had several episodes of vomiting without evidence of hematemesis. However, on 1-13-94, her abdominal pain worsened and the patient was brought to the hospital by the paramedics. While in transport, the patient vomited bright red blood. She also notes that her stool had been black after hospital discharge. The patient is now admitted and has an NG tube in place.

PAST MEDICAL HISTORY: The patient was hospitalized at Arcadia Medical Center one week ago with gallbladder disease and common bile duct obstruction, as described in the previous section. There is no history of hypertension, diabetes mellitus or heart disease.

There are no known allergies.

REVIEW OF SYSTEMS:
CENTRAL NERVOUS SYSTEM: The patient has felt dizzy during the past 24 hours.
CARDIOVASCULAR, RESPIRATORY: There has been no dyspnea or chest pain.
GASTROINTESTINAL: The patient has had severe nausea with vomiting and hematemesis, as described in the history.
GENITOURINARY: There has been no dysuria.
MUSCULOSKELETAL: There have been no joint disturbances.

VITAL SIGNS: Temperature 97.5, pulse 118, respirations 22, and blood pressure 110/80

PHYSICAL EXAMINATION:

GENERAL: Well-nourished, well-developed female, alert, somewhat apprehensive. NG tube in place draining coffee-ground material.

HEENT: Pupils are equal, round and reactive to light and accommodation. Extraocular muscles are intact. Fundi are poorly visualized.

NECK: Thyroid not palpable. No jugular venous distention.

CHEST: Breath sounds clear to auscultation bilaterally.

HEART: Regular rate and rhythm. No murmurs.

ABDOMEN: Soft, nontender. Punctate wound, secondary to laparoscopic procedure last week.

EXTREMITIES: No pitting edema.

LABORATORY RESULTS IN THE EMERGENCY ROOM: WBC 14.4, hemoglobin 10.2, hematocrit 30.1. Sodium 140, potassium 4.5, chloride 100, bicarbonate 25, BUN 23, creatinine 0.6. Random glucose 126.

IMPRESSION:

1. Upper gastrointestinal bleed; rule out secondary to Mallory-Weiss tear, rule out complications stemming from Problem No. 2.
2. Status post ERCP (endoscopic retrograde cholangiopancreatography) 3 days ago due to Problems 3 and 4.
3. Status post hospitalization last week with gallstones and common bile duct obstruction, secondary to retained stone.
4. Status post laparoscopic cholecystectomy last week, secondary to problem No. 3.

PLAN:

1. Admit.
2. NG tube to low suction.
3. Upper endoscopy by Dr. Albert Adler.
4. Follow-up.

ALFRED ACKERMAN, MD

AA: AA89
D: 1-13-94
T: 1-14-94
Document: 5555.aa

Exercise 20-17

Medical History Report 2

BILL BLAKE DOCTORS OFFICE
9000 Broadway Street
Brighton, DC 23787

HISTORY AND PHYSICAL

Patient: Bobby Bumble
93485 Bumpkiss Court
Barkingville, DC 23456

Date of Birth: 01-01-44

Patient #: 44444

Attending: Bill Blake, MD

Date: 06-23-93

History: The patient is a 49-year-old white male with chronic instability of the right ankle due to at least a 23° Taylor tilt. Patient states that 2 months ago he was running to catch a bus and the R ankle collapsed underneath him. He fell to the pavement injuring his R ankle and R wrist. He was transported to Bronson Brothers Medical Center. X-rays showed no evidence of fracture or dislocation to either the ankle or wrist. However, Taylor tilt of ankle was discovered at that time. Patient states that he has had chronic instability of the ankle for "a number of years," possibly relating to a college football injury.

There has been no history of chest pain, palpitations, shortness of breath, dizziness, or lightheadedness.

Physical Exam: Cooperative, pleasant middle-aged male who appeared in no acute distress. Mouth—pharynx not injected. Neck—supple without mass or tenderness. Chest—clear with equal breath sounds bilaterally. There was no chest wall discomfort demonstrable on compression. Heart—normal S1 and S2 without murmur. Abdomen—benign.

Diagnosis: Chronic instability, right ankle due to 23° Taylor tilt.

Plan: Anterior lateral ligamentous reconstruction of the R ankle using the peroneus brevis tendon.

Bill Blake, MD

BB: bbb46
dd: 6-23-93
dt: 6-23-93
Document: 77788.bb

Exercise 20-18

Medical History Report 3

CANYON CITY HOSPITAL
4440 Center Drive
Carson, CT 06001

GASTROINTESTINAL CONSULTATION

PATIENT: CATHY CRENSHAW

DATE: 11-6-93

ATTENDING: CARL CALLAHAN, MD

HISTORY: Patient is a middle-aged female who presents with jaundice over the past 2 weeks. The patient has had a long history of medical problems, which include the following: (1) Adult-onset diabetes mellitus, (2) Hypertension, (3) Dialysis, (4) Congestive heart failure, and also (5) Pneumonia.

The patient's recent medical history started in March of 1992, when she presented with gangrene of the left foot. She underwent a left below-the-knee amputation, which was eventually converted to a left above-the-knee amputation in March 1992. Subsequently, the patient developed cholecystitis in the same hospitalization and underwent a cholecystectomy.

Additional surgical history includes small bowel resection in 1980. Multiple vascular surgeries on the legs, left and right, and she is also status post hysterectomy.

SOCIAL HISTORY: Patient discontinued tobacco in 1982 and she has never abused alcohol.

Patient was noted to have jaundice April 1993, but this resolved and she states that she has been tested for Hepatitis B and C at the Dialysis Center and this is now positive.

REVIEW OF SYSTEMS:

HEENT: Patient does wear glasses.

CARDIOPULMONARY: Positive for pneumonia and congestive heart failure related to fluid overload.

SOCIAL HISTORY: History is positive for patient socially being a teacher and she is now retired because of the multiple medical problems. She does occasional part-time work for Creative Creations Corp. making small handicrafts. She has had periodic diarrhea and constipation and also vomiting has started over the past couple of weeks.

PHYSICAL EXAMINATION

Reveals a well-developed, fairly well-nourished female.

PULSE: 88

BLOOD PRESSURE: 150/90

RESPIRATION: 18

WEIGHT: 132 pounds

HEENT: Atraumatic and normocephalic. Obvious scleral icterius is noted.

LUNGS: Clear

CARDIAC: Normal S1 and normal S2

ABDOMEN: Soft, benign, nontender

EXTREMITIES: Without clubbing, cyanosis or edema

NEUROLOGIC: Grossly normal

The patient does not have all of her medications, so we are unable to review all of her medications.

ASSESSMENT: At this time the patient has jaundice; quite possibly this may be obstructive.
Would suggest SMA 6-12, CBS, PT, PTT, Hepatitis B, core antibody Hepatitis C antibody to evaluate for the possibility that this may be Hepatitis. The possibilities include that this may be drug-induced vs. viral-induced hepatitis. Other considerations include obstructive jaundice, possibly related to common bile duct stone vs. stricture of the common bile duct. There is also another possibility that patient may be having a neoplasm via periodic jaundice of 4-93 and now 11-93, would suggest that patient may have possible gallstone vs. Hepatitis C. Would therefore suggest the above studies including ultrasound, endoscopic retrograde cholangiopancreatography.

CARL CALLAHAN, MD

CC: CC999
d: 11-6-93
t: 11-7-93
Document: 9900099.cc

Exercise 20-19

Medical History Report 4

DUNCAN DAY HOSPITAL
4499 Door Way
Duncan, DE 15678

PATIENT NAME:	DAISY DOOLITTLE
PATIENT NUMBER:	009998
PHYSICIAN:	DAVID DAY, MD
DATE ADMITTED:	11/30/93

HISTORY AND PHYSICAL

Pt is to have surgery at Duncan Day Hospital on 12/7/93. Procedure to be performed by Dr. Donald Denny.

CHIEF COMPLAINT: Dysfunctional uterine bleeding, carcinoma of the cervix.

HISTORY OF PRESENT ILLNESS: Pt went to Duncan Day Hospital on 11/26/93 complaining of abnormal vaginal discharge & bleeding for one week. Was seen by Dr. Doris Dean. LMP Feb 93. Last intercourse Sunday 11/24/93. Pt thought she might be pregnant but didn't pass tissue. Lab test indicated she was not. Abd. x-ray taken. Numerous small masses were found in the uterus, cervix & vaginal canal.

PAST MEDICAL HISTORY: Four NSVD, 2 prior abortions Feb 92, Nov 92. 1 miscarriage requiring extraction, Mar 93.

There are no known allergies.

VITAL SIGNS: BP 120/70, Pulse 90, Resp 23

PHYSICAL EXAMINATION:

GENERAL: Well-nourished, well-developed 34 y/o H female, cooperative, nervous.

HEENT: Pupils equal, round and reactive to light and accommodation. Extraocular muscles are intact.

NECK: Thyroid not palpable. No jugular venous distention.

CHEST: Breath sounds good to auscultation bilaterally.

HEART: Regular rate and rhythm, no murmurs.

ABDOMEN: Soft, nontender. No masses palpable.

PELVIC: Vaginal vault clear, cervix showed signs of cancer that was biopsied.

EXTREMITIES: Normal, with good reflexes.

IMPRESSION:

1. Carcinoma of the cervix

PLAN:

1. Surgical procedure by Dr. Donald Denny

DAVID DAY, MD

DD: DD98
D: 11/30/93
T: 11/30/93
Document: 999440.ddd

Exercise 20-20

Medical History Report 5

EASTWOOD COMMUNITY MEDICAL CENTER
7854 East Road
Eastwood, CA 98765

PATIENT NAME: EDWARD EDMUNDS

PATIENT NUMBER: 685947-465

PHYSICIAN: ESTHER EDELMAN, MD

DATE ADMITTED: 5-10-93

HISTORY AND PHYSICAL

The patient is to have surgery on 5/10/93. Procedure is to be performed by Dr. Evelyn Elliot, orthopedic surgeon.

CHIEF COMPLAINT: Gunshot wound to both knees.

HISTORY OF PRESENT ILLNESS: This 66-year-old male, who is a retired surgeon, suffered a gunshot wound that traversed the left knee and entered the right knee, on the morning of 5/9/93. There is a bullet that is lodged in the distal right femur. Apparently wounds to both the left and right knee were caused by the same projectile. The patient had driven to a store and while walking from his car to the store entrance he was struck by the bullet. The patient saw no one near who appeared to be responsible. Thus, the bullet may have been from a stray gunshot.

The patient was seen that day in the Eastwood Community Medical Center Emergency Room by Dr. Eric Ericson. An orthopedic surgical consultant was called in and there was a discussion of possible surgical intervention.

The patient was seen by Dr. Evelyn Elliot on 5/9/93. Dr. Elliot has reviewed the x-ray films that were taken at Eastwood Community Medical Center. She has recommended surgical intervention to remove the bullet from the distal right femur. Apparently there are bone fragments in the joint space.

The patient was seen at the hospital on 5/9/93 for medical evaluation. Since suffering the gunshot wound, the patient has not had severe pain or bleeding. He has been treated with Cipro 750 mg p.o. b.i.d. The patient has not been febrile.

PAST MEDICAL HISTORY: The patient takes no medication on a regular basis. He is not being treated for hypertension, but the patient was given diuretics for about a 2-month period in 1976. Blood pressure apparently had been elevated at that time. Subsequent measurements of blood pressure have been within normal limits. There is no history of diabetes mellitus. The patient has no frank history of heart disease, but he had had abnormal EKGs done in 1976 and 1992. The record of March 16, 1992, reveals normal sinus rhythm with some nonspecific ST and T wave changes. The patient was seen at that time because of dyspepsia. He has had no chest pain in the past. There has never been dyspnea on exertion, and the patient has not been treated for heart disease. The patient has never previously been hospitalized.

PHYSICAL EXAMINATION:
GENERAL: Well-nourished, older-aged male, alert, cooperative.

HEAD, EYES, EARS, NOSE AND THROAT: Pupils equal, round and reactive to light and accommodation. Extraocular muscles intact. Fundi poorly visualized.

NECK: Thyroid not palpable. No jugular venous distention.

CHEST: Breath sounds good to auscultation bilaterally.

HEART: Regular rate and rhythm, no murmurs.

ABDOMEN: Soft, nontender.

RECTAL: Prostate normal size and symmetrical. Stool brown in color.

EXTREMITIES: Right knee with puncture wound medial aspect; moderate edema. 1+ pitting right lower leg edema. Punctate gunshot wounds on the anterior and medial left patellar area.

IMPRESSION:
1. Gunshot wound right and left knees with projectile embedded in distal right femur.
2. History of abnormal EKG, nonspecific ST and T wave changes, unchanged since March 1992.
3. History of dyspepsia.
4. Status post tonsillectomy in childhood.
5. Allergy to penicillin.

PLAN:
1. Orthopedic surgical procedure by Dr. Evelyn Elliot.

ESTHER EDELMAN, MD

EE: EE77
D: 5/9/93
T: 5/9/93
Document: 12345678.eee

Appendix 20-1

Interpretations of Medical Reports

Triage Report 1

First, transfer the patient identity information from the patient chart and the triage report to the UB-92. This includes name and address information placed in Items 12 and 13.

Next, go through the UB-92 item by item and try to locate the information that is needed to complete each box.

The name and address of the hospital (Item 1) are not listed. This information would be known by the medical biller, since it would be his or her place of employment.

The type of bill (Item 4) would be 131, since it is for a hospital outpatient admit through discharge billing. Because additional information is not available, this bill will be for the emergency services only.

The federal tax number would be listed in Item 5. This is provided by the provider of service to their medical billers.

Item 6 is the statement period. The patient was admitted to the emergency room on 1/13/94, then was subsequently admitted to a hospital room. Therefore, the statement ending date should be 1/13/94.

Insurance coverage information would be taken from the patient file that had been set up in the Introduction to Medical Claims section.

The patient is female, Item 15.

The patient's marital status is on the Patient Information Sheet. She is single, so an S would be placed in Item 16.

The patient was admitted on 13 Jan 94, so 1/13/94 would be placed in Item 17.

The patient arrived at 14:09, so this time should be placed in Item 18.

Since the patient was admitted, a 1 should be placed in Item 19 and a 7 in Item 20.

Item 21 is the discharge hour. Since the patient was not actually discharged, this information would be left blank.

Item 22 is the status at time of billing. The patient was admitted; therefore, an 09 would be placed in this box.

There would be no condition codes since the patient has not stated any special conditions associated with his condition (Items 24 through 30).

There are no occurrence codes or occurrence span codes; therefore, Items 32 through 36 would be left blank.

According to the patient chart, the responsible party is the patient. Her name and address would be listed in Item 38.

Items 39 through 41 would be left blank since there are no specific values listed in the triage report. However, it should be noted that ultrasound scanning of the gallbladder and upper abdomen was taken. Therefore, there would be a professional component involved in reading the ultrasound, so a value would need to be added for patients with Medicare or Medicaid coverage.

Item 42 would be coded with the appropriate revenue code and Item 43 with the description. There would generally be a standard charge for the Emergency Room. The coding and description would be as follows: EMERG ROOM = 450.

The information given on the triage report would need to be added with information regarding the standard fees that the hospital charges for these services to complete the billing form.

The patient chart lists Atlantic Assurance as the patient's insurance coverage. Therefore, Atlantic Assurance would be entered on Item 50.

There is no signature on file for release of information (Item 52) or for assignment of benefits (Item 53). These signatures would need to be obtained prior to filing the claim with the insurance carrier.

If the patient made any payments on the bill, this amount would be placed in Item 54. This amount would then be subtracted from the total in Item 55.

Since it is unknown whether the patient has previously paid her deductible or what amount of coinsurance is due from the patient, it is assumed that the insurance carrier is responsible for the entire amount of the bill. This amount should be placed in Item 55.

The patient is the insured on the patient chart. Therefore, her name would go on Item 58 and the code 01 (self) would be placed in Item 59.

Since no subscriber certificate number has been given, the medical biller should place the patient's Social Security number under Item 60. This will allow them to verify her policy.

The patient is employed by Artistic Aardvarks. Since there is insurance, it can be assumed that the patient is working full-time. Therefore, her employment status (Item 64) should be listed as 1.

The name Artistic Aardvarks and the address would be listed under Items 65 and 66.

Item 67 would contain the diagnosis listed in the Discharge Impression portion of the triage report. However, this patient has been admitted for further study. Therefore the chief complaint: Hematemesis would be given. This has a diagnosis code of 578.0.

There were no additional diagnoses associated with the condition, so Items 68 through 75 would be left blank.

There were no procedures performed, so Items 79 through 81 would be left blank.

The attending physician information would be taken from the bottom of the triage report and placed in Item 82. Remember to include any title designations (eg, MD).

No secondary physician was listed, so Item 83 would be left blank.

Under remarks, it would be appropriate to leave it blank.

Triage Report 2

First, transfer the patient identity information from the triage report and the patient chart to the UB-92. This includes name and address information placed in Items 10 and 11, and birth date placed in Item 12.

Next, go through the UB-92 Item by Item and try to locate the information that is needed to complete each box.

The name and address of the hospital (Item 1) are not listed. This information would be known by the medical biller, since it would be his or her place of employment.

The patient control number (Item 3) would be the admission number on the triage report and the account number on the patient admitting form. None is listed, so for now this can be left blank.

The type of bill (Item 4) would be 131 since it is for a hospital outpatient, admit through discharge.

The Federal tax number would be listed in Item 5.

Item 6 is the statement period. The patient was admitted on 06/19/93. Since the discharge time is before midnight, the discharge date would also be 06/19/93, and these would also be the statement period dates.

The patient's birth date is listed on the patient chart and it should be placed in Item 14.

The patient is male, Item 15.

The patient chart shows that the patient is married, so an M would be placed in Item 16.

The patient was admitted on 06/19/93, so this information would be placed in Item 17.

The patient arrived at 09:37, so 09 should be placed in Item 18.

Item 21 is the discharge hour, 13:01.

Item 22 is the patient's status at time of billing. The patient was sent home, therefore an 01 would be placed in this box.

There are no occurrence codes; therefore, Items 32 through 36 would be left blank.

According to the admitting form, the responsible party is the patient. His name and address would be listed in Item 38.

Item 42 would be coded with the appropriate revenue code. There is usually a standard charge for the emergency room and for the wrist and ankle x-rays. The coding would be as follows: DX XRAY/OTHER = 329, EMERG ROOM = 450. Information given on the triage report would need to be added with information regarding the standard fees that the hospital charges for these services to complete the billing form.

The patient chart lists Barkerville Assurance Company as his insurance coverage. Therefore, enter it in Item 50.

There is no signature on file for release of information (Item 52) or for assignment of benefits (Item 53). These signatures would need to be obtained prior to filing the claim with the insurance carrier.

If the patient made any payments on the bill, this amount would be placed in Item 54. This amount would then be subtracted from the total in Item 55.

The patient is listed as the insured on the patient chart. Therefore, his name would go on Item 58. The code 01 (self) would be placed in Item 59.

Since no employee number has been given, the medical biller should place the patient's Social Security number under Item 60. This will allow them to verify his insurance policy.

Since the patient has insurance through his employer, it may be assumed that he is a full-time employee. Therefore, a 1 should be placed in Item 64.

Bobby's employer is listed as Bumbling Bureaucrats. This name and the address following it on the patient chart would be listed under Items 65 and 66.

Item 67 would contain the diagnosis listed in the Discharge Impression portion of the triage report: (1) Sprain, R wrist. The diagnosis code is 842.00.

There were no additional diagnosis associated with the condition. Therefore, Items 68 through 77 would be left blank.

No surgical procedures were performed, so Items 80 through 81 would be left blank.

The attending physician information would be taken from the triage report and placed in Item 82. Remember to include any title designations (eg, MD).

No secondary physician is listed, so Item 83 would be left blank.

Under remarks (Item 84), it would be appropriate to leave it blank.

Operative Report 1

Step 1

The first step in interpreting and billing the information contained on an operative report is to determine the procedures and services that were utilized.

Operative report #1 is for an operation that utilized hospital operating room and supply services, and the services of a surgeon, an assistant surgeon, and an anesthesiologist.

Since the hospital services and supplies would be contained within a hospital record and would be billed on the UB-92, the medical biller would need the patient's entire file of supplies and services rendered. Since this information is not available from the operative report and Patient Information Sheet (and since the hospital medical billers are usually separate from those of the surgeon, assistant surgeon, and anesthesiologist), the medical biller would be unable to complete a UB-92 from the information given.

Otherwise, the doctor should bill for his services individually, using a HCFA-1500.

Step 2

Transfer the information contained in the header section of the report to the HCFA-1500. For example, transfer the information:

DATE: 1-13-9 (to Item 24A)
PATIENT: Abby Addison (Item 2)
SURGEON: Albert Adler, MD (Item 33)
PRE-OP DX: Rule out cause of upper gastrointestinal bleed.
POST-OP DX: Mallory-Weiss tear (Item 21)

This introductory information is in the header area. In particular, if a diagnosis is not provided on the claim form, it can be obtained from the Post-Op Dx field.

Step 3

Locate the additional information needed on the Patient Information Sheet and transfer it in the same manner.

Step 4

As previously indicated, an operative report is used to determine the procedures actually performed. Therefore, the next step is to break down the Operation Performed information into CPT verbiage.

Location of the operative area: Upper gastrointestinal bleed

Procedure: Upper gastrointestinal endoscopy.

As indicated, this procedure involved the upper gastrointestinal tract. Therefore, open the CPT to the digestive system, gastrointestinal, upper. Code 43235 indicates with or without duodenoscopy. Therefore this would be the correct code.

Operative Report 2

Step 1

The first step in interpreting and billing the information contained on an operative report is to determine the procedures and services that were utilized.

Operative report #2 is for an operation that utilized hospital operating room and supply services, and the services of a surgeon, an assistant surgeon, and an anesthesiologist.

Since the hospital services and supplies would be contained within a hospital record and would be billed on the UB-92, the medical biller would need the patient's entire file of supplies and services rendered. Since this information is not available from the operative report and Patient Information Sheet (and since the hospital medical billers are usually separate from those of the surgeon, assistant surgeon, and anesthesiologist), the medical biller would be unable to complete a UB-92 from the information given.

Otherwise, each of the other providers of service should bill for their services individually, each using an HCFA-1500.

Step 2

The only differences among each of the medical billings would be in the procedural section of the HCFA-1500 (Items 24E through 24H) and the charges (Items 24F and 28 through 30). Therefore, we will cover the billing of these services together.

First, transfer the information contained in the header section of the report to the HCFA-1500. For example, transfer the information:

DATE:	8/20/93 (to Item 24A)
PATIENT:	Bobby Bumble (Item 2) 93485 Bumpkiss Court (Item 5) Barkingville, DC 23456
PATIENT DOB:	1/1/44 (Item 3)
SURGEON:	Ben Bennett, MD (Item 33)*
ASSISTANT:	Brian Bradley, MD (Item 33)*
PRE-OP DX:	Chronic Anterior and Lateral Instability of the Right Ankle (Not included)
POST-OP DX:	Anterior Lateral Ligamentous Reconstruction of the Right Ankle Using the Peroneus Brevis Tendon (Item 21)
ANESTHESIOLOGIST:	Bertha Blues, MD (Item 33)*
ANESTHESIA:	Epidural

This introductory information is the header area. In particular, if a diagnosis is not provided on the claim form, it can be obtained from the Post-Op Dx field.

*NOTE: The names of the surgeon, assistant surgeon, and anesthesiologist would each be placed in Item 33 on only their own billing form.

Step 3

Locate the additional information needed on the Patient Information Sheet and transfer it in the same manner.

Step 4

As previously indicated, an operative report is used to determine the procedures actually performed. Therefore, the next step is to break down the Operation Performed information into CPT verbiage.

Location of the operative area: Anterior Lateral Ligament

Procedure: Reconstruction of the right ankle using a graft from the peroneus brevis tendon.

As indicated, this procedure involved the ankle. Therefore, open the CPT to the lower musculoskeletal system. Locate the codes therein that deal with the ankle or with the peroneus brevis tendon. There are only three appropriate codes. Since there was no repair performed on the bone, the arthroplasty can be eliminated. That leaves only two possible codes.

As a medical biller, you would need to have the physician state whether this was a primary or a secondary repair. A primary repair would probably have a higher UCR, and therefore would pay more. However, the medical biller should never assume that the procedure that pays the highest is the one that should be used. Submitting claims for procedures that were not actually done is fraud.

Therefore:

For the surgeon, if the doctor stated that the primary procedure was done, the appropriate code would be 27695. If the doctor stated that the secondary procedure was done, the appropriate code would be 27698.

If you were the claims examiner and this report came to you without an appropriate CPT code, you might not be able to determine whether this was a secondary or primary repair. However, since the secondary repair probably allows a lower UCR, that would be the procedure code (27698) probably utilized. If that code was incorrect, the doctor would be expected to contact the payor for an adjustment.

For the assistant surgeon, the appropriate code with the modifier -80 would be listed as the procedure. Both are listed in the Assistant Surgeons List, so it would be acceptable to bill the assistant surgeon's charges regardless of which procedure was performed.

For the anesthesiologist, go to the anesthesia section of the CPT and locate the "LOWER LEG (BELOW KNEE)" section. This is a procedure on the muscles and tendons (see postoperatic diagnosis). Since the procedure is not a repair of Achilles tendon (01472) nor a gastrocnemius recession (01474), the procedure is not specified. Therefore, the code 01470—Anesthesia for procedures on nerves, muscles, tendons and fascia of lower leg, ankle, and foot, not otherwise specified, would be used.

Also remember to include the total time under anesthesia on the claim form.

Diagnostic Report 1

Step 1

Determine the correct billing form to use. The bill is for provider services. Therefore, the HCFA-1500 would be used to bill for diagnostic testing reports.

Step 2

Transfer the information from the diagnostic testing report to the HCFA-1500.

Step 3

Transfer the information from the patient information sheet to the HCFA-1500.

Step 4

The procedure was a Gallbladder and Upper Abdominal Ultrasound, which has a CPT code of 76700 (Echography, abdominal, B-scan and/or real time with image documentation; complete).

Diagnostic Report 2

Step 1

Determine the correct billing form to use. The bill is for provider services. Therefore, the HCFA-1500 would be used to bill for diagnostic testing reports.

Step 2

Transfer the information from the diagnostic testing report to the HCFA-1500.

Step 3

Transfer the information from the patient information sheet to the HCFA-1500.

Step 4

The procedures were an x-ray of AP & LAT right ankle, which has a CPT code of 73600 and another x-ray of AP & LAT right wrist, which has a CPT code of 73100.

Medical History Report 1

Step 1

Determine the correct billing form to use. The bill is for services rendered by a physician. Therefore, the HCFA-1500 would be used to bill for medical history reports.

Step 2

Transfer the information from the medical history report to the HCFA-1500.

Step 3

Transfer the information from the Patient Information Sheet to the HCFA-1500.

Step 4

The service provided was an inpatient visit with a history and physical, which has a CPT code of 99221.

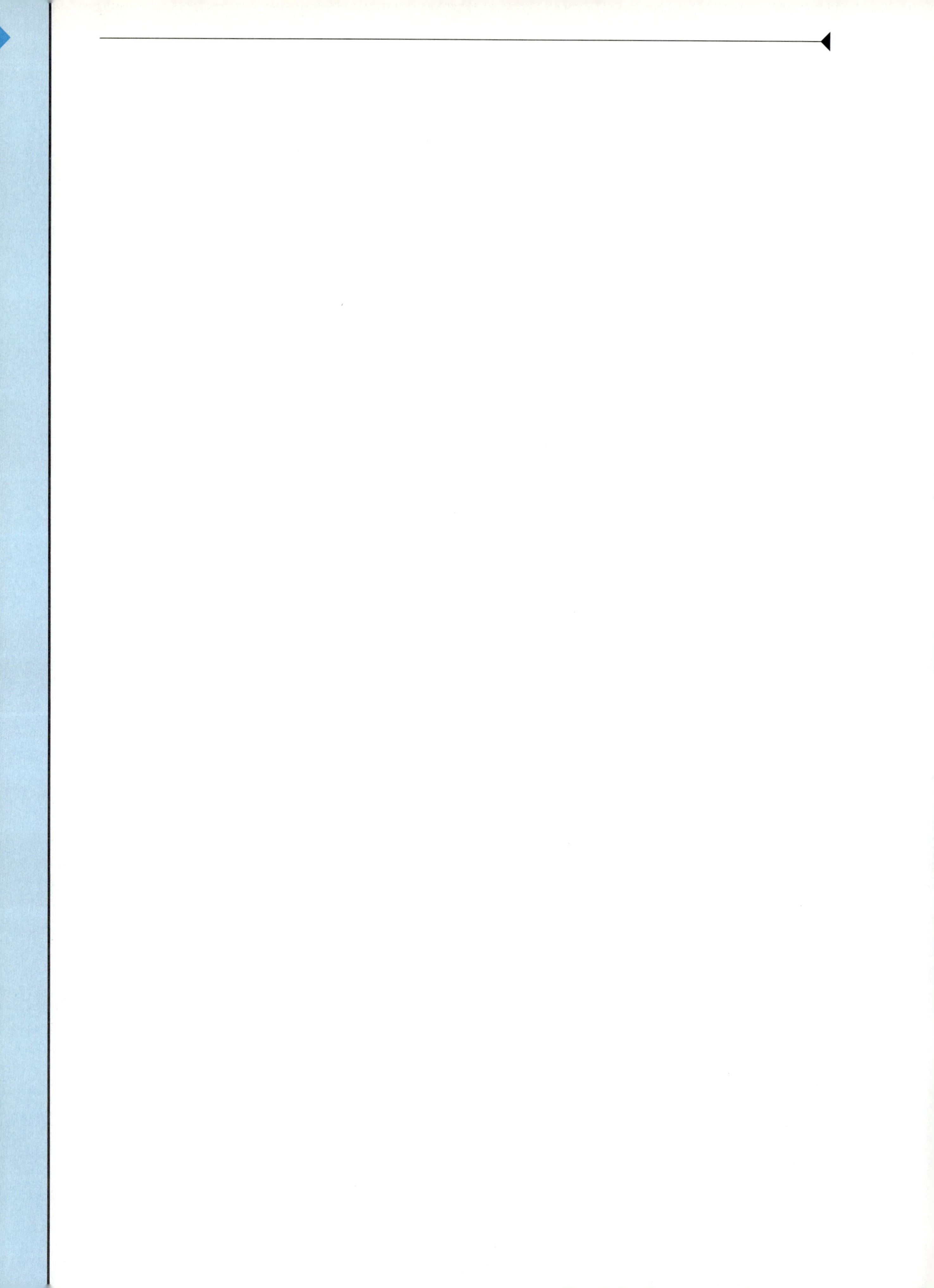

Index

N

O

P

R

S

T

U

V

W